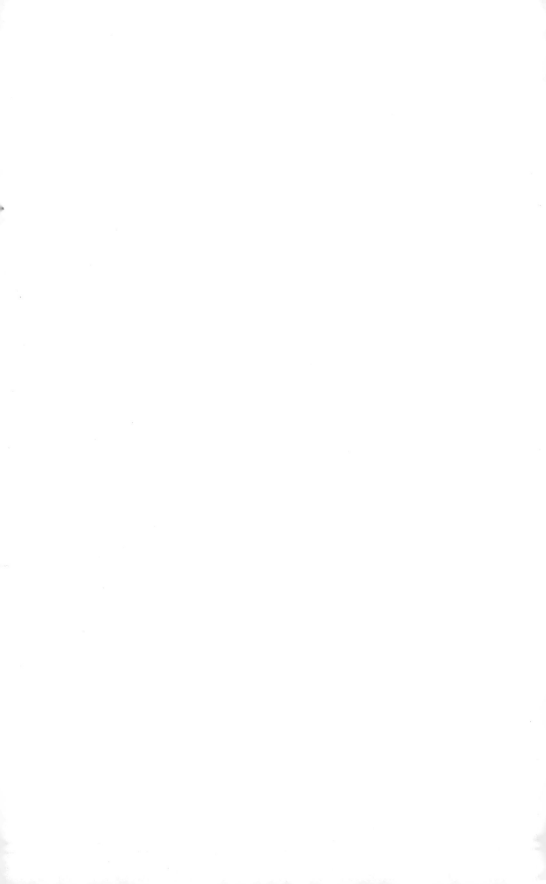

Cognitive Impairment in Schizophrenia

Characteristics, Assessment, and Treatment

Cognitive Impairment in Schizophrenia

Characteristics, Assessment, and Treatment

Edited by

Philip D. Harvey, PhD
Professor of Psychiatry and Behavioral Sciences,
University of Miami Miller School of Medicine,
Miami, FL, USA

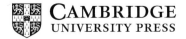

CAMBRIDGE
UNIVERSITY PRESS

University Printing House, Cambridge CB2 8BS, United Kingdom

Cambridge University Press is part of the University of Cambridge.

It furthers the University's mission by disseminating knowledge in the pursuit of education, learning and research at the highest international levels of excellence.

www.cambridge.org
Information on this title: www.cambridge.org/9781107013209

© Cambridge University Press 2013

First published 2013
Reprinted 2014

Printed in the United States of America by Sheridan Books, Inc.

A catalogue record for this publication is available from the British Library

Library of Congress Cataloguing in Publication data

Cognitive impairment in schizophrenia : characteristics, assessment, and treatment / edited by Philip D. Harvey.
　　p.　cm.
　Includes bibliographical references and index.
　ISBN 978-1-107-01320-9 (Hardback)
　I. Harvey, Philip D., 1956–
[DNLM: 1. Schizophrenia–complications.　2. Cognition Disorders–etiology. WM 203]
　616.89′8–dc23

2012024803

ISBN 978-1-107-01320-9 Hardback

Contents

Contributors

André Aleman
Department of Cognitive Neuropsychiatry, University of Groningen, Groningen, the Netherlands

Narmeen Ammari
Department of Psychology, York University, Toronto, Ontario, Canada

Alan Anticevic
Department of Psychiatry, Yale University School of Medicine; NIAAA Center for the Translational Neuroscience of Alcoholism; Abraham Ribicoff Research Facilities, Connecticut Mental Health Center, New Haven, CT, USA

Deanna M. Barch
Departments of Psychology and Radiology, Washington University in St. Louis, St. Louis, MO, USA

Christopher R. Bowie
Departments of Psychology and Psychiatry, Queen's University, Kingston, Ontario, Canada

Katherine E. Burdick
Department of Psychiatry, Mount Sinai School of Medicine, New York, NY, USA

Sara J. Czaja
Department of Psychiatry and Behavioral Sciences, Center on Aging, University of Miami Miller School of Medicine, Miami, FL, USA

Anthony S. David
Department of Cognitive Neuropsychiatry, Institute of Psychiatry, King's College London, London, UK

Colin A. Depp
Department of Psychiatry, University of California San Diego; San Diego Veterans Healthcare System, San Diego, CA, USA

Dwight Dickinson
Genes, Cognition and Psychosis Program, and Clinical Brain Disorders Branch, IRP, NIMH, NIH, Bethesda; the Lieber Institute for Brain Development, Johns Hopkins Medical Campus, Baltimore, MD, USA

Gary Donohoe
Neuropsychiatrics Genetics Research Group, Department of Psychiatry and Trinity College Institute of Neuroscience, Trinity College, Dublin, Ireland

Melissa Fisher
Department of Psychiatry, University of California San Francisco; San Francisco Department of Veteran Medical Affairs Center, San Francisco, CA, USA

Benjamin Glicksberg
Department of Psychiatry, Mount Sinai School of Medicine, New York, NY, USA

Michael F. Green
Semel Institute for Neuroscience and Human Behavior, David Geffen School of Medicine at University of California Los Angeles; Department of Veterans Affairs, Desert Pacific Mental Illness Research, Education, and Clinical Center, Los Angeles, CA, USA

Maya Gupta
Departments of Psychology and Psychiatry, Queen's University, Kingston, Ontario, Canada

Philip D. Harvey
Department of Psychiatry and Behavioral Sciences, University of Miami Miller School of Medicine, Miami, FL, USA

R. Walter Heinrichs
Department of Psychology, York University, Toronto, Ontario, Canada

Katherine Holshausen
Departments of Psychology and Psychiatry, Queen's University, Kingston, Ontario, Canada

William P. Horan
Semel Institute for Neuroscience and Human Behavior, David Geffen School of Medicine at University of California Los Angeles; Department of Veterans Affairs, Desert Pacific Mental Illness Research, Education, and Clinical Center, Los Angeles, CA, USA

Daniel C. Javitt
Department of Psychiatry and Neuroscience, Division of Experimental Therapeutics, Columbia University College of Physicians and Surgeons; Schizophrenia Research, Nathan Kline Institute for Psychiatric Research, Orangeburg, NY, USA

Richard Keefe
Department of Psychiatry, Duke University Medical Center, Durham, NC, USA

John H. Krystal
Department of Psychiatry, Yale University School of Medicine; NIAAA Center for the Translational Neuroscience of Alcoholism; Abraham Ribicoff Research Facilities, Connecticut Mental Health Center, New Haven, CT, USA

David Loewenstein
Department of Psychiatry and Behavioral Sciences, Center on Aging, University of Miami Miller School of Medicine, Miami, FL, USA

Susan R. McGurk
Center for Psychiatric Rehabilitation, Department of Occupational Therapy, Boston University, Boston, MA, USA

Kristopher I. Mathis
Department of Veterans Affairs, Desert Pacific Mental Illness Research, Education, and Clinical Center, Los Angeles, CA, USA

Brent Mausbach
Department of Psychiatry, University of California, San Diego, CA, USA

Ashley A. Miles
Department of Psychology, York University, Toronto, Ontario, Canada

Kim T. Mueser
Center for Psychiatric Rehabilitation, Department of Occupational Therapy, Boston University, Boston, MA, USA

Eva Muharib
Department of Psychology, York University, Toronto, Ontario, Canada

Robin Murray
Department of Psychosis Studies, Institute of Psychiatry, King's College London, London, UK

Akshay Nair
South London and Maudsley NHS Foundation Trust, London, UK

Rogerio Panizzutti
Instituto de Ciências Biomédicas, Universidade Federal do Rio de Janeiro, Rio de Janeiro, RJ, Brazil

Thomas Patterson
Department of Psychiatry, University of California San Diego, San Diego, CA, USA

Amy E. Pinkham
Department of Psychology, Southern Methodist University, Dallas, TX, USA

Abraham Reichenberg
Department of Psychosis Studies, Institute of Psychiatry, King's College London, London, UK

Manuela Russo
Department of Psychosis Studies, Institute of Psychiatry, King's College London, London, UK

Jonathan Schaefer
Genes, Cognition and Psychosis Program and Clinical Brain Disorders Branch, IRP, NIMH, NIH, Bethesda; the Lieber Institute for Brain Development, Johns Hopkins Medical Campus, Baltimore, MD, USA

Karuna Subramaniam
Department of Psychiatry, University of California San Francisco; San Francisco Department of Veteran Medical Affairs Center, San Francisco, CA, USA

Laura Vergel de Dios
Department of Psychiatry, University of California San Diego, San Diego, CA, USA

Sophia Vinogradov
Department of Psychiatry, University of California San Francisco; San Francisco Department of Veteran Medical Affairs Center, San Francisco, CA, USA

Daniel R. Weinberger
Genes, Cognition and Psychosis Program and Clinical Brain Disorders Branch, IRP, NIMH, NIH, Bethesda; Lieber Institute for Brain Development, Johns Hopkins Medical Campus, Baltimore, MD, USA

Jonathan K. Wynn
Semel Institute for Neuroscience and Human Behavior, David Geffen School of Medicine at University of California Los Angeles; Department of Veterans Affairs, Desert Pacific Mental Illness Research, Education, and Clinical Center, Los Angeles, CA, USA

Preface

This book contains the latest information about cognition in schizophrenia, focusing on the causes, characteristics, importance of, and treatments for this most important feature of the illness. This book is published 13 years after a similar edited book that reviewed the state of the art up to the year 2000. There are many new developments including a more detailed focus on treatment and much more sophisticated examinations of the correlates of cognitive impairments. Similar to the last book, the chapters contained here are written by the highest level of experts in the field, many of whom have been collaborating with each other (and with me) for the past 25 years or more.

There are several developments that have received increased attention in the last decade. They include the genetics of cognitive deficits, pharmacological treatment of cognitive deficits, the importance of social cognition, the notion of functional capacity as a potential mediator of the influence of cognition on everyday functioning, sophisticated strategies for the measurement of cognitive change in treatment studies, and more sophisticated analyses of neurobiological and neuroimaging correlates of cognitive deficits. Similar in topic, but broader in scope, are considerations of the centrality of cognition in the illness, evaluations of the impact of cognition on everyday outcomes, the effects of aging on cognition in schizophrenia, and dimensions of symptoms in the illness.

There have been huge developments in the last decade. The Measurement and Treatment Research to Improve Cognition in Schizophrenia (MATRICS) initiative has brought cognition to the center of interest for treatment of disability. Multiple treatments have been tested and a few have had some success. Others have failed and some pharmaceutical companies have stopped trying to develop treatment for central nervous system diseases, which is short-sighted on their part and potentially hurtful to our patients. Other parties have entered the field and attempted to step into the gap from which some of the large companies have fled. The next few years will also be critical.

This book has the potential to tell you just about everything you need to know about the current state of cognition in schizophrenia. The coverage is broad, the writing is clear, and the excitement felt by these authors comes through when you read their writing. This is not bland and pedestrian; it is state of the art and very well presented. There is information for people interested in causes and cures. There is information for people who are interested in symptom structure and cognitive impairments, and there is information on the developmental course of cognition in schizophrenia over the lifespan. The latest and most exciting treatments are described, as are the efforts of researchers who are attempting to refine the assessment of schizophrenia, still an important task 115 years after the definition of the concept.

Thanks are in order to many people. I would like to thank the authors for their hard work, both in these chapters and in producing the data before that led to these chapters. I would like to thank the thousands of patients who have volunteered their time to participate in these research studies, mine included. I would like to thank the donors and philanthropists who support research on cognition in schizophrenia, and I would also like to thank the readers who are interested in this important topic.

In the past year while this book was being compiled, we lost one of the pioneers of research on cognition in schizophrenia, John M. Neale, who died last fall. He had recently won the Society for Research in Psychopathology's inaugural Sustained Mentorship Award and was clearly the most important educator in the field of cognition in schizophrenia. Consistent with his influence, the authors of four of the chapters in this book are members of his academic lineage. His studies of the interface between cognition, emotion, and clinical symptoms influence the field still and his mentorship has resulted in an enduring legacy. We will not forget you, John.

Abbreviations

AD Alzheimer's disease

ADHD attention deficit hyperactivity disorder

AMPA α-amino-3-hydroxy-5-methyl-4-isoxazole propionic acid

AVLT Auditory Verbal Learning Test

BACS Brief Assessment of Cognition in Schizophrenia

BADE bias against disconfirmatory evidence

BADS Behavioural Assessment of the Dysexecutive Syndrome

BCA Brief Cognitive Assessment

B-CATS Brief Cognitive Assessment Tool for Schizophrenia

BDNF brain-derived neurotrophic factor

BOLD blood oxygenation level-dependent

CAI Cognitive Assessment Interview

CAINS Clinical Assessment Interview for Negative Symptoms

CANTAB Cambridge Neuropsychological Test Automated Battery

CC cognitive control

CCE Contrast–Contrast Effect Task

CDR Cognitive Drug Research

CET Cognitive Enhancement Therapy

CG computer games (condition)

CNTRICS Cognitive Neuroscience Treatment Research to Improve Cognition in Schizophrenia

CNV copy number variants

COMT catechol-o-methyl transferase

CONSIST Cognitive and Negative Symptoms in Schizophrenia Trial

CPT Continuous Performance Test

CSGI clinically significant cognitive impairment

CVLT California Verbal Learning Test

DAFS Direct Assessment of Functional Status (scale)

DLPFC dorsolateral prefrontal cortex

DMN default mode network

DPX Dot Probe Expectancy Task

DRS Dementia Rating Scale

DS degraded stimulus

DSM Diagnostic and Statistical Manual of Mental Disorders

DTI diffusion tensor imaging

EFB Everyday Functioning Battery

EM episodic memory

ERN error-related negativity

ERP evoked response potential/event-related potential

ES effect sizes

EST enriched supportive therapy

FDA U.S. Food and Drug Administration

FEP first-episode psychosis

fMRI functional magnetic resonance imaging

FRN feedback-related negativity

GABA gamma-aminobutyric acid

GAD glutamic acid decarboxylase

GAT GABA transporter

GWAS genome-wide association studies

HF hippocampal formation

HVLT Hopkins Verbal Learning Test

ICC intraclass correlation

ILS Independent Living Scales

ILSS Independent Living Skills Survey

IPS individual placement and support

IP identical pairs

IQ intelligence quotient

ITAQ Insight and Treatment Attitudes Questionnaire

JOVI Jitter Orientation Visual Integration Task

JTC jump to conclusions

LGN lateral geniculate nucleus

LTD long-term depression

LTP long-term potentiation

MASC Maryland Assessment of Social Competence

MATRICS Measurement and Treatment Research to Improve Cognition in Schizophrenia

MCCB MATRICS Consensus Cognitive Battery

MCI mild cognitive impairment

MEG magnetoencephalography

METT Micro-Expressions Training Tool

MHC major histocompatibility complex

MMAA Medication Management Ability Assessment

MMLT Micro-Module Learning Test

MMN mismatch negativity

MMSE Mini-Mental State Examination

MMT Medication Management Test

MSCEIT Mayer–Salovey–Caruso Emotional Intelligence Test

MSE Modified Six Elements Test

NAB Neuropsychological Assessment Battery

NART National Adult Reading Test

NEAR neuropsychological and educational approach to remediation

NET Neurocognitive Enhancement Therapy

NIH National Institutes of Health

NIMH National Institute of Mental Health

NMDA N-methyl-D-aspartate

PANSS Positive and Negative Syndrome Scale – insight item G12

PCP phencyclidine

PD Parkinson's disease

ph-fMRI pharmacological neuroimaging

QLS Quality of Life Survey

QWB Quality of Well-Being status

RBANS Repeatable Battery for the Assessment of Neuropsychological Status

RDoC research domain criteria

RISE Relational and Item Specific Encoding Task

RMBT Rivermead Behavioural Test

ROC receiver operator curve

ROI region of interest

SAI Schedule for Assessment of Insight

SCIT social cognitive interaction training

SCoRS Schizophrenia Cognition Rating Scale

SCT social cognition training

SETT Subtle Expressions Training Tool

SLOF Specific Levels of Functioning Scale

SNP single nucleotide polymorphism

SSPA Social Skills Performance Assessment

SUMD Scale to Assess Unawareness of Mental Disorder

TABS Test of Adaptive Behavior in Schizophrenia

TAR training of affect recognition

THC (delta-9-)tetrahydrocannabinol

ToM theory of mind

MT Trail Making Test (part B only)

TURNS Treatment Units for Research on Neurocognition and Schizophrenia

UPSA University of California performance skills assessment

VALERO Validating Real-World Outcomes

VBM voxel-based morphometry

VIM Validation of Intermediate Measures

WAIS Wechsler Adult Intelligence Scale

WCST Wisconsin Card Sorting Test

WHODAS World Health Organization Disability Assessment Schedule

WM working memory

WMS Wechsler Memory Test

WRAT Wide Range Achievement Test

Cognition as a central illness feature in schizophrenia

R. Walter Heinrichs, Ashley A. Miles, Narmeen Ammari, and Eva Muharib

Introduction

Schizophrenia is a loose and heterogeneous syndrome defined by implausible and peculiar beliefs and sensory experiences, social withdrawal, restricted or inappropriate emotional expression, and disorganized behavior. These positive and negative symptoms were described clearly and comprehensively in Kraepelin's (1896, 1919) seminal accounts of dementia praecox. It is perhaps less well appreciated that a range of cognitive deficits were also considered characteristic of the illness (Table 1.1). Indeed, another pioneer, Bleuler (1943, 1950), argued that impairments in "associative" thinking were "fundamental" abnormalities in schizophrenia whereas delusions and hallucinations were only "accessory" symptoms. Nevertheless, for several decades psychotic symptoms were used to define the disorder and impairments in basic cognitive processes were neglected, excluded, or viewed as peripheral treatment artifacts (Randolph et al., 1993). Over the last 20 years this situation has changed and cognition has re-emerged as a core domain of schizophrenia research and intervention initiatives. Yet determining the meaning and significance of cognitive performance and impairment in the disorder remains both a challenge and an opportunity. Is an understanding of cognition essential to advance schizophrenia science and treatment or is it a secondary problem, an interesting sideline that addresses a correlate, but not a determinant of the disorder? This chapter considers evidence from both perspectives and argues for a critical appraisal of the role of cognition in psychotic illness.

Early research on cognition in schizophrenia

The psychiatric pioneers of schizophrenia research considered a variety of cognitive problems in their clinical case descriptions, but these efforts were limited by the questionable validity of interviews and subjective data and observations as well as by sampling biases. For example, dementia praecox was regarded initially as a deteriorative disorder associated with poor outcome in the majority of cases (Kraepelin, 1919). Yet this poor prognosis probably reflected, in part, the nature of psychiatric caseloads in the early twentieth century. Patients with favorable outcomes were omitted or not followed and study samples were seldom representative of the patient population (Riecher-Rössler & Rössler, 1998).

Another limitation was the estimation of cognitive profiles on the basis of clinical experience and observation alone. Thus Bleuler (1943) maintained that patients with schizophrenia had preserved or even superior memory for events and personal material

Table 1.1.

Kraepelin's (1919) psychic symptoms of dementia praecox	
1. Perception	19. Impulsive actions
2. Attention	20. Catatonic excitement
3. Hallucinations	21. Stereotyped attitudes, movement
4. Orientation	22. Mannerisms
5. Consciousness	23. Parabulia (illogical actions)
6. Memory	24. Negativism
7. Retention (pseudomemories)	25. Personality
8. Train of thought	26. Practical efficiency
9. Association	27. Movements of expression
10. Stereotypy (repetitive ideas)	28. Incoherence
11. Paralogia, evasion	29. Stereotypy (sentence repetitions)
12. Constraint of thought	30. Negativism (mutism, evasion)
13. Mental efficiency	31. Derailments in word-finding
14. Judgment	32. Paraphasia
15. Delusions	33. Neologisms
16. Emotional dullness	34. Akataphasia (peculiar language)
17. Weakening of volitional impulse	35. Syntax
18. Automatic obedience	36. Derailments in train of thought

and were forgetful only on occasion due to "disorganization." This conclusion was based on responses to questions posed during clinical interviews. Bleuler typically assessed autobiographical memory through the process of obtaining a patient's life history. In contrast, "memory for experiences during the examination" was assessed by asking for an account of what had been discussed at the beginning of the interview. Although the importance of cooperation and comprehension of instruction was recognized, there was no standard stimulus material or objective scoring, no validity checks, no normative comparison, and little reference to or appreciation of findings from memory research. Not surprisingly, therefore, Bleuler's assertion about preserved memory has been contradicted by subsequent documentation of relatively severe memory problems in schizophrenia, including episodic and autobiographical deficits (Aleman et al., 1999; Berna et al., 2011; Heinrichs & Zakzanis, 1998). Interview and self-report data continue to yield poor or marginal validity in the estimation of cognitive ability (Johnson et al., 2011; Ventura et al., 2010). However, impairment is demonstrated readily and reliably through application of a variety of psychometric and experimental tasks that are informed by cognitive and neuropsychological research. These tasks measure performance objectively in terms of accuracy, error rates, and completion times as well as in deviations from general population norms. The transition from observation and interview to measurement and performance was an essential precondition for an accurate understanding of cognition in schizophrenia. Yet, by itself, this methodological advance did not ensure that cognitive studies were considered central to schizophrenia science.

The first systematic research application of objective methods to cognition in schizophrenia was developed by Shakow (1962, 1963). This ground-breaking research was concerned primarily with preparatory intervals and reaction time performance and the concept of "set." Set involves the ability to respond adaptively and appropriately to a stimulus situation. Schizophrenia patients found it difficult to "maintain" set and tended to respond to parts and irrelevant aspects of the situation. The concept of set maintenance lives on in measures like the Wisconsin Card Sorting Test and has also been integrated into the study of attention (Cautin, 2008; Mirsky et al., 1992). Unfortunately, the research approach and findings developed by Shakow remained peripheral to the understanding of psychotic illness for many years. More recently, his legacy and the application of methods grounded in experimental psychology to schizophrenia have gained new strength and impact through the development of cognitive neuroscience.

Nevertheless, it is largely through a parallel development, the introduction and use of neuropsychological test batteries designed for clinical assessment of large numbers of schizophrenia patients and comparison subjects, that evidence of cognitive impairment has become overwhelming. By the 1970s it was apparent that the Halstead–Reitan and Luria–Nebraska test batteries were able to discriminate heterogeneous neurological patients from healthy controls (Kane et al., 1985). Hit rates and group discrimination were often greater than 90% (Golden, 1981). However, the scores of neurological and schizophrenia patients overlapped and discrimination was lower or difficult to replicate (Heaton et al., 1978). Initially this score overlap was interpreted as evidence of instrument invalidity or alternately as evidence for the existence of a subset of schizophrenia patients with both "brain damage" and psychosis. Distinguishing between schizophrenia and brain damage was regarded as a difficult diagnostic challenge for clinical neuropsychologists. Then with the rapid expansion and extension of neuroscience theory and methods to psychiatry, views shifted and cognitive impairment in psychotic disorders increasingly "made sense" and came to be expected. Impairment could be understood as a reflection of underlying disturbances in neural systems that mediated the disorder (Flor-Henry, 1990). Hence the inclusion of neuropsychological measures in schizophrenia research became relatively routine during the 1990s. In tandem with these developments and a burgeoning literature, the first meta-analyses became feasible, quantifying results from hundreds of studies and thousands of patients and healthy comparison subjects (Aleman et al., 1999; Heinrichs & Zakzanis, 1998). Thus cognitive impairment, initially viewed as essential to schizophrenia, only to be relegated to the periphery by mid-twentieth century research and clinical lore, has returned as a "core" feature of the disorder and a key target of treatment efforts. Consider the evidence in support of this rediscovered importance.

Criteria for judging the importance of cognition in schizophrenia

There are at least four ways in which cognition may represent a primary and essential feature of schizophrenia and related psychotic illnesses. First, the illness may express itself pervasively and reliably in cognitive performance in the same way that, say, parkinsonism expresses itself in resting tremor or Alzheimer's disease expresses itself in rapid forgetting.

It follows that cognitive abnormalities and traits should occur at extremely high rates in patients with the diagnosis. Second, an essential and primary illness feature is one that is intrinsic and not peripheral to the disorder. Impaired cognitive performance should not be reducible to secondary or iatrogenic influences that reflect treatments, prolonged illness burden, hospitalization, or associated stresses and state influences. In other words, cognitive impairments should be inherent in the disease process and not by-products of receiving a diagnosis. Third, insofar as the symptoms of schizophrenia result from underlying defects in cognitive operations and their neural substrates, it should be possible to index these operations and therefore predict symptom occurrence and severity. If this holds true, the clinical illness cannot be understood without reference to cognition. Fourth, it stands to reason that cognitive processes are essential for adaptive transactions with the environment and impairment limits these transactions, giving rise to inadequate life skills, dependency, unemployment, and other aspects of low functional status. Thus cognitive performance should be a powerful predictor of functionality in schizophrenia patients. Understanding functional outcome in the disorder should require cognitive theory and data. Moreover, cognition may be more than a predictor and correlate of functionality; it may be a causal determinant. If this is the case, then changing a patient's cognitive status should lead to changes in functional status and improvements in outcome that would not otherwise be possible. Successful functionally oriented treatment may require the enhancement of cognitive performance.

Do all patients with schizophrenia have cognitive impairment?

Meta-analytic quantification of cognitive data in schizophrenia patients and non-psychiatric subjects shows unequivocally that very large standardized differences in group means exist across a variety of tests and constructs (Aleman et al., 1999; Forbes et al., 2009; Heinrichs & Zakzanis, 1998; Johnson-Selfridge & Zalewski, 2001; Mesholam-Gately et al., 2009). The magnitude of these differences reliably approaches 1.5 pooled standard deviation units for processing speed and aspects of sensory, verbal, and working memory and averages 1.0 standard deviation unit across tests of attention, executive function, language, motor and spatial abilities, as well as general intelligence. More refined syntheses indicate that measures of processing speed may be the single most sensitive cognitive indicator of schizophrenia, but the broadly based nature of the impairment has continued to receive support (Dickinson et al., 2007). An interpretive reference point for these averaged group differences is provided by Cohen's (1988) idealized distribution overlap percentages. Thus a standardized mean difference of 1.5 corresponds to an estimated overlap between schizophrenia and control distributions of less than 30%, and even 1.0 separates a large majority (65%) of patients and healthy people.

For a comparative perspective, consider the selection of standardized schizophrenia–healthy control group differences presented in Table 1.2 in relation to findings in other areas of the brain and behavior. The magnitude of differences in cognition equal or exceed effect sizes (ES) for moderate–severe traumatic brain injury and composite cognition measures (ES=0.92±0.17; Schretlen & Shapiro, 2003), right cerebral hemisphere stroke effects and nonverbal memory (ES=1.20±0.40; Gillespie et al., 2006), preclinical and subsequent Alzheimer's disease and memory scores (ES=1.06±0.21; Schmand et al., 2010), and attention deficit hyperactivity disorder and executive function (ES=0.54±0.03; Willcutt et al., 2005). In addition, Table 1.2 shows that within the schizophrenia literature,

Table 1.2. Selected meta-analytical findings and abnormalities in schizophrenia patients

Finding: Effect size	Distribution	Separation (%)[1]
1. Neurological soft signs (sensory and motor)[2]	1.59±0.21	73
2. Impaired coding (processing speed)[3]	1.57±0.09	72
3. Reduced letter–number span (working memory)[4]	1.36±0.14	67
4. Reduced semantic word fluency[5]	1.34±0.22	67
5. Backward visual masking[6]	1.27±0.24	64
6. Impaired learning of word lists[3]	1.25±0.20	64
7. Impaired general intellectual ability[3]	1.19±0.29	63
8. Impaired executive ability (WCST)[3]	1.00±0.19	55
9. P50 sensory gating ratio[7]	0.93±0.35	52
10. Maintenance gain in eye tracking[8]	0.87±0.12	50
11. Reduced P300 amplitude[9]	0.85±0.20	50
12. Increased dopamine receptors (PET)[6]	0.70±0.54	43
13. Reduced hippocampal volume (MRI)[10]	0.55±0.19	36
14. Hypofrontality during activation (PET)[10]	0.37±0.08	25

Note: the table shows average effect sizes (standardized mean differences) from schizophrenia patient–healthy control group comparisons, 95% confidence intervals, and estimated joint distribution separation (non-overlap). WCST, Wisconsin card sorting test; PET, positron emission tomography; MRI, magnetic resonance imaging.
[1] Cohen, 1988
[2] Chan et al., 2010
[3] Dickinson et al., 2007
[4] Forbes et al., 2009
[5] Doughty & Done, 2009
[6] Heinrichs, 2001
[7] Chang et al., 2011
[8] O'Driscoll & Callahan, 2008
[9] Bramon et al., 2004
[10] Davidson & Heinrichs, 2003

effect magnitudes for cognitive impairment are larger than effects reported for regional frontal and temporal lobe brain volumes and reduced prefrontal lobe activation in the illness and also exceed effects reported for dopamine receptor densities. Moreover, confidence intervals for averaged cognitive effects consistently exclude 0 (zero) and compare favorably with or exceed margins of error found with neurobiological data (Heinrichs, 2001). This stability reflects the highly reproducible nature of group differences in cognitive performance. Overall, the strength and stability of the evidence supports assertions that the psychotic disease process expresses itself very frequently in cognitive aspects of brain function (Heinrichs, 2005).

Nonetheless, despite this wealth of robust evidence, it may be a mistake to conclude that cognitive impairment truly is pervasive and inevitable across the patient population. Meta-analytic quantification implies that 70%–75% of schizophrenia patients perform below general population values on many standard cognitive tasks. Therefore, a significant

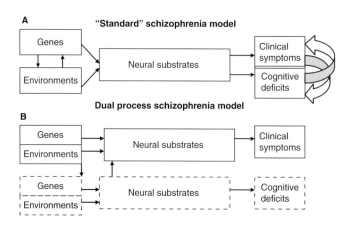

Figure 1.1. Diagram illustrating the distinction between "standard" disease models assuming common neural substrates and pathologies for both psychotic symptoms and cognitive deficits and dual process models that posit independent or weakly correlated psychotic and cognitive substrates in schizophrenia.

minority, 20%–25%, must overlap with healthy people on many ability indicators. A much smaller but potentially important minority may even perform above the healthy mean on these tasks.

The existence of cognitively exceptional schizophrenia patients, or those with task performance at or above normal control values, challenges prevailing assumptions of obligatory deficit and may have major consequences and value for understanding the illness. In particular, preserved and proficient cognitive ability occurring in the presence of a psychotic process implies a dissociation and duality of pathophysiologies underpinning the schizophrenia syndrome. "Standard" models of schizophrenia (see Figure 1.1A) assume that cognitive impairments are inherently tied to the disease process, perhaps preceding the expression of psychosis and persisting with symptom remission, but reflecting the same underlying matrix of neural substrates and genetic and environmental variables. In contrast, a dual process model (Figure 1.1B) holds that cognitive performance deficits index a disturbed system that is partly to completely dissociable from the process underpinning psychotic symptoms. Indeed, from this alternate perspective, cognitive impairment is a secondary process that occurs frequently and in combination with the primary (psychotic) disease process, but remains biologically and behaviorally distinct and not reducible to the psychotic process.

Evidence of relative performance normality in a small portion of patients has been reported occasionally since standard neuropsychological test batteries were first applied to schizophrenia in the 1970s (Golden et al., 1982; Silverstein & Zerwic, 1985). Yet interest in these patients as a potentially valuable resource for understanding psychotic illness has developed slowly and only in the last decade. True neurocognitive normality in the disorder, not to mention giftedness or exceptionality, is a controversial idea and requires careful validation. There are striking case examples of the co-occurrence of psychosis and intellectual or artistic brilliance, but these may be exceptions that prove the rule (see Figure 1.2). It is a challenge to determine the breadth, validity, and possible limits of exceptionality in the patient population in part because of the large number and diversity of measures used in neuropsychological research. The neuropsychological literature on schizophrenia comprises hundreds of studies, thousands of patients and comparison participants, and dozens of tasks and experimental paradigms indexing aspects of intelligence and reasoning, memory and

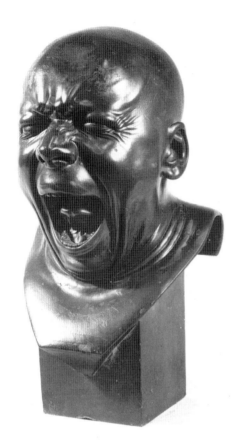

Figure 1.2. Illustration demonstrates the co-existence of psychosis and highly developed artistic and constructional skill in the work of Franz Xaver Messerschmidt (1735–1783). Messerschmidt was a Bavarian sculptor who developed schizophrenia and continued to produce technically accomplished pieces, but strongly influenced by delusions and hallucinations (Heinrichs, 2003). The sculpture shown was given the title *The Yawner* not by the artist, but by later observers and critics. (Reproduced with permission of the Museum of Fine Arts, Budapest, 2012.)

learning, language, attention, and executive and spatial ability. The most frequently used measures include standardized tests like the Wechsler Adult Intelligence Scale (WAIS) (Wechsler, 2008), Wisconsin Card Sorting Test (WCST) (Heaton et al., 1993), and Wechsler Memory Scale (WMS) (Pearson Education, 2008), but there are also batteries of composite and specially constructed measures including the Measurement and Treatment Research to Improve Cognition in Schizophrenia (MATRICS) (Nuechterlein et al., 2008) combination of tasks selected specifically for schizophrenia. Moreover, there is no single definition of normality or exceptionality in psychometric terms.

One frequently used definition of normality involves average-level performance as determined by published general population norms on a selection of standard ability measures. Norm-referenced approaches are sometimes augmented or alternated with expert ratings of individual patient test profiles. The validity of normality definitions is then evaluated by comparing putatively normal patient and healthy groups directly on a battery of tasks. However, average or even above-average scores on a subset of ability measures do not guarantee equivalent levels of performance across all possible neurocognitive tests. Thus Palmer et al. (1997) used a combination of expert ratings and normative criteria to identify 27.5% of their sample of schizophrenia patients as neuropsychologically normal. This subgroup was statistically indistinguishable from a healthy control group on a comprehensive test battery except for a mild deficiency on learning tasks. An even smaller subgroup comprising 11% of the patients also performed normally in learning. Several later investigations supported a 20%–30% overall prevalence of performance normality in schizophrenia (Allen et al., 2003; Holtahusen et al., 2002; Kremen et al., 2000; Weickert et al., 2000). Nevertheless, direct comparison of putatively normal patient and healthy control groups has often found differences in specific abilities including abstraction and executive cognition (Allen et al., 2003; Kremen et al., 2000; Weickert et al., 2000), attention (Kremen et al., 2000; Weickert et al., 2000), and motor skill (Allen et al., 2003; Holtausen et al., 2002; Kremen et al., 2001). Moreover, average-range performance on norms-based summary indices like IQ may mask abnormal ability patterns in patient groups. For example, Wilk et al. (2005) studied schizophrenia patients matched to healthy people with average IQs and found that subtest profiles differed, with patients showing relative deficiencies on memory and processing speed tasks and relative superiority in verbal comprehension and nonverbal reasoning. This study is also notable because it reported data on 13 patients and 13 controls with IQs in the "high-average" range. Group differences in cognitive performance were observed even in these higher functioning patients. Accordingly, patients may score in a norms-defined "average range" on a battery of measures or on a composite score like IQ, but still demonstrate abnormalities or deficiencies on specific tasks when compared directly with a healthy control group.

An additional criterion for normality used by some researchers requires equivalence between current and estimated premorbid levels of performance. The logic underlying this criterion is that intellectual performance in the average population range may reflect deterioration from even higher or above-average ability prior to illness. Oral reading tests are used to provide estimates of premorbid intellectual ability insofar as visual word recognition seems to resist diffuse and multifocal neurological processes (Nuechterlein et al., 2004; Strauss et al., 2006). Weickert et al. (2000) found no difference in the Wide Range Achievement Test (WRAT) reading scores between healthy controls and intellectually "preserved" schizophrenia patients. In contrast, and consistent with a "deterioration" hypothesis, Kremen et al. (2000) reported significantly higher reading scores in neuropsychologically normal patients relative to healthy controls. The premorbid level-of-performance issue remains both infrequently researched and unresolved. In addition, the validity of the idea that a true period of premorbidity exists in a disorder that already expresses itself neurodevelopmentally in childhood and adolescence is questionable.

In a recent study of patients and healthy people with superior verbal ability, our group (Heinrichs et al., 2008) used vocabulary scaled scores ≥ 14 (90th percentile) from the WAIS-III as the criterion for exceptionality. The use of individual rather than composite ability scores like IQ as exceptionality markers has advantages that include efficiency and validity, while also preventing the kind of performance masking described by Wilk et al. (2005). Vocabulary scores are believed to reflect longstanding cognitive traits and are excellent estimators of general ability. Nonetheless, superior range vocabulary scores do not guarantee this level of performance across all tasks. It is noteworthy that verbally exceptional patients in this study scored within average-high-average rather than superior ranges in terms of nonverbal reasoning, working memory, processing speed, verbal learning, word generation, and response inhibition. However, the same pattern of high verbal relative to other abilities was seen in healthy people, and we found no statistically significant group differences across these tasks. Therefore, a pronounced relative strength in verbal skill, with more average or high-average performance in other abilities, is probably a normal pattern in the general population. This study also found no evidence of current versus estimated premorbid functioning discrepancies based on reading scores. The lack of such a discrepancy argues strongly against the idea that verbally superior patients were functioning at even higher levels prior to illness and subsequently declined into the superior range. Nevertheless, the battery of measures used was relatively brief and lacked data for two of the eight separable ability factors identified for schizophrenia (Nuechterlein et al., 2004). These unrepresented abilities include visual learning and memory, and social cognition. Thus the possibility remains that verbally exceptional patients are impaired relative to exceptional controls on these missing ability factors.

It seems reasonable to conclude that cognitive impairment reliably occurs at very high rates in schizophrenia, typically approaching 75% of the patient population, which equals or exceeds the prevalence of impairment in many neurological disorders. However, the existence of even relatively small proportions of neuropsychologically normal or gifted patients makes it hard to answer with an unequivocal "yes" to the question of whether impairment is universal in the illness. To be sure, apparently normal patients may have subtle deficits relative to healthy comparison groups even when test scores are within norm-referenced limits and conventionally defined "average" ranges. Yet until the possibility of preserved cognition in schizophrenia is resolved, impairment should be regarded as probable and highly prevalent, but not obligatory in the illness.

Cognitive impairment in schizophrenia: essence or artifact?

Averaged patient–control group differences in cognitive impairment may be relatively large, but do these differences express the underlying disease process or are they products of powerful medications, years of chronic stress and social disadvantage, and poor motivation? Perhaps surprisingly, meta-analyses and longitudinal studies show that antipsychotic medications have a mildly beneficial rather than adverse effect on cognition in chronic patients (Harvey & Keefe, 2001; Keefe et al., 2007; Mishara & Goldberg, 2004; Thornton et al., 2006). A recent clinical trial comparing first- and second-generation medications in first-episode patients found that all treatments yielded standardized mean differences ranging from ES=0.33 to ES=0.56 relative to baseline at six-month follow-up on a composite cognition measure (Davidson et al., 2009). Moreover, there is evidence that these findings hold up cross-culturally, at least in terms of patients assessed relatively early in their illness (Guo et al., 2011). It is unclear to what extent practice effects may contribute to these improvements in performance, but some recent data suggest this contribution is fairly small (Keefe et al., 2011).

Against this evidence of mild–moderate cognitive benefits for antipsychotic medication there are occasional findings of adverse effects. For example, coding and symbol substitution tasks that require processing speed but also manual dexterity and fine control are highly sensitive to schizophrenia (Dickinson et al., 2007). However, a recent meta-analytic report suggests that a substantial proportion of this effect may be due to adverse motor effects of a chlorpromazine-equivalent medication dose (Knowles et al., 2010). The report found that studies reporting data from highly medicated patients yielded significantly larger impairments in processing speed than studies on less medicated patients. In contrast, other aspects of cognitive performance did not vary with medication dose across studies. One conjecture that may account for such findings involves interference with basal ganglia motor systems due to dopamine receptor blockade. Presumably these dopamine-containing systems contribute to the motor and learning components of processing speed tasks and cannot function normally in the presence of this blockade. Yet a small number of studies suggest that antipsychotic medication may affect task performance even in the absence of a motor task component. For example, there are data indicating that different aspects of nondeclarative memory are reduced as a function of whether schizophrenia patients are treated with first- or second-generation medications (Beninger, 2006; Beninger et al., 2003). In addition, spatial working memory deficits have been reported in first-episode patients treated with risperidone (Reilly et al., 2007). At the same time, it is noteworthy that secondary medications used to treat or reduce the side effects of therapeutic drugs may have negative effects on cognition. McDermid Vaz & Heinrichs (2002) found that memory-impaired patients were more likely to be receiving anticholinergic medication relative to unimpaired patients. Recent evidence confirms this association and suggests that anti-cholinergic drugs reduce the effectiveness of cognitive training (Vinogradov et al., 2009). Moreover, discontinuing anticholinergic drugs can lead to cognitive improvements (Drimer et al., 2004). Taken together, reports in the literature suggest that antipsychotic drugs may yield mild performance-enhancing benefits for many cognitive tasks, but also some adverse effects. These adverse effects are especially indicated in relation to adjunct anticholinergic medication. However, there is no compelling evidence that the breadth and magnitude of cognitive impairment in schizophrenia is attributable to the use of these medications.

Apart from medication, many patients with schizophrenia endure years of chronic illness, social disadvantage, and recurrent hospitalization. There is evidence that stress has physiological and structural effects, and impairs cognitive operations associated with the prefrontal cortex (Hains et al., 2009). Perhaps enduring a socially stigmatized chronic illness rather than the intrinsic schizophrenic disease process itself gives rise to lowered cognitive performance. Against this, it is important to note that cognitive deficits are present in patients with first-episode psychosis (Mesholam-Gately et al., 2009), as well as in attenuated form during the prodrome prior to symptom onset (Seidman et al., 2010) and in adolescents with elevated genetic risk for the illness (Fusar-Poli et al., 2007; Lewandoski et al., 2011). In addition, deficits found in first-episode patients are broadly based but somewhat larger in processing speed and verbal memory, thereby underscoring similarities with data obtained from more chronic samples. Bozikas and Andreou (2011) report that cognitive impairment was stable for up to 10 years in first-episode patients, with possible deterioration noted only in some aspects of verbal memory. Moreover, cross-sectional studies comparing first-episode and chronic psychosis patients provide further evidence that cognitive impairment occurs early and persists rather than developing slowly over the course of illness and treatment (Mesholam-Gately et al., 2009; Sponheim et al., 2010). In light of such findings it is difficult to maintain that the experience of becoming a chronic psychiatric patient rather than the underlying condition is the primary influence on cognitive performance in schizophrenia.

Do cognitive deficits produce the psychopathology of schizophrenia?

Cognitive impairment may be prevalent and largely intrinsic to schizophrenia, but can cognitive theory and data account for delusions, hallucinations, disorganized speech and behavior, withdrawal, and restricted emotion? The interface between cognition and psychosis is a longstanding puzzle that stems in part from the search for neuropsychological correlates of symptom states during the 1990s. Numerous investigations showed that negative symptoms vary moderately with standard cognitive tasks requiring learning and rapid response generation whereas positive symptoms and cognitive performance are usually independent. For example, O'Leary et al. (2000) studied psychotic, negative, and disorganization symptoms in relation to 20 different neuropsychological test scores. Nine of 20 correlations between negative symptoms and cognitive scores primarily indexing verbal memory, attention, and fluency measures were significant, but with a very modest average coefficient of r=0.26. Three correlations including IQ measures were significant in the disorganization symptom data, also with an average of r=0.26. Only two out of 20 correlations were significant in the psychotic symptoms data, with an average of r=0.24. Moreover, these two significant results were from visual memory trials wherein *better* memory performance was associated with *increased* severity of psychotic symptoms.

More recent reviews and empirical reports have confirmed that relations between symptom severity, especially psychotic symptoms, and standard cognitive performance measures are weak and often absent across many clinical samples (Andreasen et al., 2005; Dibben et al., 2009; Ragland et al., 2007). Thus Dominguez et al. (2009) synthesized symptom–cognition correlations from 58 studies published between 1986 and 2007 and found that cognitive measures accounted for only 1%–8% of the variance in disorganization and negative symptom dimensions and no significant positive symptom variance. Another and independently conducted meta-analysis largely confirmed these findings (Ventura et al., 2010). Such weak or absent cognition–psychopathology associations are difficult to accommodate within views that a single disease process gives rise to both psychosis and impaired cognitive performance. Instead, the lack of association implies dual- or multi-process disease models wherein cognitive deficits may occur frequently in the presence of psychosis but also in its absence, and conversely, psychosis should be observable in the absence of cognitive impairment.

If cognitive impairment and psychosis reflect independent disease processes that may co-occur in the way that, say, parkinsonism and dementia often co-occur, then cognitively intact schizophrenia patients should be as symptomatic as those with impairments. Indeed, the small number of patients with above-average abilities should not differ in psychotic symptom severity from patients with average or impaired abilities. Few studies have addressed the psychopathology–cognition relationship by studying patients with above-average relative to lower-ability levels, perhaps because there are so few of them. However, in terms of those with relatively normal or preserved cognitive ability, Palmer et al. (1997) reported positive and negative symptom severities that were indistinguishable from those found in cognitively impaired patients. This finding was supported by Holthausen et al. (2002), Kremen et al. (2000), and Wexler et al. (2009). In contrast, Goldstein et al. (2005) found that patients with relatively preserved cognition were more likely to have paranoid symptoms and McDermid Vaz and Heinrichs (2002) reported broadly elevated symptoms in memory-impaired relative to unimpaired patients. Ammari et al. (2010) found no differences in positive symptoms between intellectually and memory-impaired and average ability-range patients, but did report differences in negative symptoms. However, no differences in psychotic, negative, or mood-related symptoms were found in our study of patients with and without superior-range verbal abilities (Heinrichs et al., 2008).

Thus far it appears that the severity of symptoms associated with schizophrenia is largely if not completely dissociable from performance on standard cognitive measures used in neuropsychological assessment. However, these measures may not be the most suitable probes for investigating the cognition–psychopathology interface. A common criticism of standard cognitive and neuropsychological measures developed for clinical assessment is that they involve more than one process and fail to specify operations that may be selectively impaired or preserved in schizophrenia and other disorders. Moreover, many of these measures were designed to assess deficits in neurological patients with space-occupying brain lesions or to assess school and special education populations rather than patients with psychotic disorders. Hence, the small number of research reports that apply more specific measures to the study of symptoms partially address this criticism. For example, the cognitive analysis of thought and language disorganization symptoms in schizophrenia was advanced by Harvey and associates in the 1980s and 1990s (Harvey, 1985; Harvey et al., 1990; Harvey & Serper, 1990). This literature included experimental paradigms that related the severity of thought and language disorder to processing resources in attention and "reality" monitoring, whereby patients were required to discriminate between their own thoughts and speech. More recent work on disorganization symptoms has shown that context processing as indexed by the AX version of the Continuous Performance Test predicts symptom severity (Barch et al., 2003; MacDonald et al., 2005). It appears then that carefully designed and theoretically driven measurement paradigms may yet uncover connections between cognition and at least some aspects of psychopathology.

As a further case in point, several British psychologists have hypothesized cognitive mechanisms as an essential link in the pathophysiology-to-psychosis sequence. These mechanisms include an inability to integrate and modify current sensory data in light of stored representations and regularities, giving rise to anomalous experiences like delusions (Gray et al., 1991; Hemsley, 1993, 2005). Alternatively, psychotic symptoms may result from a breakdown in cognitive monitoring whereby self-generated thoughts and actions are experienced as alien and external (Frith, 1992, 2005). On the other hand, psychosis may be more related to biases than to outright impairments in cognitive processing. Thus a persistent attribution bias that assigns the causes of negative personal events to the external world may lead to the construction of paranoid phenomenology (Bentall et al., 2001). At the same time, a bias toward premature decision making about event probabilities may contribute to the development of delusions (Garety & Freeman, 1999; Speechley et al., 2010). These proposed cognitive mechanisms and theories do not exclude the influence of environmental stressors, neurobiology, or genes in the development of psychotic illness. However, they assign cognition a central role in the causal pathway leading from neural disturbance to symptom expression. Is the importance assigned to cognition in these theories justified?

There is a section of the literature referred to as "cognitive neuropsychiatry" that has developed to explore and test these ideas, especially in relation to delusions. Perhaps the most frequently studied effect derives from the observation that patients with persecutory delusions are prone to "jump to conclusions" (JTC) and make decisions after a single trial in probabilistic reasoning tasks (Corcoran et al., 1995; Fine et al., 2007; Garety et al., 2005). Here then is a cognitive process directly linked to a positive symptom. However, recent studies suggest that many delusional patients fail to show the bias (Colbert et al., 2010). In addition, although JTC occurs in first-episode patients it does not associate with delusions or other specific symptoms (Dudley et al., 2011). Recent evidence also suggests that JTC may vary with general intellectual ability, thereby undermining arguments that it represents a reasoning bias rather than simply impairment (Lincoln et al., 2010).

Delusional patients also tend to demonstrate belief rigidity or a bias against disconfirmatory evidence (BADE) (Woodward et al., 2006). However, like JTC, this bias is equally prevalent in patients without delusions (Woodward et al., 2008). Aspects of social cognition under investigation include an "externalizing" attribution tendency in blaming other people for negative events (Kaney & Bentall, 1989; Langdon et al., 2010) as well as theory of mind deficits. Externalizing attribution findings have recently been extended to first-episode and high-risk participants with persecutory thinking (An et al., 2010). Nonetheless, like the JTC effect, the specificity of the externalizing bias to patients with persecutory delusions remains in doubt (Jolley et al., 2006). Similarly, the theory of mind construct has generated partially successful investigations into the cognitive basis of persecutory beliefs. Difficulty inferring the intentions of other people would seem to be a strong candidate for a cognitive mechanism underlying paranoia. However, support is decidedly mixed, with some studies finding links between theory of mind deficits and persecutory delusions (Mehl et al., 2010). Yet demonstrating symptom specificity remains a challenge, and a meta-analysis reported deficits in all symptom groups and especially in those with disorganization (Sprong et al., 2007).

The nature of the psychopathology–cognitive interface is also implicated in light of evidence that cognitive impairment persists in patients after successful symptomatic treatment with antipsychotic medication (Elvevåg & Goldberg, 2000; Ma et al., 2007). This persistence, despite symptom remission, also applies to the JTC effect, which further weakens its putative link to delusions. On the other hand, belief rigidity observed in patients with delusions may improve in step with symptom reduction (So et al., 2010). For the most part, however, declines in the severity of psychotic and negative symptoms seem to occur with minimal or no corresponding change in cognitive status. Still, it is not clear whether cognitive impairments always persist in symptomatically remitted patients and the evidence is uneven, especially when rigorous requirements for remission status are applied. Consensus guidelines propose low benchmark ratings of key positive and negative symptoms across a six-month interval as the criterion for remission (Andreasen et al., 2005). Studies by Helldin et al. (2006) and Kopelowicz et al. (2005) support the idea that cognitive impairment and remission failure go hand in hand. In contrast, Krishnadas et al. (2007) found impairment in remitted patients, and Buckley et al. (2007) reported no relationship between neuropsychological deficits and remission status, although a portion of remitted patients did experience neuropsychological improvement.

On balance, although schizophrenia is characterized by severe and apparent disturbances in the *content* of thought and perception, as well as by slowed processing and reduced communication, these disturbances associate minimally or not at all with impaired performance on standard cognitive ability tests. Thought disorder and disorganization symptoms seem to lend themselves more readily than delusions to cognitive analysis, but receive only intermittent research attention. The cognitive psychiatry approach stresses the measurement of specific cognitive operations that may underpin psychotic symptoms. Yet the data do not provide consistent or convincing evidence, thus far, that reasoning and belief biases are essential to delusions. These biases instead may be essential to psychosis in general. The weight of evidence bearing on the cognition–symptom relationship is still based disproportionately on the use of standard neuropsychological tests. Until this situation changes and consistent and strong findings emerge from cognitive neuropsychiatry, the conclusion that cognitive performance and psychosis are largely independent remains tenable.

Is cognitive performance a primary and essential determinant of functional outcome in schizophrenia?

The understanding of outcome in prolonged psychotic illness has become more sophisticated over the past two decades. Spurred by several persuasive and influential articles, outcome has broadened beyond old benchmarks like symptom reduction and hospital discharge to include degree of independence in community living, occupational development, social relationships, and quality of life. Cognitive performance has emerged as a key predictor and perhaps mediator of this broader and more functionally oriented definition of outcome.

Since the publication of a paper by Green (1996), a large increase has occurred in the number of publications investigating relations between cognitive impairments and community adjustment and independence. Evidence accrued over the past decade has shown consistently that cognitive ability is a significant predictor of critical aspects of functional status including work performance and independent living skills. Moreover, some studies indicate that functional deficits are more strongly related to impaired cognition than to either positive or negative symptoms (Keefe & Fenton, 2007). In other reports, no relationship between symptoms and functional status is observed, but significant links are seen between specific cognitive domains (e.g., verbal learning) and outcome (Kurtz et al., 2008). Previous review articles have argued that deficits in cognition account for significant proportions of variance in social skills, community independence, and skill acquisition in outpatient rehabilitation programs (e.g., Green et al., 2000, 2004). For example, McGurk and Mueser (2004) found that impaired mental flexibility, learning and memory, and processing speed were associated with poor work performance. Additional research has shown a relationship between impaired cognitive functioning and poor financial competence (Niekawa et al., 2007). Furthermore, Schutt et al. (2007) found that executive functioning predicted self-care, better verbal memory predicted more positive social contacts, and sustained attention predicted communication skills. Early reviews of the literature (e.g., Green, 1996; Green et al., 2000) reported mean effect sizes of the relationship between individual cognitive abilities and functional outcome in the medium range (i.e., ES=0.50; r=0.30), and larger effects when composite indicators of cognitive functioning are used (Green et al., 2004).

The validity of cognitive measures as predictors of outcome dimensions was the subject of a recent meta-analysis that synthesized data from 52 studies published between 1991 and 2008, and 12 cognitive and four outcome domains (Fett et al., 2011). The amount of outcome variance accounted for by cognitive measures ranged from approximately 4% in the case of attention measures predicting social outcomes to 23% in the theory of mind tasks predicting community functioning. For comparative purposes consider these fairly modest validities in relation to medical and behavioral meta-analytic data compiled by Meyer et al. (2001). For example, stress electrocardiograms account for about 5% of the variance in coronary artery disease, intelligence test scores account for 6% of job effectiveness ratings, and screening mammogram results account for about 9% of cancer morbidity at one year follow-up. On the other hand, validities are not always so modest. Neuropsychological test scores account for more than 18% of the variance in the driving ability of dementia patients (Reger et al., 2004), IQ scores capture 19% of the variance in educational achievement, and ultrasound tests capture almost 69% of the variance in peripheral artery disease. The average variance for data on 63 medical tests compiled by Meyer et al. (2001) was 13%, whereas 26 psychological and cognitive measures averaged 12%. It seems reasonable to conclude that commonly used cognitive measures vary with functional outcome measures in schizophrenia about as much as many measures used in medicine and other applied psychology contexts vary with their criteria. At best, cognitive measures capture perhaps a quarter of the variance in any given outcome dimension, but average validities are more modest and similar to findings in other fields. Not surprisingly, even strong advocates of the validity of cognitive measurements as outcome indicators in schizophrenia acknowledge that many variables influence patients' behavior and adjustment in real-life settings (Green, 2006).

Apart from the ability of cognitive measures to predict important aspects of functional status, there is the question of whether cognitive *change* necessarily or even often leads to functional change. Cognitive performance may be an important predictor of outcome without actually mediating functionality in any way. A preliminary review (Matza et al., 2006) of the little literature relevant to this question (six longitudinal treatment and three non-treatment studies) indicated that outcome changes vary significantly with changes in memory, processing speed, and executive ability. Moreover, the complementary change relationship was demonstrable for both pharmacological and psychosocial treatments. However, the specific findings were heterogeneous across studies and the adequacy of functional outcome measures was questioned. In addition, change relationships were not quantified or presented as effect sizes. Another study using cognitive remediation showed that improvements in working memory related to improved social functioning six months later (Wykes et al., 2007). Fiszdon et al. (2008) examined cognition in relation to life quality over a 12-month period in 151 schizophrenia patients engaged in work therapy programs. Improvements in immediate recall of prose material and *declines* in the conceptual level percentage on the WCST were modestly associated with overall quality of life changes. It is not clear why increased concreteness should associate with improved life quality, although this finding may reflect the nature of work therapy, client populations, and their regimen of activities. More supportive evidence was reported in a study of cognitive enhancement therapy and functional outcome (Eack et al., 2010). Improved cognitive and social–cognitive performance associated with improved functional outcome, with data indicating that Part B of the Trail Making Test uniquely mediated the relationship. Unfortunately, data on variance accounted for were not provided, making assessment of the magnitude of the cognitive change–functional change relationship difficult to estimate.

In aggregate, the literature on cognitive performance and functional outcome supports the validity of cognition as an important but modest predictor, which nonetheless compares favorably with validities reported in many fields of medicine and applied psychology. However, most of the variance in outcome remains unaccounted for by cognitive measures and a key corollary issue remains barely addressed. For instance, there are few data bearing on the extent to which changes in cognitive performance are preconditions or even predictors of meaningful changes and improvements in functional status and adjustment. In view of the very large resources being assigned to the enhancement of cognition in schizophrenia, a clearer understanding of the link between cognitive and functional change seems imperative.

How important is cognition in schizophrenia?

The study of attention, learning and memory, problem solving and language, and other aspects of cognition has emerged, receded, and shifted from the center to the periphery and back again over the history of schizophrenia. In many ways it is difficult to imagine an understanding of a psychotic illness not being built on a foundation of cognition and neuropsychology. Yet does the evidence support the view that cognitive processes and impairment are so pervasive, so intrinsic, so tied to the defining psychopathology and functional consequences of schizophrenia that the illness is best understood as a disorder of cognition?

Given the uncertain validity of the diagnostic category of schizophrenia in the *Diagnostic and Statistical Manual of Mental Disorders*, DSM-IV and prospective DSM-V systems, it is probably unrealistic to expect every patient to demonstrate a normative or control-referenced deficit in cognitive performance. The estimated prevalence of impairment using the most sensitive neuropsychological tests approximates 75% of the patient population and there is little evidence that this impairment is reducible to treatment artifacts. Antipsychotic medications seem to have a mildly beneficial influence on performance, whereas drugs used to lessen side-effects may compound but do not create the cognitive deficits observed in most patients. At the same time, the possibility of preserved cognition in a significant minority of people with schizophrenia has not been resolved and this challenges the assertion that cognitive impairment is a truly defining characteristic of the illness. It may be that patients with apparently preserved abilities have subtle or more selective deficits. This is an empirical question that can be addressed through more systematic and sustained research attention. However, even if cognitively high-functioning patients demonstrate subtle deficits, the weak or absent association between psychotic symptoms and cognitive performance signals a major challenge to disease models and theories that assign cognition a key role in the transition from neural events to psychopathology. To be sure, this lack of association may reflect the use of relatively blunt measures and inappropriate constructs not designed to uncover the hidden cognitive operations that promote psychosis. Yet the more specific and refined methods used in cognitive neuropsychiatry have, thus far, not provided compelling and consistent data to link symptoms and several candidate cognitive mechanisms. Could this mean that cognition and psychosis reflect independent processes that often but not necessarily occur together?

The neurological literature furnishes a perspective on this question by documenting disorders where cognitive impairment and psychosis co-occur at widely divergent frequencies. Thus, by definition, cognitive impairment is highly prevalent in frontotemporal dementia, but psychosis is rare (Mendez et al., 2008). The majority of patients with Parkinson's disease eventually develop cognitive deficits, but psychosis is much less common and largely a by-product of medication (Friedman, 2010). Similarly, cognition is impaired in close to 80% of patients with systemic lupus erythematosis, whereas only 5% develop psychosis (Brey et al., 2002). In contrast, psychosis is much more prevalent in both Alzheimer's disease and vascular dementia and occurs most frequently when cognitive impairment is severe (Ostling et al., 2010). On the other hand, psychosis also exceeds population base rates following traumatic brain injury but it appears regardless of injury severity, whereas cognitive impairment exceeds psychosis in prevalence and is linked to severity (Kim et al., 2007). None of this proves that cognitive impairment and psychosis are independent disease processes. However, the data do imply that psychosis is not proportionately, directly, or invariably associated with cognitive impairment in central nervous system disorders.

Whatever the outcome of the debate regarding neuropsychological normality in schizophrenia, patients with relatively preserved abilities also offer a perspective on the cognition–functional outcome interface. Those with apparently intact abilities and no evidence of decline from putative premorbid levels have presumably benefited from these abilities over their lifespans. This situation contrasts with cognitively impaired patients demonstrating performance gains in response to pharmacologically or behaviorally based cognitive enhancement. These treated patients may translate their enhanced cognition into outcome gains to a moderate degree and over an extended period of time. However, surely the functional benefit of cognition is maximal for patients with relatively preserved and lifelong abilities. In this regard, it is sobering to note that even the most cognitively advantaged patients remain severely disadvantaged in terms of community adjustment when compared to healthy people at the same ability level. Effect sizes (standardized mean difference) between 2.0 and 3.0 are reported for group comparisons in community independence (Ammari et al., 2010; Heinrichs et al., 2008). It is thereby difficult to escape the conclusion that cognitive performance is only one possible mediator of functionality and may even play a minor role.

In conclusion, there is no doubt that schizophrenia typically involves impaired cognitive performance across a variety of measures. Moreover, there is little doubt that this impairment is largely intrinsic to the illness. The possibility of preserved cognition and its implications for understanding the illness, along with questions of whether cognition truly mediates functional outcome and underpins psychotic symptoms, remain relatively open. These unanswered questions provide rich avenues for further investigation into schizophrenia as a cognitive disorder.

References

Aleman, A., Hijman, R., de Haan, E. H., et al. (1999). Memory impairment in schizophrenia: a meta-analysis. *American Journal of Psychiatry*, **156**, 1358–1366.

Allen, D. N., Goldstein, G., & Warnick, E. (2003). A consideration of neuropsychologically normal schizophrenia. *Journal of the International Neuropsychological Society*, **9**, 56–63.

Ammari, N., Heinrichs, R. W., & Miles, A. A. (2010). An investigation of 3 neurocognitive subtypes in schizophrenia. *Schizophrenia Research*, **121**, 32–38.

An, S. K., Kang, J. I., Park, J. Y., et al. (2010). Attribution bias in ultra-high risk for psychosis and first-episode schizophrenia. *Schizophrenia Research*, **118**, 54–61.

Andreasen, N. C., Carpenter, W. T. Jr., Kane, J. M., et al. (2005). Remission in schizophrenia: proposed criteria and rationale for consensus. *American Journal of Psychiatry*, **162**, 441–449.

Barch, D. M., Carter, C. S., MacDonald, A. W. 3rd., et al. (2003). Context-processing deficits in schizophrenia: diagnostic specificity, 4-week course, and relationships to clinical symptoms. *Journal of Abnormal Psychology*, **112**, 132–143.

Beninger, R. J. (2006). Dopamine and incentive learning: a framework for considering antipsychotic medication effects. *Neurotoxicity Research*, **10**, 199–209.

Beninger, R. J., Wasserman, J., Zanibbi, K., et al. (2003). Typical and atypical antipsychotic medications differentially affect two nondeclarative memory tasks in schizophrenic patients: a double dissociation. *Schizophrenia Research*, **61**, 281–292.

Bentall, R. P., Corcoran, R., Howard, R., et al. (2001). Persecutory delusions: a review and theoretical integration. *Clinical Psychology Review*, **21**, 1143–1192.

Berna, F., Bennouna-Greene, M., Potheegadoo, J., et al. (2011). Impaired ability to give a meaning to personally significant events in patients with schizophrenia. *Consciousness and Cognition*, **20**, 703–711.

Bleuler, E. (1943). *Lehrbuch der Psychiatrie*. Berlin: Springer.

Bleuler, E. (1950). *Dementia praecox, or the group of schizophrenias*. (J. Zinkin, Trans.). New York, NY: International Universities Press. (Original work published 1911.)

Bozikas, V. P. & Andreou, C. (2011). Longitudinal studies of cognition in first episode psychosis: a systematic review of the literature. *Australian and New Zealand Journal of Psychiatry*, **45**, 93–108.

Bramon, E., Rabe-Hesketh, S., Sham, P., et al. (2004). Meta-analysis of the P300 and P50 waveforms in schizophrenia. *Schizophrenia Research*, **70**, 315–329.

Brey, R. L., Holliday, S. L., Saklad, A. R., et al. (2002). Neuropsychiatric syndromes in lupus: prevalence using standardized definitions. *Neurology*, **58**, 1214–1220.

Buckley, P. F., Harvey, P. D., Bowie, C. R., et al. (2007). The relationship between symptomatic remission and neuropsychological improvement in schizophrenia patients switched to treatment with ziprasidone. *Schizophrenia Research*, **94**, 99–106.

Cautin, R. L. (2008). David Shakow and schizophrenia research at Worcester State Hospital: the roots of the scientist-practitioner model. *Journal of the History of the Behavioral Sciences*, **44**, 219–237.

Chan, R. C., Xu, T., Heinrichs, R. W., et al. (2010). Neurological soft signs in schizophrenia: a meta-analysis. *Schizophrenia Bulletin*, **36**, 1089–1104.

Chang, W. P., Arfken, C. L., Sangal, M. P., et al. (2011). Probing the relative contribution of the first and second responses to sensory gating indices: a meta-analysis. *Psychophysiology*, **48**, 980–992.

Cohen, J. (1988). *Statistical Power Analysis for the Behavioral Sciences*. (2nd edn.). New York, NY: Academic Press.

Colbert, S. M., Peters, E., & Garety, P. (2010). Jumping to conclusions and perceptions in early psychosis: relationship with delusional beliefs. *Cognitive Neuropsychiatry*, **15**, 422–440.

Corcoran, R., Mercer, G., & Frith, C. D. (1995). Schizophrenia, symptomatology and social inference: investigating "theory of mind" in people with schizophrenia. *Schizophrenia Research*, **17**, 5–13.

Davidson, L. & Heinrichs, R. W. (2003). Quantification of brain imaging findings on the frontal and temporal lobes in schizophrenia: a meta-analysis. *Psychiatry Research: Neuroimaging*, **122**, 69–87.

Davidson, M., Galderisi, S., Weiser, M., et al. (2009). Cognitive effects of antipsychotic drugs in first-episode schizophrenia and schizophreniform disorder: a randomized, open-label clinical trial (EUFEST). *American Journal of Psychiatry*, **166**, 675–682.

Dibben, C. R., Rice, C., Laws, K., et al. (2009). Is executive impairment associated with schizophrenic syndromes? A meta-analysis. *Psychological Medicine*, **39**, 381–392.

Dickinson, D., Ramsey, M. E., & Gold, J. M. (2007). Overlooking the obvious: a meta-analytic comparison of digit symbol coding tasks and other cognitive measures in schizophrenia. *Archives of General Psychiatry*, **64**, 532–542.

Dominguez, Mde G., Viechtbauer, W., Simons, C. J. P., et al. (2009). Are psychotic psychopathology and neurocognition orthogonal? A systematic review of their associations. *Psychological Bulletin*, **135**, 157–171.

Doughty, O. J. & Done, D. J. (2009). Is semantic memory impaired in schizophrenia? A systematic review and meta-analysis of 91 studies. *Cognitive Neuropsychiatry*, **14**, 473–509.

Drimer, T., Shahal, B., & Barak, Y. (2004). Effects of discontinuation of long-term anticholinergic treatment in elderly schizophrenia patients. *International Clinical Psychopharmacology*, **19**, 27–29.

Dudley, R., Shaftoe, D., Cavanagh, K., et al. (2011). 'Jumping to conclusions' in first-episode psychosis. *Early Intervention in Psychiatry*, **5**, 50–56.

Eack, S. M., Pogue-Geile, M. F., Greenwald, D. P., et al. (2010). Mechanisms of functional improvement in a 2-year trial of cognitive enhancement therapy for early schizophrenia. *Psychological Medicine*, **22**, 1–9.

Elvevåg, B. & Goldberg, T. E. (2000). Cognitive impairment in schizophrenia is the core of the disorder. *Critical Reviews in Neurobiology*, **14**, 1–21.

Fett, A. K., Viechtbauer, W., Dominguez, M. D., et al. (2011). The relationship between neurocognition and social cognition with functional outcomes in schizophrenia: a meta-analysis. *Neuroscience and Biobehavioral Reviews*, **35**, 573–588.

Fine, C., Gardner, M., Craigie, J., et al. (2007). Hopping, skipping or jumping to conclusions? Clarifying the JTC bias in delusions. *Cognitive Neuropsychiatry*, **12**, 46–77.

Fiszdon, J. M., Choi, J., Goulet, J., et al. (2008). Temporal relationship between change in cognition and change in functioning in schizophrenia. *Schizophrenia Research*, **105**, 105–113.

Flor-Henry, P. (1990). Neuropsychology and psychopathology: a progress report. *Neuropsychology Review*, **1**, 103–123.

Forbes, N. F., Carrick, L. A., McIntosh, A. M., et al. (2009). Working memory in schizophrenia: a meta-analysis. *Psychological Medicine*, **39**, 889–905.

Friedman, J. H. (2010). Parkinson's disease psychosis 2010: a review article. *Parkinsonism and Related Disorders*, **16**, 553–560.

Frith, C. (1992). *The Cognitive Neuropsychology of Schizophrenia*. Hove: Lawrence Erlbaum.

Frith, C. (2005). The neural basis of hallucinations and delusions. *Comptes Rendus Biologies*, **328**, 169–175.

Fusar-Poli, P., Perez, J., Broome, M., et al. (2007). Neurofunctional correlates of vulnerability to psychosis: a systematic review and meta-analysis. *Neuroscience and Biobehavioral Reviews*, **31**, 465–484.

Garety, P. & Freeman, D. (1999). Cognitive approaches to delusions: a critical review of theories and evidence. *British Journal of Clinical Psychology*, **38**, 113–154.

Garety, P. A., Freeman, D., Jolley, S., et al. (2005). Reasoning, emotions, and delusional conviction in psychosis. *Journal of Abnormal Psychology*, **114**, 373–384.

Gillespie, D. C., Bowen, A., & Foster, J. K. (2006). Memory impairment following right hemisphere stroke: a comparative meta-analytic and narrative review. *Clinical Neuropsychologist*, **20**, 59–75.

Golden, C. J. (1981). The Luria-Nebraska Neuropsychological Battery: theory and research. In P. McReynolds (ed.), *Advances in Psychological Assessment*. (vol. **5**). San Francisco, CA: Jossey-Bass, pp. 191–235.

Golden, C. J., MacInnes, W. D., Ariel, R. N., et al. (1982). Cross-validation of the ability of the Luria-Nebraska Neuropsychological Battery to differentiate chronic schizophrenics with and without ventricular enlargement. *Journal of Consulting and Clinical Psychology*, **50**, 87–95.

Goldstein, G., Shemansky, W. J., & Allen, D. N. (2005). Cognitive function in schizoaffective disorder and clinical subtypes of schizophrenia. *Archives of Clinical Neuropsychology*, **20**, 153–159.

Gray, J. A., Feldon, J., Rawlins, J. N. P., et al. (1991). The neuropsychology of schizophrenia. *Behavioural and Brain Sciences*, **14**, 1–84.

Green, M. F. (1996). What are the functional consequences of neurocognitive deficits in schizophrenia? *American Journal of Psychiatry*, **153**, 321–330.

Green, M. F. (2006). Cognitive impairment and functional outcome in schizophrenia and bipolar disorder. *Journal of Clinical Psychiatry*, **67**, 36–42.

Green, M. F., Kern, R. S., Braff, D. L., et al. (2000). Neurocognitive deficits and functional outcome in schizophrenia: are we measuring the right stuff? *Schizophrenia Bulletin*, **26**, 119–136.

Green, M. F., Kern, R. S., & Heaton, R. K. (2004). Longitudinal studies of cognition and functional outcome in schizophrenia: implications for MATRICS. *Schizophrenia Research*, **72**, 41–51.

Guo, X., Zhai, J., Wei, Q., et al. (2011). Neurocognitive effects of first- and second-generation antipsychotic drugs in early-stage schizophrenia: a naturalistic 12-month follow-up study. *Neuroscience Letters*, **503**, 141–146.

Hains, A. B., Vu, M. A., Maciejewski, P. K., et al. (2009). Inhibition of protein kinase C signaling protects prefrontal cortex dendritic spines and cognition from the effects of chronic stress. *Proceedings of the National Academy of Sciences of the United States of America*, **106**, 17957–17962.

Harvey, P. D. (1985). Reality monitoring in mania and schizophrenia. The association of thought disorder and performance. *Journal of Nervous and Mental Disease*, **173**, 67–73.

Harvey, P. D., Docherty, N. M., Serper, M. R., et al. (1990). Cognitive deficits and thought disorder: II. An 8-month followup study. *Schizophrenia Bulletin*, **16**, 147–156.

Harvey, P. D. & Keefe, R. S. (2001). Studies of cognitive change in patients with schizophrenia following novel antipsychotic treatment. *American Journal of Psychiatry*, **158**, 176–184.

Harvey, P. D. & Serper, M. R. (1990). Linguistic and cognitive failures in schizophrenia. A multivariate analysis. *Journal of Nervous and Mental Disease*, **178**, 487–493.

Heaton, R. K., Baade, L. E., & Johnson K. L. (1978). Neuropsychological test results associated with psychiatric disorders in adults. *Psychological Bulletin*, **85**, 141–162.

Heaton, R. K., Chelune, G. J., Talley, J. L., et al. (1993). *Wisconsin Card Sorting Test Manual-Revised and Expanded*. Odessa, FL: Psychological Assessment Resources, Inc.

Heinrichs, R. W. (2001). *In Search of Madness: Schizophrenia and Neuroscience*. New York, NY: Oxford University Press.

Heinrichs, R. W. (2005). The primacy of cognition in schizophrenia. *American Psychologist*, **60**, 229–242.

Heinrichs, R. W., Miles, A., Smith D., et al. (2008). Cognitive, clinical, and functional characteristics of verbally superior schizophrenia patients. *Neuropsychology*, **22**, 321–328.

Heinrichs, R. W. & Zakzanis, K. K. (1998). Neurocognitive deficit in schizophrenia: a quantitative review of the evidence. *Neuropsychology*, **12**, 426–445.

Helldin, L., Kane, J. M., Karilampi, U., et al. (2006). Remission and cognitive ability in a cohort of patients with schizophrenia. *Journal of Psychiatric Research*, **40**, 738–745.

Hemsley, D. R. (1993). A simple (or simplistic?) cognitive model for schizophrenia. *Behaviour Research and Therapy*, **31**, 633–646.

Hemsley, D. R. (2005). The development of a cognitive model of schizophrenia: placing it in context. *Neuroscience and Biobehavioral Reviews*, **29**, 977–988.

Holthausen, E. A, Wiersma, D., Sitskoorn, M. M., et al. (2002). Schizophrenic patients without neuropsychological deficits: subgroup, disease severity or cognitive compensation? *Psychiatry Research*, **112**, 1–11.

Johnson, I., Tabbane, K., Dellagi, L., et al. (2011). Self-perceived cognitive functioning does not correlate with objective measures of cognition in schizophrenia. *Comprehensive Psychiatry*, **52**, 688–692.

Johnson-Selfridge, M. & Zalewski, C. (2001). Moderator variables of executive functioning in schizophrenia: meta-analytic findings. *Schizophrenia Bulletin*, **27**, 305–316.

Jolley, S., Garety, P., Bebbington, P., et al. (2006). Attributional style in psychosis: the role of affect and belief type. *Behaviour Research and Therapy*, **44**, 1597–1607.

Kane, R. L., Parsons, O. A., & Goldstein, G. (1985). Statistical relationships and discriminative accuracy of the Halstead-Reitan, Luria-Nebraska, and Wechsler IQ scores in the identification of brain damage. *Journal of Clinical and Experimental Neuropsychology*, **7**, 211–223.

Kaney, S. & Bentall R. P. (1989). Persecutory delusions and attributional style. *British Journal of Medical Psychology*, **62**, 191–198.

Keefe, R. S., Bilder, R. M., Davis, S. M., et al. (2007). Neurocognitive effects of antipsychotic medications in patients with chronic schizophrenia in the CATIE Trial. *Archives of General Psychiatry*, **64**, 633–647.

Keefe, R. S. & Fenton, W. S. (2007). How should DSM-V criteria for schizophrenia include cognitive impairment? *Schizophrenia Bulletin*, **33**, 912–920.

Keefe, R. S., Fox, K. H., Harvey, P. D., et al. (2011). Characteristics of the MATRICS Consensus Cognitive Battery in a 29-site antipsychotic schizophrenia clinical trial. *Schizophrenia Research*, **125**, 161–168.

Kim, E., Lauterbach, E. C., Reeve, A., et al. (2007). Neuropsychiatric complications of traumatic brain injury: a critical review of the literature (a report by the ANPA Committee on Research). *Journal of Neuropsychiatry and Clinical Neurosciences*, **19**, 106–127.

Knowles, E. E., David, A. S., & Reichenberg, A. (2010). Processing speed deficits in schizophrenia: reexamining the evidence. *American Journal of Psychiatry*, **167**, 828–835.

Kopelowicz, A., Liberman, R. P., Ventura, J., et al. (2005). Neurocognitive correlates of recovery from schizophrenia. *Psychological Medicine*, **35**, 1165–1173.

Kraepelin, E. (1896). *Psychiatrie: ein lehrbuch für studierende und arzte.* (5th edn.). Leipzig: Barth.

Kraepelin, E. (1919). *Dementia praecox and paraphrenia* (R. M. Barclay, Trans.). Edinburgh: Livingstone.

Kremen, W. S., Seidman, L. J., Faraone, S. V., et al. (2000). The paradox of normal neuropsychological function in schizophrenia. *Journal of Abnormal Psychology*, **109**, 743–752.

Kremen, W. S., Seidman, L. J., Faraone, S. V., et al. (2001). Intelligence quotients and neuropsychological profiles in patients with schizophrenia and healthy volunteers. *Biological Psychiatry*, **50**, 453–462.

Krishnadas, R., Moore, B. P., Nayak, A., et al. (2007). Relationship of cognitive function in patients with schizophrenia in remission to disability: a cross-sectional study in an Indian sample. *Annals of General Psychiatry*, **6**, 19.

Kurtz, M. M., Wexler, B. E., Fujimoto, M., et al. (2008). Symptoms versus neurocognition as predictors of change in life skills in schizophrenia after outpatient rehabilitation. *Schizophrenia Research*, **102**, 303–311.

Langdon, R., Ward, P. B., & Coltheart, M. (2010). Reasoning anomalies associated with delusions in schizophrenia. *Schizophrenia Bulletin*, **36**, 321–330.

Lewandoski, K. E., Cohen, B. M., & Ongur, D. (2011). Evolution of neuropsychological dysfunction during the course of schizophrenia and bipolar disorder. *Psychological Medicine*, **41**, 225–241.

Lincoln, T. M., Ziegler, M., Mehl, S., et al. (2010). The jumping to conclusions bias in delusions: specificity and changeability. *Journal of Abnormal Psychology*, **119**, 40–49.

Ma, X., Wang, Q., Sham, P. C., et al. (2007). Neurocognitive deficits in first-episode schizophrenic patients and their first-degree relatives. *American Journal of Medical Genetics Part B: Neuropsychiatric Genetics*, **144**B, 407–416.

MacDonald A. W. 3rd., Carter, C. S., Kerns, J. G., et al. (2005). Specificity of prefrontal dysfunction and context processing deficits to schizophrenia in never-medicated patients with first-episode psychosis. *American Journal of Psychiatry*, **162**, 475–484.

Matza, L. S., Buchanan, R., Purdon, S., et al. (2006). Measuring changes in functional status among patients with schizophrenia: the link with cognitive impairment. *Schizophrenia Bulletin*, **32**, 666–678.

McDermid Vaz, S. & Heinrichs, R. W. (2002). Schizophrenia and memory impairment: evidence for a neurocognitive subtype. *Psychiatry Research*, **113**, 93–105.

McGurk, S. R. & Mueser, K. T. (2004). Cognitive functioning, symptoms, and work in supported employment: a review and heuristic model. *Schizophrenia Research*, **70**, 147–173.

Mehl, S., Rief, W., Lüllmann, E., et al. (2010). Are theory of mind deficits in understanding intentions of others associated with persecutory delusions? *Journal of Nervous and Mental Disease*, **198**, 516–519.

Mendez, M. F., Shapira, J. S., Woods, R. J., et al. (2008). Psychotic symptoms in frontotemporal dementia: prevalence and review. *Dementia and Geriatric Cognitive Disorders*, **25**, 206–211.

Mesholam-Gately, R. I., Giuliano, A. J., Goff, K. P., et al. (2009). Neurocognition in first-episode schizophrenia: a meta-analytic review. *Neuropsychology*, **23**, 315–336.

Meyer, G. J., Finn, S. E., Eyde, L. D., et al. (2001). Psychological testing and psychological assessment. A review of evidence and issues. *American Psychologist*, **56**, 128–165.

Mirsky, A. F., Lochhead, S. J., Jones, B. P., et al. (1992). On familial factors in the attentional deficit in schizophrenia: a review and report of two new subject samples. *Journal of Psychiatric Research*, **26**(4), 383–403.

Mishara, A. L. & Goldberg, T. E. (2004). A meta-analysis and critical review of the effects of conventional neuroleptic treatment on cognition in schizophrenia: opening a closed book. *Biological Psychiatry*, **55**, 1013–1022.

Niekawa, N., Sakuraba, Y., Uto, H., et al. (2007). Relationship between financial competence and cognitive function in patients with schizophrenia. *Psychiatry and Clinical Neuroscience*, **61**, 455–461.

Nuechterlein, K. H., Barch, D. M., Gold, J. M., et al. (2004). Identification of separable cognitive factors in schizophrenia. *Schizophrenia Research*, **72**, 29–39.

Nuechterlein, K. H., Green, M. F., Kern, R. S., et al. (2008). The MATRICS Consensus Cognitive Battery, part 1: test selection, reliability, and validity. *American Journal of Psychiatry*, **165**, 203–213.

O'Driscoll, G. A. & Callahan, B. L. (2008). Smooth pursuit in schizophrenia: a meta-analytic review of research since 1993. *Brain and Cognition*, **68**, 359–370.

O'Leary, D. S., Flaum, M., Kesler, M. L., et al. (2000). Cognitive correlates of the negative, disorganized, and psychotic symptom dimensions of schizophrenia. *Journal of Neuropsychiatry Clinical Neurosciences*, **12**, 4–15.

Ostling, S., Gustafson, D., Blennow, K., et al. (2010). Psychotic symptoms in a population-based sample of 85-year-old individuals with dementia. *New England Journal of Medicine*, **328**, 153–158.

Palmer, B. W., Heaton, R. K., Paulsen, J. S., et al. (1997). Is it possible to be schizophrenic yet neuropsychologically normal? *Neuropsychology*, **11**, 437–446.

Pearson Education. (2008). *Wechsler Memory Scale,* 4th edn.: *Clinical Features of the New Edition.* New York, NY: Pearson Education.

Ragland, J. D., Yoon, J., Minzenberg, M. J., et al. (2007). Neuroimaging of cognitive disability in schizophrenia: search for a pathophysiological mechanism. *International Review of Psychiatry*, **19**, 417–427.

Randolph, C., Goldberg, T. E., & Weinberger, D. R. (1993). The neuropsychology of schizophrenia. In K. M. Heilman & E. Valenstein (eds.), *Clinical Neuropsychology.* (3rd edn.). New York, NY: Oxford University Press, pp. 499–522.

Reger, M. A., Welsh, R. K., Watson, G. S., et al. (2004). The relationship between neuropsychological functioning and driving ability in dementia: a meta-analysis. *Neuropsychology*, **18**, 85–93.

Reilly, J. L., Harris, M. S., Khine, T. T., et al. (2007). Antipsychotic drugs exacerbate impairment on a working memory task in first-episode schizophrenia. *Biological Psychiatry*, **62**, 818–821.

Riecher-Rössler, A. & Rössler, W. (1998). The course of schizophrenic psychoses: what do we really know? A selective review from an epidemiological perspective. *European Archives of Psychiatry and Clinical Neuroscience*, **248**, 189–202.

Schmand, B., Huizenga, H. M., & van Gool, W. A. (2010). Meta-analysis of CSF and MRI biomarkers for detecting preclinical Alzheimer's disease. *Psychological Medicine*, **40**, 135–145.

Schretlen, D. J. & Shapiro, A. M. (2003). A quantitative review of the effects of traumatic brain injury on cognitive functioning. *International Review of Psychiatry*, **15**, 341–349.

Schutt, R. K., Seidman, L. J., Caplan, B., et al. (2007). The role of neurocognition and social context in predicting community functioning among formerly homeless seriously mentally ill persons. *Schizophrenia Bulletin*, **33**, 1388–1396.

Seidman, L. J., Giuliano, A. J., Meyer, E. C., et al. (2010). Neuropsychology of the prodrome to psychosis in the NAPLS consortium: relationship to family history and conversion to psychosis. *Archives of General Psychiatry*, **67**, 578–588.

Shakow, D. (1962). Segmental set. *Archives of General Psychiatry*, **6**, 1–17.

Shakow, D. (1963). Psychological deficit in schizophrenia. *Behavioral Science*, **8**, 275–305.

Silverstein, M. L. & Zerwic, M. J. (1985). Clinical psychopathologic symptoms in neuropsychologically impaired and intact schizophrenics. *Journal of Consulting and Clinical Psychology*, **53**, 267–268.

So, S. H., Garety, P. A., Peters, E. R., et al. (2010). Do antipsychotics improve reasoning biases? A review. *Psychosomatic Medicine*, **72**, 681–693.

Speechley, W. J., Whitman, J. C., & Woodward, T. S. (2010). The contribution of hypersalience to the "jumping to conclusions" bias associated with delusions in schizophrenia. *Journal of Psychiatry and Neuroscience*, **35**, 7–17.

Sponheim, S. R., Jung, R. E., Seidman, L. J., et al. (2010). Cognitive deficits in recent-onset and chronic schizophrenia. *Journal of Psychiatric Research*, **44**, 421–428.

Sprong, M., Schothorst, P., Vos, E., et al. (2007). Theory of mind in schizophrenia: meta-analysis. *British Journal of Psychiatry*, **191**, 5–13.

Strauss, E., Sherman, E. M., & Spreen, O. (2006). *A Compendium of Neuropsychological Tests.* (3rd edn.). New York, NY: Oxford University Press.

Thornton, A. E., Van Snellenberg, J. X., Sepehry, A. A., et al. (2006). The impact of atypical antipsychotic medications on long-term memory dysfunction in schizophrenia spectrum disorder: a quantitative review. *Journal of Psychopharmacology*, **20**, 335–346.

Ventura, J., Reise, S. P., Keefe, R. S., et al. (2010). The Cognitive Assessment Interview (CAI): development and validation of an empirically derived, brief interview-based measure of cognition. *Schizophrenia Research*, **121**, 24–31.

Vinogradov, S., Fisher, M., Warm, H., et al. (2009). The cognitive cost of anticholinergic burden: decreased response to cognitive training in schizophrenia. *American Journal of Psychiatry*, **166**, 1055–1062.

Wechsler, D. (2008). *Wechsler Adult Intelligence Scale.* (4th edn.). San Antonio, TX: Psychological Corporation.

Weickert, T. W., Goldberg, T. E., Gold, J. M., et al. (2000). Cognitive impairments in patients with schizophrenia displaying preserved and compromised intellect. *Archives of General Psychiatry*, **57**, 907–913.

Wexler, B. E., Zhu, H., Bell, M. D., et al. (2009). Neuropsychological near normality and brain structure abnormality in schizophrenia. *American Journal of Psychiatry*, **166**, 189–195.

Wilk, C. M., Gold, J. M., McMahon, R. P., et al. (2005). No, it is not possible to be schizophrenic yet neuropsychologically normal. *Neuropsychology*, **19**, 778–786.

Willcutt, E. G., Doyle, A. E., Nigg, J. T., et al. (2005). Validity of the executive function theory of attention-deficit/hyperactivity disorder: a meta-analytic review. *Biological Psychiatry*, **57**, 1336–1346.

Woodward, T. S., Moritz, S., Cuttler, C., et al. (2006). The contribution of a cognitive bias against disconfirmatory evidence (BADE) to delusions in schizophrenia. *Journal of Clinical and Experimental Neuropsychology*, **28**, 605–617.

Woodward, T. S., Moritz, S., Menon, M., et al. (2008). Belief inflexibility in schizophrenia. *Cognitive Neuropsychiatry*, **13**, 267–277.

Wykes, T., Reeder, C., Landau, S., et al. (2007). Cognitive remediation therapy in schizophrenia: randomised controlled trial. *British Journal of Psychiatry*, **190**, 421–427.

Chapter

2

The multi-faceted, "global" cognitive impairment profile in schizophrenia

Dwight Dickinson, Jonathan Schaefer, and Daniel R. Weinberger

Acknowledgments

We gratefully acknowledge the contributions of Jody Mozersky to data analyses in this chapter. This work was supported by the Intramural Research Program, National Institute of Mental Health, NIH.

Introduction

Conceptualization of cognitive impairment in schizophrenia has shifted in recent years, responding to the vast expansion of biological knowledge about the illness. Schizophrenia is now well-recognized as a neurodevelopmental disorder with a trajectory that begins in utero, that evolves in the first decades of life through a multidirectional interplay among genetic, environmental, and stochastic influences, and that results at maturity in disturbed patterns of brain structure, connectivity, and activation (Lewis & Levitt, 2002; Marenco & Weinberger, 2000; Weinberger, 1995). These abnormalities are often subtle (relating, for example, to cell migration, dendritic complexity, or experience-dependent remodeling of microcircuitry) and are highly variable from one affected individual to the next. However, they affect widely acting neurotransmitter systems (e.g., dopamine, glutamate, GABA) and abnormalities are over-represented in critical neural hubs, including the prefrontal cortex and hippocampal formation (Callicott et al., 2000; Meyer-Lindenberg et al., 2005; Weinberger et al., 1992). In short, during the full course of premorbid development, schizophrenia is woven deep into the fabric of the brain – gradually, intricately, and microscopically. After the onset of illness, many facets of the brain's behavioral output are altered fundamentally. Schizophrenia can result in dramatic symptomatology, including auditory hallucinations, paranoid and bizarre delusions, and disordered language, but also in reduced motivation, emotional expression, social interest, and activity level. In everyday terms, people with the illness often experience disability spanning decades, with low rates of employment and marriage, poor somatic health and quality of life, and even markedly reduced life expectancy.

Given the neurodevelopmental nature of schizophrenia, and the extensive evidence of brain and behavioral disturbance in adulthood, it is no surprise that cognitive performance is also broadly disrupted. At present, several things about this disruption are clear. First, cognitive differences are among the first behavioral manifestations of the disorder, with mild cognitive impairments often evident in early childhood, many years before other prodromal

---

Cognitive Impairment in Schizophrenia, ed. Philip D. Harvey. Published by Cambridge University Press. © Cambridge University Press 2013.

signs, frank psychotic symptoms, or exposure to schizophrenia pharmacology (Cannon et al., 2000a; Cannon et al., 2002; Lewandowski et al., 2011; Niendam et al., 2003; Reichenberg et al., 2010). These very different developmental trajectories in schizophrenia for classical symptom dimensions and cognition are reflected in adulthood in surprisingly modest cognition/symptom correlations (Dominguez et al., 2009; Ventura et al., 2010). Moreover, pharmacological treatments that improve positive and disorganized symptoms of the illness do very little to improve cognitive performance (Hughes et al., 2003; Rund et al., 2004). Second, the illness results in a generalized or "global" impairment of cognitive performance in affected individuals – at least when assessed using traditional neuropsychological and IQ measures – with many measures and domains affected to a similar degree (we will use the terms "global" and "generalized" interchangeably in this chapter). Across datasets, this impairment relative to community comparison groups is generally at or above one standard deviation. These impairments are present in patients in every clinical state and at every time period of the illness and emerge from studies using widely varying assessment batteries. They are well-established at first episode (Hill et al., 2004) and remain fairly stable through late middle age (Albus et al., 2002; Hughes et al., 2003; Hyde et al., 1994). Although a considerable factor, analytical literature has highlighted somewhat separable cognitive domains (e.g., attention, working memory) (Dickinson & Gold, 2008; Nuechterlein et al., 2004), and some reviews have suggested especially pronounced impairments in schizophrenia for measures within domains of verbal episodic memory (Heinrichs & Zakzanis, 1998; Reichenberg & Harvey, 2007), executive functioning (Reichenberg & Harvey, 2007), and processing speed (Dickinson et al., 2007), the saw-tooth profile of relative strengths and weaknesses on different traditional neuropsychological measures and in different domains is far less reliable and striking than the overall schizophrenia impairment (Dickinson et al., 2004; Dickinson et al., 2008; Dickinson et al., 2011; Keefe et al., 2006). Third, cognitive impairment is seen in attenuated form in the siblings and parents of individuals with schizophrenia (Dickinson et al., 2007; Dickinson et al., 2011; Goldberg et al., 1995; Snitz et al., 2006) and some studies indicate that the cognitive effect among relatives diminishes for those who are less closely related (Glahn et al., 2007; Toulopoulou et al., 2007; Tuulio-Henriksson et al., 2003). Fourth, various reports associate these performance impairments with the range of schizophrenia brain abnormalities mentioned earlier (Weinberger & Harrison, 2011) and a fast-emerging but inconsistent literature extends the association findings to suspected genetic markers of the illness, including COMT (Egan et al., 2001b), DISC1 (Porteous et al., 2006), DTNBP1 (Burdick et al., 2007), and ZNF804A (Walters et al., 2010). Finally, more so than classical symptomatology, the cognitive impairments in schizophrenia are associated with better or worse functioning in societal roles (e.g., employment, independent living), family and case manager ratings of functional status, psychiatric rehabilitation success, self-reported quality of life, and other indices of expected and desired adaptive behavior in the everyday world (Bowie et al., 2006; Goldberg et al., 1995; Green 1996; Green et al., 2004). Moreover, an important finding in this literature is that broad composites of neuropsychological performance predict everyday functioning more strongly than individual measures (Green et al., 2000; Harvey et al., 1998; Velligan et al., 1997).

Most of the findings reviewed in the previous paragraph have emerged from analyses using standardized, often orally administered, paper-and-pencil cognitive tests of the sort that comprise standard IQ and neuropsychological batteries, some of which have been used for decades (Boake, 2002). In the past decade, an alternative approach to the measurement of cognitive performance in schizophrenia, drawing on cognitive neuroscience tasks and techniques, has matured (Carter & Barch, 2007) (see Chapter 12 of this book). The cognitive neuroscience approach advocates adaptation of cognitive neuroscience paradigms for: (1) measurement of specific cognitive processes or mechanisms underlying domains; (2) identification of associated neural systems, including through the use of noninvasive imaging technologies; (3) work that translates directly between humans and animal models (Carter & Barch, 2007). One hope for this approach is that it will avoid problems with traditional neuropsychological assessment, including concerns that such measures are multi-factorial and nonspecific, that putative cognitive domains based on factor analyses of data from such measures do not map onto discrete biological systems, and that this measurement approach may obscure the relative importance of particular cognitive processes and neural substrates, failing to elucidate illness etiology and slowing development of targeted intervention strategies. The cognitive neuroscience approach is theoretically compelling and very much in vogue – it is being actively pursued in one National Institute of Mental Health (NIMH) initiative, Cognitive Neuroscience Treatment Research to Improve Cognition in Schizophrenia (CNTRICS) (Carter & Barch, 2007), and has been extended far beyond the schizophrenia context in a broad, new NIMH initiative, Research Domain Criteria (RDoC), seeking to base mental illness classification on objective biology rather than classical mental illness symptoms and phenomenology (Insel et al., 2010; Sanislow et al., 2010).

An important question for advocates of this approach, however, is whether it fosters a unrealistically reductionistic and modular view of cognition in assuming that there are fairly clear dissociations among key cognitive "component processes" and underlying circuits and that the field will progress most briskly by making these its central focus (Karmiloff-Smith, 2006; Kendler, 2005). There has been progress in adapting cognitive neuroscience paradigms to target selected component processes in schizophrenia (Barch et al., 2011; Gold et al., 2010; Ragland et al., 2011; Silverstein et al., 2011), but this literature is still fairly sparse, and it remains to be seen whether an account of broad cognition in schizophrenia can be built on this sort of foundation. Another question is whether, using this approach, target processes are experimentally constrained in ways that leave their relationships to important everyday behaviors and outcomes difficult to decipher (Gold et al., 2011). Hopefully, we will learn more as work progresses under the CNTRICS and RDoC initiatives. However, the emergence of the cognitive neuroscience perspective also raises interesting questions about the utility of neuropsychological assessment in this disorder, about the nature and meaning of the generalized cognitive impairment, and about the value of further research in this area. More concretely, cognitive neuroscience challenges us to consider whether generalized impairment interpretations of neuropsychological findings in schizophrenia mainly reflect limitations of existing measures rather than revealing something fundamental about the structure of cognition in this disorder. One possibility is that traditional neuropsychological tasks and indices of global impairment are such blunt instruments – so inherently multifactorial and nonspecific, so subject to motivation issues, medication effects, and other epiphenomena – that their utility for understanding schizophrenia etiology and advancing its treatment is sharply limited (Carter, 2005; Gold et al., 2009; Jonides & Nee, 2005; MacDonald & Carter, 2002). Another possibility is that generalized cognitive impairment, historically and perhaps most readily indexed through neuropsychological assessment, is a fundamental and expected product of abnormal neurodevelopment in schizophrenia that needs to be a central consideration in the search for cognition enhancing treatments (Dickinson, 2008; Dickinson & Harvey, 2009).

The current chapter offers several lines of analysis in support of the latter view. We begin with some elaboration about the nature of the generalized cognitive impairment in schizophrenia. A number of large meta-analyses have provided clarifying evidence about the breadth of this deficit (Aleman et al., 1999; Dickinson et al., 2007; Heinrichs & Zakzanis, 1998) and, in the first section, we offer an update of earlier reviews. In the following section we explore other senses in which the schizophrenia cognitive impairment is global. We examine consistencies and inconsistencies in the patterns of impairment over time, across geographic regions, within families, and across groups. Finally, we discuss facets of global cognitive impairment in schizophrenia that reach beyond cognitive testing and the likely role of this dimension of schizophrenia in future research.

Global cognitive impairment as reflected in schizophrenia meta-analyses

In 1998, Heinrichs and Zakzanis published the first large-scale meta-analysis of cognitive deficit findings in schizophrenia, drawing on more than 200 studies conducted between 1980 and 1997 (Heinrichs & Zakzanis, 1998) and documenting a far-reaching cognitive impairment with an overall mean of 0.92 standard deviations relative to community comparison groups (Heinrichs, 2005). Various smaller reviews followed, generally focused on a particular cognitive domain (Aleman et al., 1999) or set of measures (Bokat & Goldberg, 2003). Although narrower in focus than the Heinrichs review, our 2007 meta-analysis (Dickinson et al., 2007) offered the closest thing to a comprehensive update for studies completed in the following decade through 2006, and with a similar outcome. Across measures and samples, this later analysis found a grand mean effect size of schizophrenia on cognitive performance of 0.98 standard deviations. Although the time since that last review has been short, a number of quite large datasets have entered the literature, driven in part by the power requirements of genetics analyses and increasing "internationalization" of schizophrenia research. On the strength of these recent, large sample studies, we have undertaken a further investigation, fully independent of the earlier analyses.

Meta-analysis methods

As in the earlier analyses, we focused on individual measures rather than on broader cognitive constructs (e.g., executive functioning, attention), avoiding assumptions about the structure and constituents of broader cognitive abilities. In contrast to Heinrichs and Zakzanis (1998), but consistent with Dickinson et al. (2007), we limited selection to studies that used broad selections of cognitive measures, which could be described as "full neuropsychological batteries." To further limit analyses to the most informative studies, we selected only large sample studies (all schizophrenia numbers $\geq$ 89). Articles for the meta-analysis were located through key word searches in PubMed for the period 2006 to 2011. Further, we searched the reference lists from these articles to identify additional publications.

Standard criteria were used to select studies/samples for review: (1) the study must have contrasted cognitive performance in schizophrenia patients and healthy controls; (2) the study must have based schizophrenia diagnoses on contemporary diagnostic criteria (e.g., DSM-III-R, DSM-IV, ICD-9 or later); (3) results must have been reported with sufficient detail to allow calculation of effect sizes; (4) finally, the study must have been reported in

English. From several hundred studies identified in initial searches, 32 articles were retained for examination in greater detail. Of these, 24 non-overlapping studies met all selection criteria and were retained for the meta-analysis. While our general approach was to combine data on an individual test-by-test basis, in some instances we combined data across very similar tests. For example, we combined data across different word list learning tests, different sets of prompts for letter and category fluency tasks, and digit symbol coding variants. Additionally, full battery IQ scores and estimates based on IQ battery short forms were also combined, as were reading scores from the Wide Range Achievement Test (WRAT) and National Adult Reading Test (NART). We also recorded information about a number of potential moderator variables, including mean sample age, illness chronicity, and geographical location of study.

Effect sizes for each cognitive variable from each study were calculated as the mean difference between schizophrenia and healthy control performance divided by the pooled standard deviation, adjusted for small sample bias (Hedges' g) (Hedges & Olkin, 1985). The direction of these numerous effect sizes was uniformly negative, reflecting worse performance by people with schizophrenia than by comparison subjects. These values were weighted and combined for each variable using a random effects model (Raudenbush, 1994; Shaddish & Haddock, 1994). This conservative estimation method yields more generalizable parameter estimates than would be obtained using a fixed effects model, evident in larger standard errors and smaller z-scores (Raudenbush, 1994).

Meta-analysis results

Across these studies, cognitive results were analyzed for 5006 schizophrenia patients and 5125 community comparison subjects. Schizophrenia cases, on average, were 37.6 years of age (SD=9.0), compared to 37.8 years for the controls (SD=10.5). Mean education for cases was 12.4 years (SD=2.79) and 14.0 (SD=2.59) for controls. Duration of illness averaged 14 (SD=9.78) years for 11 studies that reported this information. Table 2.1 displays the results of meta-analyses of schizophrenia and comparison group differences in cognitive performance on 31 variables for which we had at least three separate samples.

Cohen's criteria – 0.20 for a small effect, 0.50 for a medium effect, and 0.80 for a large effect – guided interpretation of the effect sizes (Cohen, 1988). As shown in Table 2.1, cognitive performance is significantly impaired in schizophrenia across performance domains, with a grand mean effect size of g=1.01. All effects are statistically significant. The largest effect size obtained was g=1.55 for story memory, nearly double Cohen's convention for a large effect, while the smallest was g=0.51 for digit span forward. These effect sizes can also be interpreted in terms of the percentage of non-overlap between the distributions of test scores for the schizophrenia and healthy control groups (Cohen, 1988). The grand mean effect size denotes approximately 55% non-overlap between the schizophrenia and control distributions. The story memory effect indicates 73% non-overlap between distributions. Verbal memory measures as a group showed the largest effects, followed by composite measures derived from IQ tests or specialized neuropsychological batteries such as the Brief Assessment of Cognition in Schizophrenia (BACS) (Keefe et al., 2004) and the Measurement and Treatment Research to Improve Cognition in Schizophrenia (MATRICS) Consensus Cognitive Battery (MCCB) (Nuechterlein et al., 2008). Measures of crystallized verbal intelligence (word reading and vocabulary) showed

Table 2.1. Summary of results of a meta-analysis of cognition from 24 studies and 5006 people with schizophrenia

	Studies (n)	Controls (n)	Schizophrenia patients (n)	Effect size (g)	SE	95% Up	95% Down
Broad cognitive performance							
Full scale IQ or estimated FSIQ	8	2500	2248	1.20	0.11	1.41	0.98
Verbal IQ	3	987	608	1.21	0.10	1.41	1.00
Performance IQ	3	986	614	1.38	0.10	1.59	1.18
Neuropsychological composite (e.g., BACS, MCCB)	5	699	713	1.37	0.15	1.66	1.09
Premorbid IQ/crystallized intelligence							
Word reading	8	1950	1352	0.62	0.13	0.88	0.35
Vocabulary	5	1299	706	0.60	0.12	0.84	0.35
Processing speed							
Digit–symbol	12	3424	2910	1.40	0.15	1.69	1.11
Trails A	9	1905	1450	0.90	0.15	1.19	0.62
Trails B	11	2530	1791	0.98	0.14	1.25	0.70
Verbal episodic memory							
List learning–total words learned	13	2642	2813	1.25	0.16	1.56	0.95
List learning–delayed recognition	8	1210	889	1.21	0.17	1.55	0.88
Story learning	6	2094	1460	1.41	0.11	1.63	1.20
Story memory	5	1960	1336	1.55	0.10	1.75	1.35
Visual episodic memory							
Figure learning	8	2347	1412	0.99	0.13	1.23	0.74
Figure memory	7	2169	1278	1.03	0.13	1.29	0.77
Reasoning/problem solving							
WCST categories	7	2011	1296	1.09	0.14	1.36	0.82
WCST perseverative errors	7	2054	1270	1.01	0.13	1.25	0.76
Stroop color–word	6	1162	809	0.84	0.15	1.13	0.55
Matrix reasoning	3	739	389	0.90	0.12	1.13	0.67
Tower tasks	7	1087	942	0.70	0.14	0.98	0.43
Similarities	4	2026	975	0.73	0.09	0.90	0.56
Block design	6	2420	1910	0.65	0.09	0.83	0.47
Short-term and working memory							
Digit span forward	4	1752	958	0.51	0.01	0.54	0.49
Digit span backward	5	1515	989	0.78	0.14	1.05	0.51
Letter–number sequencing	4	1243	827	1.13	0.14	1.41	0.85
N-back (1-back)	3	1086	770	1.05	0.11	1.26	0.84
N-back (2-back)	3	1085	770	1.06	0.11	1.27	0.85

Table 2.1. (cont.)

	Studies (n)	Controls (n)	Schizophrenia patients (n)	Effect size (g)	SE	95% Up	95% Down
Fluency							
Letter fluency	10	1820	1450	1.06	0.16	1.39	0.74
Category fluency	12	2768	1833	1.08	0.15	1.37	0.79
Design fluency	3	488	309	1.00	0.14	1.28	0.71
Simple motor							
Grooved pegboard– dominant hand	3	382	276	0.60	0.18	0.95	0.25
Grand mean				1.009			

FSIQ, Full Scale IQ; BACS, brief assessment of cognition in schizophrenia; MCCB, MATRICS consensus cognitive battery; WCTS, Wisconsin card sorting test.

smaller effects than most other measures, as they did in earlier meta-analyses (Dickinson et al., 2007; Heinrichs & Zakzanis, 1998), but these effects were nevertheless of a magnitude that calls into question the practice of viewing the measures as indices of premorbid IQ (Harvey et al., 2006). Visual episodic memory variables and fluency variables grouped very near g=1.0. Other variable groupings included mixtures of higher and lower effect sizes.

Comment on meta-analysis

Although we stress global cognitive impairment in this chapter, it is clear from the literature (reviewed in [Gold et al., 2009; Reichenberg & Harvey, 2007]) and from current and previous meta-analyses that cognitive deficits in schizophrenia are not uniform. One example of this is the more limited evidence of impairment in non-conscious procedural learning (Goldberg et al., 1993), which is not routinely assessed in neuropsychological evaluations. Similarly, it has been difficult to document schizophrenia deficits in a number of relatively automatic processes relating to the allocation of attentional resources and selection of targets (Gold et al., 2009). Hence, an important qualification of global impairment is that this impairment is most evident among the effortful, consciously guided cognitive processes that are the main focus of clinical neuropsychology. Even in the arena of effortful cognition, however, impairment effect sizes vary. In the current analysis, as in earlier analyses (Dickinson et al., 2007; Heinrichs & Zakzanis, 1998), the largest effect sizes, for story learning and memory, digit symbol coding, and performance IQ, are more than twice the magnitude of the smallest effect sizes, for crystallized verbal ability (word reading, vocabulary), simple short-term memory (digit span forward), and motor speed. Non-overlapping confidence intervals indicate that these differences in effect size magnitude are significant.

Such findings are not at odds with a global impairment interpretation, for several reasons. Use of the term "global impairment" does not imply that all domains of performance should be affected uniformly. An early, low-level neural insult (e.g., in cell migration or dendritic arborization) would be expected, over developmental time, to have different impacts on different cognition domains. Relatively "preserved" performance – even apparent "sparing" – may simply indicate areas where the shape and timing of neurodevelopmental

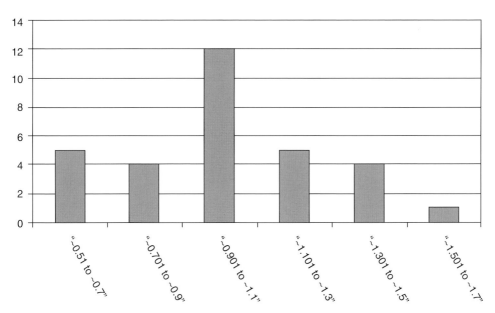

Figure 2.1. Frequency of effect sizes of different magnitudes from those reported in Table 2.1. Effect sizes are concentrated around the grand mean effect size of 1.01 standard deviations.

irregularities work differently or where compensation in an abnormal system is particularly effective. Word-reading and vocabulary findings in current and past meta-analyses are a strong case in point. These are considered measures of accumulated, "crystallized" verbal ability, in contrast to more "fluid" abilities involved in novel problem solving (Cattell, 1967; Horn & Cattell, 1967), and are thought to be relatively stable and resistant to brain insult in adulthood (Russell, 1980). In euthymic bipolar disorder, despite generalized cognitive impairment averaging two-thirds of a standard deviation on other traditional neuropsychological variables, word-reading and vocabulary are almost entirely preserved (Mann-Wrobel et al., 2011). Yet, across analyses, impairments on these same variables in schizophrenia samples are typically 0.60 standard deviations or more. Therefore, rather than calling into question the generality of the illness effect on cognition in schizophrenia, these findings may in fact be particularly good evidence of a broad disruption of normal development and knowledge acquisition beginning quite early in life (Reichenberg & Harvey, 2007). In other words, these measures might be better described as pre-acute than premorbid, reflecting impairments that arise and crystallize during the insidious phase of illness but which are less affected than more fluid abilities by brain changes that accompany the emergence of full-blown psychosis. Additionally, the overall impairment level across measures is simply far more impressive than the variation from effect size to effect size. In the current analysis, the grand mean effect size (1.01) is almost four times the standard deviation of the effects (0.27). Figure 2.1 shows the frequencies of different effect sizes from the current analyses and depicts the concentration of values around the midpoint even more clearly.

Confidence intervals around the effect size point estimates tend to be large and some of the variation probably reflects measurement error. Furthermore, some differences may relate to the measurement properties of different instruments rather than their cognitive targets per se (Chapman & Chapman, 1973; Miller et al., 1995). Thus, it may be that meta-analyses regularly highlight verbal memory and digit symbol coding variables, not only because these measures tap domains that are somewhat more strongly affected in schizophrenia, but also because the measures are simple and reliable relative to other measures, such as card sorting tasks. Differences in the impairments observed for coding tasks relative to trail making tasks, although all are within the broader domain of processing speed, may support this argument.

In summary, the current meta-analysis, quite consistently with earlier analyses, describes a broad impairment of effortful cognitive processing in schizophrenia cases relative to community comparison groups. Inevitably, given the challenges of measuring cognition and the host of interacting factors influencing development, the impairment is not uniform across indices of cognitive performance or invariant in profile from individual to individual with the disorder. Nevertheless, effect sizes across a range of measures – verbal memory, processing speed, reasoning and problem solving, working memory, and summary or composite scores like Full-Scale IQ – point to a one-standard deviation disadvantage in people with the illness. This broad impairment is a predictable by-product of a subtle but widespread neurodevelopmental disruption.

Other senses in which the cognitive impairment in schizophrenia is global

While global or generalized characterizations may first evoke an idea of substantial impairment across a battery of cognitive measures, there are other respects in which these descriptors are apt. In this section, we review meta-analytic and other data suggesting that: (1) the generalized deficit findings are robust over thirty years of intensive research involving well in excess of 10 000 people with schizophrenia; (2) they are robust in different regions around the world; (3) they are robust within families; (4) cognitive structure in people with this disorder is more intercorrelated or unitary than it is in comparison groups.

Generalized deficits over the past three decades

In the previous section, several references were made to consistencies in the findings of different meta-analyses.

In Table 2.2, comparable results for three meta-analytic samples are arranged side-by-side (results for the first sample were presented in two publications [Heinrichs & Zakzanis, 1998; Zakzanis et al., 1999]). Together, they survey neuropsychological and intellectual assessment findings from 1980 to 2011. There are, however, important differences among the analyses. The first meta-analysis, covering the longest period, attempted to locate all studies reporting schizophrenia/control comparisons from traditional cognitive assessment instruments that were also published in English and that met substantive and standard meta-analysis study selection criteria. The second and third study samples were limited. Dickinson et al. included a special focus on digit symbol coding tasks in the context of a broad meta-analysis, thus studies were only retained for that analysis if they used assessment batteries that included a version of this measure (Dickinson et al., 2007). The current meta-analysis did not include a narrow substantive focus, but was limited to large battery and large sample studies in order to make the review more manageable. There are other obvious differences. Relatively modern diagnostic criteria, narrowing the boundaries of

Table 2.2. Side-by-side comparison of results from three meta-analysis samples comparing schizophrenia patients' cognitive performance to that of controls, covering the years 1980 to 2011

		Heinrichs & Zakzanis (1998); Zakzanis et al. (1999)	Dickinson et al. (2007)	Current analysis
Time period covered		1980–1997	1995–2006	2006–2011
Schizophrenia mean (SD) age (yr)		34.4 (10.0)	31.5 (7.3)	37.6 (9.0)
Schizophrenia % males		82.4	. . .	67.8
Schizophrenia mean (SD) education (yr)		12.0 (1.1)	12.3 (1.1)	12.4 (2.8)
Mean (SD) duration of illness (yr)		12.7 (7.6)	9.1 (5.9)	14.0 (2.6)
Overall number of studies included		204	37	24
Mean (SD) sample size per study		36.1 (30.2)	53 (33.9)	208.6 (214)
Meta-analysis grand mean	ES	0.92	0.98	1.01
	SZ	7420	1961	5006
Full scale or estimated IQ	ES	1.1	1.19	1.2
	SZ	1018	863	2248
Word reading (premorbid IQ)	ES	0.42	0.59	0.61
	SZ	1069	450	1352
WAIS vocabulary	ES	0.53	0.9	0.6
	SZ	2046	586	706
WAIS block design	ES	0.46	0.84	0.65
	SZ	1166	607	1910
Combined verbal learning	ES	1.41	. . .	. . .
	SZ	1088	. . .	. . .
Story learning	ES	. . .	1.19	1.41
	SZ	. . .	863	1460
List learning	ES	. . .	1.25	1.25
	SZ	. . .	1254	2813
Nonverbal/figure learning	ES	0.74	0.82	0.99
	SZ	379	544	1412
WCST categories	ES	1.01	0.81	1.09
	SZ	1387	1018	1296
WCST perseverative errors	ES	1.06	0.79	1.01
	SZ	1387	1295	1270
Coding/digit symbol	ES	1.11	1.57	1.4
	SZ	1204	1961	2910
Trail making test, form A	ES	0.7	0.88	0.9
	SZ	1204	1081	1450

Table 2.2. (cont.)

		Heinrichs & Zakzanis (1998); Zakzanis et al. (1999)	Dickinson et al. (2007)	Current analysis
Trail making test, form B	ES	0.8	0.92	0.98
	SZ	1387	1190	1791
WAIS digit span forward	ES	0.69	0.73	0.51
	SZ	440	175	958
WAIS digit span backward	ES	0.82	0.86	0.78
	SZ	440	155	989
Combined verbal fluency	ES	1.15	. . .	. . .
	SZ	1020	. . .	. . .
Letter fluency	ES	. . .	0.83	1.06
	SZ	. . .	1213	1450
Category fluency	ES	. . .	1.41	1.08
	SZ	. . .	462	1833

WAIS, Wechsler adult intelligence scale; WCST, Wisconsin card sorting test; ES, effect size; SZ, number of schizophrenia patients.

schizophrenia considerably, were introduced in 1980 with the third edition of the *Diagnostic and Statistical Manual of Mental Disorders* (DSM), but have evolved through three revisions of the DSM since then (Association, 2000). Similarly, the cognitive measures have changed considerably during this period. To take one example, in 1980 the original Wechsler Adult Intelligence Scale (WAIS) was still in use – in 2008 the fourth edition of this battery was released (Wechsler, 2008). Demographics for the schizophrenia cases reflected in the three meta-analysis samples also differ: the sample of studies reviewed in Heinrichs and Zakzanis was heavily male, the Dickinson et al. sample was younger and less chronic, whereas the current sample was older and more chronic across studies (Table 2.2).

Despite the differences in meta-analysis characteristics and samples, and the evolution over time of diagnostic criteria and assessment measures, the similarities in the pattern of effect sizes across the three reviews are striking. As a group, effect sizes for the verbal memory measures are higher than most others across analyses. Consistently, the word-reading and digit span measures are at the lower end of the distribution of effect sizes. Differences from analysis to analysis, with few exceptions, are quite small relative to the effects derived. Another point worth emphasizing is that the variables that show the greatest consistency across analyses are the approximations of generalized cognitive ability. Some variation from review to review is apparent for the specific, individual measures; however– across studies spanning thirty years and thousands of people with schizophrenia and despite variation in diagnostic and assessment practices – the composite measures of global cognitive ability are remarkably stable. The range for grand mean effects is 0.09 standard deviations, while the range for IQ is 0.10 standard deviations, in both cases less than one-tenth of the documented impairment.

Generalized deficits around the globe

Increasing numbers of large, neuropsychological battery studies in recent years make it possible to compare schizophrenia cognitive deficits in different global regions using the same or very similar cognitive tests. From the current meta-analysis, we divided studies into those based on samples from either North America, Europe, or Asia and examined effect sizes for which there was at least one study reporting an effect size in each region. One difficulty arose. As a group, the North American samples included subjects who were considerably older than the European and Asian samples (an average of 45.3 years for North America, compared to 32.2 and 32.5 years for Europe and Asia, respectively). To avoid confounding the comparison with age differences, we used only the "youngest" North American sample, which was also the largest – from the NIMH/CBDB Study of Schizophrenia Genetics (D. R. Weinberger, PI, summarized in Dickinson et al., 2011), with an average age of 35.5 years. The results of this comparison are presented in Table 2.3.

With fewer studies per effect size estimate, there is more variation region to region than was evident in the comparisons over time (see Table 2.2), and some outlying values are apparent – extremely low Trail Making Test (TMT) impairments in one Asian study, very high story memory values from one European study, higher than expected digit symbol coding impairment in the NIMH/CBDB sample, and substantial variability across regions in nonverbal/figure learning and memory performance. However, given the cultural and language differences, and the vagaries of test translation, the more striking impression, again, is of strong consistency from geographic region to geographic region. As in the comparison over time (Table 2.2), memory and symbol coding values are consistently high, word-reading values are consistently low, and effect sizes for card sorting variables generally hover near 1.0. Estimates of Full Scale IQ are high but somewhat more variable than in the comparisons over time (Table 2.2). Again, however, the grand means of the region by region effects are among the least variable indices, with a range from the largest to the smallest one-fifth as large as the typical impairment.

Pattern of cognitive deficits within families

Although the literature on familial deficits is not nearly as extensive as that summarized in earlier sections, various reviews have reported a pattern of attenuated but still generalized cognitive deficits in the close relatives of people with schizophrenia (Dickinson et al., 2007; Sitskoorn et al., 2004; Snitz et al., 2006; Szoke et al., 2005; Trandafir et al., 2006). Effects between 0.30 and 0.60 standard deviations on a wide range of measures are frequently observed. Although the general finding of mild impairment in relatives seems reliable, the inclusion of parents in many of the studied samples confounds interpretation somewhat. Several studies have considered only unaffected siblings and these also document broad but mild impairment (Cannon et al., 1994; Egan et al., 2001a). Twin studies have refined these findings in an interesting way, showing the sensitivity of cognition to illness within monozygotic twin-pairs discordant for schizophrenia (Cannon et al., 2000b; Goldberg et al., 1990; Kremen et al., 2006). Although the samples are small, these studies demonstrate that ill twins, almost uniformly, perform worse than unaffected twins (Goldberg et al., 1990; Kremen et al., 2006). Using data from the NIMH/CBDB study, we posed a similar question regarding people with schizophrenia and their unaffected full-

Table 2.3. Side-by-side comparison of results from three global regions based on subdivision of information from the current meta-analysis

Global region		North America	Europe	Asia
Schizophrenia mean (SD) age (yr)		35.5 (10.1)	32.2 (9.73)	32.5 (9.30)
Schizophrenia % males		74.4	70.43	54.99
Schizophrenia mean (SD) education (yr)		14.0 (2.2)	13.38 (2.76)	12.08 (2.88)
Mean (SD) duration of illness (yr)		12.62 (9.38)	11.22 (10.09)	12.93 (8.77)
Overall number of studies included		CBDB only	11	6
Mean (SD) sample size per study		496	248.64 (297)	157.67 (53)
Grand mean	ES	1.2	1.13	1.01
	SZ	496	2735	946
	K	1	11	6
Full scale or estimated IQ	ES	1.46	1.095	1.31
	SZ	471	2241	347
	K	1	6	2
Word reading (premorbid IQ)	ES	0.61	0.778	0.656
	SZ	471	177	327
	K	1	1	2
Story learning	ES	1.44	1.89	1.295
	SZ	468	349	671
	K	1	1	4
Story memory	ES	1.49	1.85	1.458
	SZ	464	349	548
	K	1	1	3
List learning total words learned	ES	1.7	1.036	1.443
	SZ	394	1954	327
	K	1	7	2
Nonverbal/figure learning	ES	0.92	1.533	0.67
	SZ	462	183	561
	K	1	2	3
Nonverbal/figure memory	ES	1.174	1.236	0.738
	SZ	459	287	438
	K	1	3	2
	ES	1.5	0.866	0.944
WCST categories	SZ	447	461	324
	K	1	2	2
WCST perseverative errors	ES	0.93	0.886	0.934
	SZ	439	550	324
	K	1	3	2

Table 2.3. (cont.)

Global region		North America	Europe	Asia
Coding/digit symbol	ES	1.85	1.238	1.394
	SZ	470	1925	541
	K	1	6	3
Trails A	ES	1.04	0.884	0.254
	SZ	468	652	172
	K	1	4	1
Trails B	ES	1.2	0.982	0.541
	SZ	461	755	386
	K	1	5	2
Letter fluency	ES	0.95	1.049	0.908
	SZ	467	845	103
	K	1	6	1
Category fluency	ES	1.4	1.209	0.728
	SZ	466	895	317
	K	1	6	2

WCST, Wisconsin card sorting test; ES, effect size; SZ, number of schizophrenia patients.

siblings. We analyzed data for 278 families in which one affected and one unaffected sibling completed our broad cognitive assessment battery. Siblings were well-matched on age (schizophrenia 35.1±9 yr vs. sibling 35.5±9.3 yr), although a higher proportion of the schizophrenia sample was male (74.8% vs. 43.2%) and unaffected siblings had the expected advantage in years of education (16±2.5 vs. 14.1±2.2 yr). Figure 2.2 shows, on a group basis, schizophrenia and unaffected sibling impairments relative to community controls in performance on a verbal memory composite, a processing speed composite, and a composite representing general cognitive performance (see Dickinson et al., 2011 for composite calculation details). All of the group level differences are strongly statistically significant. Both people with schizophrenia and their siblings perform reliably worse than controls (for the three cognitive variables, P<8.0 E-74 and P<8.0 E-04, respectively). Additionally, the schizophrenia cases as a group are significantly impaired relative to their siblings (all, P<1.0 E-48).

Schizophrenia impairments are similar to those seen in the meta-analysis results in Table 2.1, whereas sibling deficits, although statistically robust, are somewhat smaller compared to reports in the literature. The milder sibling deficits may result from the fact that only age-matched siblings and not parents are included in this analysis. On a group basis, siblings with schizophrenia are far more seriously impaired than are their unaffected siblings. More importantly for present purposes, sibling pair by sibling pair, the overwhelming majority of unaffected siblings performed better than affected siblings on each variable (see Table 2.4 and Figure 2.3).

Table 2.4 shows that the deviations in these better/worse performance proportions from chance (i.e., a 50/50 split) are robust. The findings are slightly stronger for the general cognitive ability composite, but are similar for all three variables. Thus, schizophrenia appears to spare cognitive impairment in few if any affected individuals–and in this sense too, the schizophrenia effect on cognition is global.

Table 2.4. Frequency, percentage, and statistical comparison of unaffected siblings who outperform siblings with schizophrenia on common cognitive variables

		Frequency	Percent	Chi-square (1df)	P
General cognitive ability	SZ higher than SIB	27	10.0	171.840	2.93E-39
	SIB higher than SZ	242	90.0		
Verbal memory	SZ higher than SIB	39	14.1	142.964	5.99E-33
	SIB higher than SZ	238	85.9		
Processing speed	SZ higher than SIB	33	11.9	161.669	4.89E-37
	SIB higher than SZ	245	88.1		

SZ, schizophrenia patient; SIB, unaffected sibling.

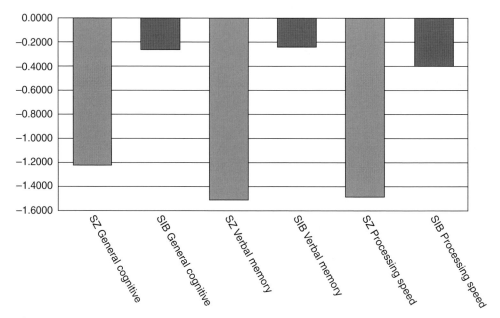

Figure 2.2. Schizophrenia and sibling cognitive impairment in 270 families (z-scores relative to community controls). Impairment z-scores are calculated using control means and standard deviations. Schizophrenia cases show substantial impairments relative to community comparison subjects, while siblings show small but reliable deficits. SZ, schizophrenia; SIB, unaffected sibling.

Similarities and differences in the domain structure of cognition between schizophrenia and comparison groups

In nonclinical groups, the extensive factor analyses of John Carroll and others have firmly established that different cognitive measures correlate with one another positively (the so-called "positive manifold") and that these data conform to a factor structure in which individual measures load on broad cognitive ability factors, such as verbal episodic memory or processing speed, which load in turn on a higher order latent factor representing general

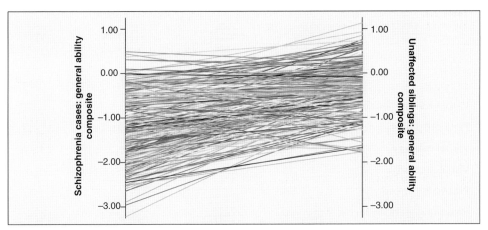

Figure 2.3. General cognitive performance in people with schizophrenia and their unaffected siblings (n=269 families). z-scores are calculated using control means and standard deviations. Each differently colored line shows the relative performance on the general cognitive ability composite of one schizophrenia case (on the left axis) and his/her unaffected sibling (on the right axis). The downward slope from right to left gives a sense of the consistency with which ill siblings underperform their unaffected siblings cognitively. (See color plate section for colored image.)

cognitive ability (Carroll, 1993; Deary, 2001; Jensen, 1998). This has been referred to as the "hierarchical" or "three-stratum" model, with individual measures forming the base of a pyramid, domain-level variables occupying an intermediate stratum, and general cognitive ability at the peak of the pyramid (Carroll, 1993, 1997). In schizophrenia, factor analyses support a sorting of cognitive test variables into cognitive domains that is largely consistent with the nonclinical literature (Allen et al., 1998; Dickinson et al., 2011; Dickinson et al., 2006; Gladsjo et al., 2004; Nuechterlein et al., 2004), thereby also supporting the assumption that these constructs have similar meaning in the context of schizophrenia. The suitability of the hierarchical model for describing relationships among neuropsychological and IQ test variables in schizophrenia data has also been demonstrated in several large datasets (Dickinson et al., 2011; Dickinson et al., 2006; Keefe et al., 2006). The hierarchical model reinforces the obvious point that there are different levels of analysis of cognitive performance. It also provides a conceptual foundation for consideration of generalized cognitive impairment in schizophrenia and for calculation of widely used global cognitive performance composites. For some purposes, such as mechanisms research (Insel et al., 2010), more disaggregated, measure-by-measure information may be most informative. For other purposes, such as predicting functional outcome, composites representing broad domains or general cognitive ability may serve better (Gold et al., 2011; Green et al., 2000).

Along with the consistencies in cognitive structure seen in schizophrenia samples and comparison groups, an interesting difference has emerged; it appears that cognitive performance is more generalized or unitary in schizophrenia than in comparison groups. The most straightforward demonstration of this is in the patterns and magnitudes of correlations among cognitive domains reported from two differently assessed, large, and entirely non-overlapping samples (Dickinson et al., 2006; Dickinson et al., 2011). For both of these samples, factor analysis was undertaken to identify empirically suitable groupings of

Table 2.5. Pearson's correlations among cognitive domain scores in two samples of schizophrenia cases and community controls

a. 2006 analysis results for healthy controls (above the diagonal; n=157) and schizophrenia group (below the diagonal; n=148)

	VC	PO	VEM	VSM	PS	RWM
Verbal comprehension		0.43	0.41	0.43	0.34	0.31
Perceptual organization	0.64		0.34	0.42	0.26	0.31
Verbal memory	0.69	0.57		0.44	0.41	0.42
Visual memory	0.64	0.73	0.63		0.15	0.20
Processing speed	0.49	0.57	0.50	0.56		0.33
Reasoning/working memory	0.64	0.65	0.64	0.69	0.64	

Controlling for age, mother's and father's education, gender, and ethnicity.

b. 2011 analysis results for healthy controls (above the diagonal; n=823) and schizophrenia group (below the diagonal; n=496)

	VEM	NB	VSM	PS	CS	SPN
Verbal memory		0.24	0.23	0.27	0.15	0.30
N-back	0.38		0.28	0.31	0.25	0.25
Visual memory	0.44	0.46		0.20	0.29	0.22
Processing speed	0.30	0.42	0.30		0.24	0.27
Card sorting	0.36	0.45	0.34	0.32		0.20
Span	0.38	0.38	0.33	0.39	0.32	

Controlling for age and gender.

VC, verbal comprehension; PO, perceptual organization; VEM, verbal memory; VSM, visual memory; PS, processing speed; RWM, reasoning/working memory; NB, N-back; CS, card sorting; SPN, span.

individual test variables into familiar cognitive domains (i.e., verbal memory, processing speed), then composite domain scores were calculated for each individual for each domain. Table 2.5 shows the bivariate correlations between pairs of domain composites for both samples.

The two studies used quite different batteries and the factor solutions share certain features, but differ in other regards. This is expected. Factor solutions vary somewhat as a function of the samples analyzed and the selection of cognitive tests and variables within tests, and are likely to be influenced by testing methodology shared between variables (Costello & Osborne, 2005; Dickinson et al., 2011). These considerations may likewise explain why the domain-level correlations also differ between studies. All correlations, for both schizophrenia and control samples, were higher in the 2006 analyses. However, the critical point for current purposes is that despite the differences in samples, cognitive measures employed, variable groupings underlying the domain composites, and the overall magnitude of domain-level correlations, the studies show the same pattern. Domain bivariate correlations are higher on average for both schizophrenia samples, and these differences compared with controls are statistically significant (P<0.001 for the 2006 analysis; P=0.027 for the 2011 analysis (Dickinson et al., 2011; Dickinson et al., 2006b)). Indeed, there is not a single instance in either study in which the control correlation exceeds the schizophrenia correlation. The 2011 analysis amplified this finding. Using multiple groups statistical modeling to test the fit of the hierarchical model of cognitive structure in people with schizophrenia, their siblings, and controls, we demonstrated that the same groupings of individual variables into domains held for all groups. However, the associations of the domain-level factors to the general cognitive ability factor were significantly stronger in the schizophrenia group than in either comparison group (Dickinson et al., 2011).

As noted, a pattern of modest but positive correlations among individual neuropsychological and IQ assessment measures and domain-level composites is firmly established for nonclinical groups and underlies interest in general cognitive ability (Carroll, 1993; Deary, 2001; Jensen, 1998). Taken together, what the schizophrenia analyses reviewed in the previous paragraph indicate is that the positive associations among cognitive measures in this illness are atypically strong. This relative strength of intercorrelation is unlikely to be a function of limitations of the measures used – within studies different groups completed the same battery of tests. Thus, there is evidence that the pattern of performance on cognitive tests in schizophrenia is more consistent from measure to measure than it is in comparison groups. The implications of these findings are not clear but they do suggest an interesting neurodevelopmental hypothesis. During early postnatal development, connectivity in the human brain expands dramatically, followed by the gradual sculpting of specialized connections and the emergence of distributed, more modularized processing in the first decades of life (Johnson, 2001). It has been proposed that certain developmental conditions (e.g., Williams syndrome) may reflect disruptions that undermine this sculpting and modularization process, leaving those affected with brains and cognitive systems that are less specialized in important respects than they are in typically developing groups (Karmiloff-Smith, 2006). In schizophrenia, some part of this effect may relate to illness-associated epiphenomena that obscure normal cognitive architecture, including psychological demoralization and medication. A more appealing hypothesis is that neurodevelopmental irregularities over many years lead to faulty and incomplete segregation of cognitive processes and give rise to an impairment that is generalized in the several respects already discussed.

General discussion of the global nature of cognitive impairments in schizophrenia

Our meta-analysis, presented in the first section of this chapter, confirmed earlier findings that cognitive impairment in schizophrenia is substantial, amounting to a one-standard deviation disadvantage relative to controls and generally cutting across various neuropsychological and IQ assessment measures, with some variation but a strong central tendency. We then presented evidence that the cognitive impairment in schizophrenia might be considered global in other ways as well. First, as emerges from a comparison of current meta-analysis results with those going back to 1980, this general deficit pattern is highly consistent over time, despite changes in diagnostic criteria and refinement of assessment measures. Moreover, among many consistent variables, the most constant over time were the most general – Full Scale IQ and the meta-analysis grand means for the different reviews considered. Second, the global cognitive impairment is truly global in character. Around the world, despite language and many other differences, the familiar pattern of impairments emerges. Third, following a number of studies of monozygotic twins discordant for schizophrenia, we showed that cognitive impairment demonstrates very strong within-family sensitivity, sorting with illness in approximately 90% of 278 affected/unaffected sibling pairs. Such findings suggest that while the severity may vary, broad cognitive impairment is likely to be a feature of the illness for the vast majority if not all of those affected. Finally, we offered evidence that the structure of cognition (at least when measured with traditional test batteries) – that is, the way different dimensions of performance associate with one another – is more unitary in people who have this condition.

We have reviewed various ways in which cognitive test performance reveals generalized cognitive impairment in schizophrenia. Other parts of the case for global impairment emerge from disparate arenas of schizophrenia research. To a considerable degree, the strength of the arguments emphasizing generalized deficits rests on the neurodevelopmental nature of this illness and, although far from being the only influence on development, genetics are obviously central. At this level too, global effects on cognition loom large. Genetics are likely to influence low-level and wide-acting mechanisms (e.g., dendritic arborization, synaptic plasticity) that support the emergence and refinement of a range of cognitive abilities over the course of development. From the study of single gene or single locus developmental disorders, such as Fragile X and Williams syndromes, it is abundantly clear that even circumscribed genetic abnormalities can have wide-ranging neural and behavioral effects (Karmiloff-Smith et al., 2002). Indeed, the hypothesis that Williams syndrome is an example of a condition with a quite selective profile of cognitive strengths and weaknesses has given way to the identification of more or less subtle but still pervasive cognitive abnormalities (Laing et al., 2001; Laing et al., 2002). Although evidence of major single gene effects is lacking in schizophrenia, the cascade of consequences from the large number of loci expected to figure in schizophrenia etiology seems likely to be no less all-encompassing.

More generally, twin studies and other work have demonstrated that genetic correlations among diverse cognitive measures are quite high (~0.60–0.80), suggesting that developmentally mediated gene effects on mature cognition are broadly focused (Alarcon et al., 1999; Butcher et al., 2006; Haworth et al., 2009; Kovas & Plomin, 2006; Plomin & Kovas, 2005). Furthermore, this generalized genetic effect appears to increase substantially during the phase of development from childhood to young adulthood (Haworth et al., 2010). Moving beyond nonclinical groups, Toulopoulou and colleagues studied twins concordant and discordant for schizophrenia (Toulopoulou et al., 2007). Modeling differences in twin correlations on IQ indices as a function of twin type (monozygotic vs. dizygotic) and illness concordance, they quantified the strength of the relationship between performance and illness, finding extensive overlap (genetic $r=-0.75$) in the genes that contribute to intelligence and schizophrenia. Additionally, they showed high heritability for IQ in this sample (70%) and that cognitive impairment was greater and more dispersed in those analyzed the greater their genetic loading for illness. Taken as a whole, the evidence shows that genetic influences on cognition tend to be generalized and that, in schizophrenia, the set of genes influencing illness overlaps substantially with the set of genes influencing cognition.

In recent years, one powerful motivation for research on cognitive impairment in schizophrenia has been the search for targeted pro-cognitive treatments. However, narrowly targeted agents (Buchanan et al., 2011; Freedman et al., 2008) have fared no better than antipsychotics (Keefe et al., 2007) in clinical trials for cognitive enhancement (if as well), and in general, trials of cognitive enhancing drugs have been disappointing (Goff et al., 2011). It is worth noting that many of the most efficacious psychotropic medications interact promiscuously with different neurotransmitter systems (e.g., clozapine, lithium) and/or that single agents (e.g., selective serotonin reuptake inhibitors, atypical antipsychotics) may be effective for a range of neuropsychiatric conditions (Young, 2006). Psychostimulants, the most effective treatment for the broad cognitive impairment in attention deficit disorders (and widely effective in improving cognitive performance in other populations) share these characteristics. The broad therapeutic profiles of these medications and discouraging results in various pro-cognitive treatment trials in recent years challenge the assumption that more targeted approaches will necessarily prove more successful. It may be that, in the context of complex effects on behavior and cognition arising through disruptions of normal development, it is not disadvantageous for medicines to act more generally.

Conclusions

Current evidence and an extensive literature indicate that cognitive performance impairment in schizophrenia is global in many important respects and is, more so than other characteristics of the illness, related to everyday outcomes like independent living and work. One way this global impairment is documented is through depressed performance on traditional cognitive assessment measures–across measures, across decades, within families, and around the globe. Such measures have been criticized on psychometric grounds and more precise instrumentation, drawing on cognitive neuroscience paradigms, is under development. However, the psychometric limitations of traditional cognitive tests do not account for the range of factors suggesting global impairment, which extend far beyond test performance to genetics and pharmacology, among other factors bearing on the disorder. Nor will the global impairment be reduced to a collection of readily dissociable processes that combine in a simple additive way. Systems in the brain develop in concert and they emit behavior as parts of individualized, complexly integrated, and dynamically shifting assemblies. It may be that the "grain size" for the neuropsychological and IQ measures, which seem to assay integrated assemblies of cross-talking components rather than individual components in isolation, is more relevant for assessing invariably complex real-world behavior. In short, the generalized nature of this impairment is a fundamental reflection of the lifelong, developmental process through which the syndrome of schizophrenia emerges and will continue to be an important focus for work aimed at improving the lives of people living with this condition.

References

Alarcon, M., Plomin, R., Fulker, D. W., et al. (1999). Molarity not modularity: multivariate genetic analysis of specific cognitive abilities in parents and their 16-year-old children in the Colorado Adoption Project. *Cognitive Development*, 14, 175–193.

Albus, M., Hubmann, W., Scherer, J., et al. (2002). A prospective 2-year follow-up study of neurocognitive functioning in patients with first-episode schizophrenia. *European Archives Psychiatry Clinical Neuroscience*, 252, 262–267.

Aleman, A., Hijman, R., de Haan, E. H., et al. (1999). Memory impairment in schizophrenia: a meta-analysis. *American Journal of Psychiatry*, 156, 1358–1366.

Allen, D. N., Huegel, S. G., Seaton, B. E., et al. (1998). Confirmatory factor analysis of the

WAIS-R in patients with schizophrenia. *Schizophrenia Research*, **34**, 87–94.

Association, A. P. (2000). *Diagnostic and Statistical Manual of Mental Disorders.* (4th edn., text rev.). Washington, DC: American Psychiatric Publishing.

Barch, D. M., Carter, C. C., Dakin, S. C., et al. (2011). The clinical translation of a measure of gain control: the contrast-contrast effect task. *Schizophrenia Bulletin*, **38**, 135–143.

Boake, C. (2002). From the Binet-Simon to the Wechsler-Bellevue: tracing the history of intelligence testing. *Journal of Clinical Experimental Neuropsychology*, **24**, 383–405.

Bokat, C. E. & Goldberg, T. E. (2003). Letter and category fluency in schizophrenic patients: a meta-analysis. *Schizophrenia Research*, **64**, 73–78.

Bowie, C. R., Reichenberg, A., Patterson, T. L., et al. (2006). Determinants of real-world functional performance in schizophrenia subjects: correlations with cognition, functional capacity, and symptoms. *American Journal of Psychiatry*, **163**, 418–425.

Buchanan, R. W., Keefe, R. S., Lieberman, J. A., et al. (2011). A randomized clinical trial of MK-0777 for the treatment of cognitive impairments in people with schizophrenia. *Biological Psychiatry*, **69**, 442–449.

Burdick, K. E., Goldberg, T. E., Funke, B., et al. (2007). DTNBP1 genotype influences cognitive decline in schizophrenia. *Schizophrenia Research*, **89**, 169–172.

Butcher, L. M., Kennedy, J. K., & Plomin, R. (2006). Generalist genes and cognitive neuroscience. *Current Opinion in Neurobiology*, **16**, 145–151.

Callicott, J. H., Bertolino, A., Mattay, V. S., et al. (2000). Physiological dysfunction of the dorsolateral prefrontal cortex in schizophrenia revisited. *Cerebral Cortex*, **10**, 1078–1092.

Cannon, M., Caspi, A., Moffitt, T. E., et al. (2002). Evidence for early childhood, pan-developmental impairment specific to schizophreniform disorder: results from a longitudinal birth cohort. *Archives of General Psychiatry*, **59**, 449–456.

Cannon, T. D., Bearden, C. E., Hollister, J. M., et al. (2000a). Childhood cognitive functioning in schizophrenia patients and their unaffected siblings: a prospective cohort study. *Schizophrenia Bulletin*, **26**, 379–393.

Cannon, T. D., Huttunen, M. O., Lonnqvist, J., et al. (2000b). The inheritance of neuropsychological dysfunction in twins discordant for schizophrenia. *American Journal of Human Genetics*, **67**, 369–382.

Cannon, T. D., Zorrilla, L. E., Shtasel, D., et al. (1994). Neuropsychological functioning in siblings discordant for schizophrenia and healthy volunteers. *Archives of General Psychiatry*, **51**, 651–661.

Carroll, J. B. (1993). *Human Cognitive Abilities: A Survey of Factor-Analytic Studies.* New York, NY: Cambridge University Press.

Carroll, J. B. (1997). The three-stratum theory of cognitive abilities. In D. P. Flanagan, J. L. Genshaft, & P. L. Harrison (eds.), *Contemporary Intellectual Assessment*. New York, NY: Guilford Press, pp. 122–130.

Carter, C. S. (2005). Applying new approaches from cognitive neuroscience to enhance drug development for the treatment of impaired cognition in schizophrenia. *Schizophrenia Bulletin*, **31**, 810–815.

Carter, C. S. & Barch, D. M. (2007). Cognitive neuroscience-based approaches to measuring and improving treatment effects on cognition in schizophrenia: the CNTRICS initiative. *Schizophrenia Bulletin*, **33**, 1131–1137.

Cattell, R. B. (1967). The theory of fluid and crystallized general intelligence checked at the 5–6 year-old level. *British Journal of Educational Psychology*, **37**, 209–224.

Chapman, L. J. & Chapman, J. P. (1973). Problems in the measurement of cognitive deficit. *Psychology Bulletin*, **79**, 380–385.

Cohen, J. D. (1988). *Statistical Power for the Behavioral Sciences*. Hillsdale, NJ: Lawrence Earlbaum.

Costello, A. B. & Osborne, J. W. (2005). Best practices in exploratory factor analysis: four recommendations for getting the most from your analysis. *Practical Assessment Research and Evaluation*, **10**, 1–9.

Deary, I. J. (2001). Human intelligence differences: a recent history. *Trends in Cognitive Sciences*, **5**(3), 127–130.

Dickinson, D. (2008). Digit symbol coding and general cognitive ability in schizophrenia: worth another look? *British Journal of Psychiatry*, **193**, 354–356.

Dickinson, D. & Gold, J. M. (2008). Less unique variance than meets the eye: overlap among traditional neuropsychological dimensions in schizophrenia. *Schizophrenia Bulletin*, **34**, 423–434.

Dickinson, D., Goldberg, T. E., Gold, J. M., et al. (2011). Cognitive factor structure and invariance in people with schizophrenia, their unaffected siblings, and controls. *Schizophrenia Bulletin*, **37**, 1157–1167.

Dickinson, D. & Harvey, P. D. (2009). Systemic hypotheses for generalized cognitive deficits in schizophrenia: a new take on an old problem. *Schizophrenia Bulletin*, **35**, 403–414.

Dickinson, D., Iannone, V. N., Wilk, C. M., et al. (2004). General and specific cognitive deficits in schizophrenia. *Biological Psychiatry*, **55**, 826–833.

Dickinson, D., Ragland, J. D., Calkins, M. E., et al. (2006). A comparison of cognitive structure in schizophrenia patients and healthy controls using confirmatory factor analysis. *Schizophrenia Research*, **85**, 20–29.

Dickinson, D., Ragland, J. D., Gold, J. M., et al. (2008). General and specific cognitive deficits in schizophrenia: Goliath defeats David? *Biological Psychiatry*, **64**, 823–827.

Dickinson, D., Ramsey, M., & Gold, J. M. (2007). Overlooking the obvious: a meta-analytic comparison of digit symbol coding tasks and other cognitive measures in schizophrenia. *Archives of General Psychiatry*, **64**, 532–542.

Dominguez Mde, G., Viechtbauer, W., Simons, C. J., et al. (2009). Are psychotic psychopathology and neurocognition orthogonal? A systematic review of their associations. *Psychology Bulletin*, **135**, 157–171.

Egan, M. F., Goldberg, T. E., Gscheidle, T., et al. (2001a). Relative risk for cognitive impairments in siblings of patients with schizophrenia. *Biological Psychiatry*, **50**, 98–107.

Egan, M. F., Goldberg, T. E., Kolachana, B. S., et al. (2001b). Effect of COMT Val108/158 Met genotype on frontal lobe function and risk for schizophrenia. *Proceedings of the National Academy of Sciences of the United States of America*, **98**, 6917–6922.

Freedman, R., Olincy, A., Buchanan, R. W., et al. (2008). Initial phase 2 trial of a nicotinic agonist in schizophrenia. *American Journal of Psychiatry*, **165**, 1040–1047.

Gladsjo, J. A., McAdams, L. A., Palmer, B. W., et al. (2004). A six-factor model of cognition in schizophrenia and related psychotic disorders: relationships with clinical symptoms and functional capacity. *Schizophrenia Bulletin*, **30**, 739–754.

Glahn, D. C., Almasy, L., Blangero, J., et al. (2007). Adjudicating neurocognitive endophenotypes for schizophrenia. *American Journal of Medical Genetics. Part B, Neuropsychiatric Genetics*, **144**B, 242–249.

Goff, D. C., Hill, M. & Barch, D. (2011). The treatment of cognitive impairment in schizophrenia. *Pharmacology, Biochemistry and Behavior*, **99**, 245–253.

Gold, J. M., Barch, D. M., Carter, C. S., et al. (2011). Clinical, functional, and intertask correlations of measures developed by the Cognitive Neuroscience Test Reliability and Clinical Applications for Schizophrenia Consortium. *Schizophrenia Bulletin*, **38**, 144–152.

Gold, J. M., Hahn, B., Strauss, G. P., et al. (2009). Turning it upside down: areas of preserved cognitive function in schizophrenia. *Neuropsychology Review*, **19**, 294–311.

Gold, J. M., Hahn, B., Zhang, W. W., et al. (2010). Reduced capacity but spared precision and maintenance of working memory representations in schizophrenia. *Archives of General Psychiatry*, **67**, 570–577.

Goldberg, T. E., Ragland, J. D., Torrey, E. F., et al. (1990). Neuropsychological assessment of monozygotic twins discordant for schizophrenia. *Archives of General Psychiatry*, **47**, 1066–1072.

Goldberg, T. E., Torrey, E. F., Gold, J. M., et al. (1993). Learning and memory in monozygotic twins discordant for schizophrenia. *Psychology Medicine*, **23**, 71–85.

Goldberg, T. E., Torrey, E. F., Gold, J. M., et al. (1995). Genetic risk of neuropsychological impairment in schizophrenia: a study of monozygotic twins discordant and concordant for the disorder. *Schizophrenia Research*, **17**, 77–84.

Green, M. F. (1996). What are the functional consequences of neurocognitive deficits in schizophrenia? *American Journal of Psychiatry*, **153**, 321–330.

Green, M. F., Kern, R. S., Braff, D. L., et al. (2000). Neurocognitive deficits and functional outcome in schizophrenia: are we measuring the "right stuff"? *Schizophrenia Bulletin*, **26**, 119–136.

Green, M. F., Kern, R. S., & Heaton, R. K. (2004). Longitudinal studies of cognition and functional outcome in schizophrenia: implications for MATRICS. *Schizophrenia Research*, **72**, 41–51.

Harvey, P. D., Friedman, J. I., Bowie, C., et al. (2006). Validity and stability of performance-based estimates of premorbid educational functioning in older patients with schizophrenia. *Journal of Clinical and Experimental Neuropsychology*, **28**, 178–192.

Harvey, P. D., Howanitz, E., Parrella, M., et al. (1998). Symptoms, cognitive functioning, and adaptive skills in geriatric patients with lifelong schizophrenia: a comparison across treatment sites. *American Journal of Psychiatry*, **155**, 1080–1086.

Haworth, C. M., Kovas, Y., Harlaar, N., et al. (2009). Generalist genes and learning disabilities: a multivariate genetic analysis of low performance in reading, mathematics, language and general cognitive ability in a sample of 8000 12-year-old twins. *Journal of Child Psychology and Psychiatry*, **50**, 1318–1325.

Haworth, C. M., Wright, M. J., Luciano, M., et al. (2010). The heritability of general cognitive ability increases linearly from childhood to young adulthood. *Molecular Psychiatry*, **15**, 1112–1120.

Hedges, L. V. & Olkin, I. (1985). *Statistical Methods for Meta-Analysis*. Orlando, FL: Academic Press.

Heinrichs, R. W. (2005). The primacy of cognition in schizophrenia. *American Psychologist*, **60**, 229–242.

Heinrichs, R. W. & Zakzanis, K. K. (1998). Neurocognitive deficit in schizophrenia: a quantitative review of the evidence. *Neuropsychology*, **12**, 426–445.

Hill, S. K., Schuepbach, D., Herbener, E. S., et al. (2004). Pretreatment and longitudinal studies of neuropsychological deficits in antipsychotic-naive patients with schizophrenia. *Schizophrenia Research*, **68**, 49–63.

Horn, J. L. & Cattell, R. B. (1967). Age differences in fluid and crystallized intelligence. *Acta Psychologica (Amsterdam)*, **26**, 107–129.

Hughes, C., Kumari, V., Soni, W., et al. (2003). Longitudinal study of symptoms and cognitive function in chronic schizophrenia. *Schizophrenia Research*, **59**, 137–146.

Hyde, T. M., Nawroz, S., Goldberg, T. E., et al. (1994). Is there cognitive decline in schizophrenia? A cross-sectional study. *British Journal of Psychiatry*, **164**, 494–500.

Insel, T., Cuthbert, B., Garvey, M., et al. (2010). Research domain criteria (RDoC): toward a new classification framework for research on mental disorders. *American Journal of Psychiatry*, **167**, 748–751.

Jensen, A. R. (1998). *The g Factor: The Science of Mental Ability*. Westport, CN: Praeger.

Johnson, M. H. (2001). Functional brain development in humans. *Nature Reviews Neuroscience*, **2**, 475–483.

Jonides, J. & Nee, D. E. (2005). Assessing dysfunction using refined cognitive methods. *Schizophrenia Bulletin*, **31**, 823–829.

Karmiloff-Smith, A. (2006). The tortuous route from genes to behavior:

A neuroconstructivist approach. *Cognitive, Affective and Behavioral Neuroscience,* **6**, 9–17.

Karmiloff-Smith, A., Scerif, G., & Thomas, M. (2002). Different approaches to relating genotype to phenotype in developmental disorders. *Developmental Psychobiology,* **40**, 311–322.

Keefe, R. S., Bilder, R. M., Davis, S. M., et al. (2007). Neurocognitive effects of antipsychotic medications in patients with chronic schizophrenia in the CATIE Trial. *Archives of General Psychiatry,* **64**, 633–647.

Keefe, R. S., Bilder, R. M., Harvey, P. D., et al. (2006). Baseline neurocognitive deficits in the CATIE schizophrenia trial. *Neuropsychopharmacology,* **31**, 2033–2046.

Keefe, R. S., Goldberg, T. E., Harvey, P. D., et al. (2004). The brief assessment of cognition in schizophrenia: reliability, sensitivity, and comparison with a standard neurocognitive battery. *Schizophrenia Research,* **68**, 283–297.

Kendler, K. S. (2005). Toward a philosophical structure for psychiatry. *American Journal of Psychiatry,* **162**, 433–440.

Kovas, Y. & Plomin, R. (2006). Generalist genes: implications for the cognitive sciences. *Trends in Cognitive Sciences,* **10**, 198–203.

Kremen, W. S., Lyons, M. J., Boake, C., et al. (2006). A discordant twin study of premorbid cognitive ability in schizophrenia. *Journal of Clinical and Experimental Neuropsychology,* **28**, 208–224.

Laing, E., Butterworth, G., Ansari, D., et al. (2002). Atypical development of language and social communication in toddlers with Williams syndrome. *Developmental Science,* **5**, 233–246.

Laing, E., Hulme, C., Grant, J., et al. (2001). Learning to read in Williams syndrome: looking beneath the surface of atypical reading development. *Journal of Child Psychology Psychiatry,* **42**, 729–739.

Lewandowski, K. E., Cohen, B. M., & Ongur, D. (2011). Evolution of neuropsychological dysfunction during the course of schizophrenia and bipolar disorder. *Psychology Medicine,* **41**, 225–241.

Lewis, D. A. & Levitt, P. (2002). Schizophrenia as a disorder of neurodevelopment. *Annual Review of Neuroscience,* **25**, 409–432.

MacDonald, A. W. 3rd. & Carter, C. S. (2002). Cognitive experimental approaches to investigating impaired cognition in schizophrenia: a paradigm shift. *Journal of Clinical and Experimental Neuropsychology,* **24**, 873–882.

Mann-Wrobel, M. C., Carreno, J. T., & Dickinson, D. (2011). Meta-analysis of neuropsychological functioning in euthymic bipolar disorder: an update and investigation of moderator variables. *Bipolar Disorders,* **13**, 334–342.

Marenco, S. & Weinberger, D. R. (2000). The neurodevelopmental hypothesis of schizophrenia: following a trail of evidence from cradle to grave. *Development and Psychopathology,* **12**, 501–527.

Meyer-Lindenberg, A. S., Olsen, R. K., Kohn, P. D., et al. (2005). Regionally specific disturbance of dorsolateral prefrontal-hippocampal functional connectivity in schizophrenia. *Archives of General Psychiatry,* **62**, 379–386.

Miller, M. B., Chapman, J. P., Chapman, L. J., et al. (1995). Task difficulty and cognitive deficits in schizophrenia. *Journal of Abnormal Psychology,* **104**, 251–258.

Niendam, T. A., Bearden, C. E., Rosso, I. M., et al. (2003). A prospective study of childhood neurocognitive functioning in schizophrenic patients and their siblings. *American Journal of Psychiatry,* **160**, 2060–2062.

Nuechterlein, K. H., Barch, D. M., Gold, J. M., et al. (2004). Identification of separable cognitive factors in schizophrenia. *Schizophrenia Research,* **72**, 29–39.

Nuechterlein, K. H., Green, M. F., Kern, R. S., et al. (2008). The MATRICS Consensus Cognitive Battery, part 1: test selection, reliability, and validity. *American Journal of Psychiatry,* **165**, 203–213.

Plomin, R. & Kovas, Y. (2005). Generalist genes and learning disabilities. *Psychological Bulletin,* **131**, 592–617.

Porteous, D. J., Thomson, P., Brandon, N. J., et al. (2006). The genetics and biology of DISC1 – an emerging role in psychosis and cognition. *Biological Psychiatry*, **60**, 123–131.

Ragland, J. D., Ranganath, C., & Barch, D. M., (2011). Relational and item-specific encoding (RISE): task development and psychometric characteristics. *Schizophrenia Bulletin*, **38**:114–124.

Raudenbush, S. W. (1994). Random effects models. In H. Cooper & L. V. Hedges (eds.), *The Handbook of Research Synthesis*. New York, NY: Sage Publications, pp. 301–321.

Reichenberg, A., Caspi, A., Harrington, H., et al. (2010). Static and dynamic cognitive deficits in childhood preceding adult schizophrenia: a 30-year study. *American Journal of Psychiatry*, **167**, 160–169.

Reichenberg, A. & Harvey, P. D. (2007). Neuropsychological impairments in schizophrenia: integration of performance-based and brain imaging findings. *Psychological Bulletin*, **133**, 833–858.

Rund, B. R., Melle, I., Friis, S., et al. (2004). Neurocognitive dysfunction in first-episode psychosis: correlates with symptoms, premorbid adjustment, and duration of untreated psychosis. *American Journal of Psychiatry*, **161**, 466–472.

Russell, E. W. (1980). Fluid and crystallized intelligence: effects of diffuse brain damage on the WAIS. *Perceptual and Motor Skills*, **51**, 121–122.

Sanislow, C. A., Pine, D. S., Quinn, K. J., et al. (2010). Developing constructs for psychopathology research: research domain criteria. *Journal of Abnormal Psychology*, **119**, 631–639.

Shaddish, W. R. & Haddock, C. K. (1994). Combining estimates of effect size. In H. Cooper & L. V. Hedges (eds.), *The Handbook of Research Synthesis*. New York, NY: Sage Publications, pp. 261–285.

Silverstein, S. M., Keane, B. P., Barch, D. M., et al. (2011). Optimization and validation of a visual integration test for schizophrenia research. *Schizophrenia Bulletin*, **38**, 125–134.

Sitskoorn, M. M., Aleman, A., Ebisch, S. J., et al. (2004). Cognitive deficits in relatives of patients with schizophrenia: a meta-analysis. *Schizophrenia Research*, **71**, 285–295.

Snitz, B. E., Macdonald, A. W. 3rd., & Carter, C. S. (2006). Cognitive deficits in unaffected first-degree relatives of schizophrenia patients: a meta-analytic review of putative endophenotypes. *Schizophrenia Bulletin*, **32**, 179–194.

Szoke, A., Schurhoff, F., Mathieu, F., et al. (2005). Tests of executive functions in first-degree relatives of schizophrenic patients: a meta-analysis. *Psychological Medicine*, **35**, 771–782.

Toulopoulou, T., Picchioni, M., Rijsdijk, F., et al. (2007). Substantial genetic overlap between neurocognition and schizophrenia: genetic modeling in twin samples. *Archives of General Psychiatry*, **64**, 1348–1355.

Trandafir, A., Meary, A., Schurhoff, F., et al. (2006). Memory tests in first-degree adult relatives of schizophrenic patients: a meta-analysis. *Schizophrenia Research*, **81**, 217–226.

Tuulio-Henriksson, A., Arajarvi, R., Partonen, T., et al. (2003). Familial loading associates with impairment in visual span among healthy siblings of schizophrenia patients. *Biological Psychiatry*, **54**, 623–628.

Velligan, D. I., Mahurin, R. K., Diamond, P. L., et al. (1997). The functional significance of symptomatology and cognitive function in schizophrenia. *Schizophrenia Research*, **25**, 21–31.

Ventura, J., Thames, A. D., Wood, R. C., et al. (2010). Disorganization and reality distortion in schizophrenia: a meta-analysis of the relationship between positive symptoms and neurocognitive deficits. *Schizophrenia Research*, **121**, 1–14.

Walters, J. T., Corvin, A., Owen, M. J., et al. (2010). Psychosis susceptibility gene ZNF804A and cognitive performance in schizophrenia. *Archives of General Psychiatry*, **67**, 692–700.

Wechsler, D. (2008). *Wechsler Adult Intelligence Test.* (4th edn.). San Antonio, TX: PsychCorp.

Weinberger, D. R. (1995). From neuropathology to neurodevelopment. *Lancet*, **346**, 552–557.

Weinberger, D. R., Berman, K. F., Suddath, R., et al. (1992). Evidence of dysfunction of a prefrontal-limbic network in schizophrenia: a magnetic resonance imaging and regional cerebral blood flow study of discordant monozygotic twins. *American Journal of Psychiatry*, **149**, 890–897.

Weinberger, D. R. & Harrison, P. J. (eds.). (2011). *Schizophrenia*. (3rd edn.). Hoboken, NJ: Wiley-Blackwell.

Young, L. T. (2006). Fewer classes of drugs for more and more psychiatric disorders. *Journal of Psychiatry and Neuroscience*, **31**, 82–83.

Zakzanis, K. K., Leach, L., & Kaplan, E. (1999). *Neuropsychological Differential Diagnosis*. Exton, PA: Swets & Zeitlinger.

Chapter

3

Comparative impairments across schizophrenia and bipolar disorder

Christopher R. Bowie, Katherine Holshausen,
and Maya Gupta

Introduction

One could make a reasonable argument that schizophrenia spectrum and bipolar disorders have more shared characteristics than dissimilarities. Commonalities are found in historical definitions, genetics, neuropathophysiology, endophenotypes, symptom presentation, course of illness, and functional outcomes. Historically, the perceived overlap of these conditions was such that among the most noteworthy works in psychiatric nosology is Kraepelin's proposal of elements that distinguish the two.

Diagnostic criteria

Current diagnostic criteria distinguish the primary psychotic (i.e., schizophrenia) and primary affective disorders (i.e., bipolar disorders) on the basis of the presence, prominence, and co-occurrence of psychotic and mood symptoms. Individuals with bipolar disorders need not experience psychosis, but when they do, psychotic symptoms occur only during mood episodes such as manic or depressive episodes. Individuals with schizophrenia may have mood symptoms but they do not meet full symptom or duration criteria for a mood episode. One historical difference in the diagnoses was the episodic nature of affective disorders compared to a chronic and progressively debilitating course in schizophrenia. Current views increasingly recognize the heterogeneous presentation and course of symptoms in schizophrenia and a number of studies find chronic impairment in the bipolar disorders.

Thus, the boundaries of the schizophrenia spectrum and bipolar disorders are blurred – most people with schizophrenia experience some form of mood disturbance at various times and over 50% of those with bipolar disorder experience psychotic symptoms (Goodwin & Jamison, 2006). Cognitive functions have been considered a core feature of these two disorders and we have seen a dramatic increase in the study of cognition in schizophrenia and, more recently, bipolar disorder (Figure 3.1). However, this domain of cognitive functioning continues to escape diagnostic criteria. In this chapter, we will discuss how the overlap and distinction of the primary psychotic (i.e., schizophrenia) and primary affective disorders (i.e., bipolar disorders) may be understood in the context of cognition.

Cognitive Impairment in Schizophrenia, ed. Philip D. Harvey. Published by Cambridge University Press. © Cambridge University Press 2013.

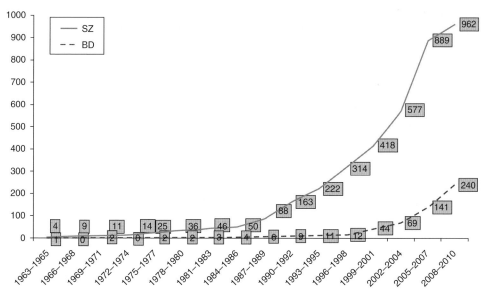

Figure 3.1. Number of publications indexed in PubMed from 1963 to 2010, during three-year intervals, with reference to cognition in schizophrenia versus bipolar disorder. BD, bipolar disorder; SZ, schizophrenia. Search terms for the schizophrenia search: ("1963"^{2} [Entrez Date]: "1965"^{2} [Entrez Date]) AND schizophr* [Title/Abstract]) AND (neuropsychol* [Title/Abstract] OR neurocog* [Title/Abstract] OR memory[MeSH Major Topic] OR executive functioning [MeSH Major Topic]). For the bipolar search: ("1963"^{2} [Entrez Date]: "1965"^{2} [Entrez Date]) AND (bipolar disorder[Title/Abstract] OR mania [Title/Abstract] OR manic depressi* [Title/Abstract])) AND (neuropsychol* [Title/Abstract] OR neurocog* [Title/Abstract] OR memory[MeSH Major Topic] OR executive functioning [MeSH Major Topic]).

Profile and course of cognitive deficits

The pattern of cognitive impairments in schizophrenia and bipolar disorders can be viewed from four dimensions: prevalence, breadth, magnitude, and course.

Prevalence of impairments

It has been argued that cognitive impairment is universal in schizophrenia, if not from a pure psychometric deviation from normal performance then at least relative to premorbid functioning (Reichenberg et al., 2002), global average performance scores that mask large relative deficits (Wilk et al., 2005), or monozygotic twin performance (Goldberg et al., 1990). Impairments are less prevalent in bipolar disorders. Using a cut-off of one standard deviation unit as the criterion for impairment, approximately 80%–84% of individuals with schizophrenia demonstrate significant impairment on cognitive tests, where almost 40% and 58% of those with remitted and psychotic bipolar disorder, respectively, perform in the impaired range (Reichenberg et al., 2009). Indeed, given the high prevalence and relative disruptions in functioning as a by-product of cognitive dysfunction, many argue that cognitive impairments should be included in future iterations of the diagnostic manuals (Keefe & Fenton, 2007).

Breadth of impairments

Cognitive impairments in schizophrenia, as reviewed in Chapter 2, appear to be generalized, leaving very few domains spared. Impairments are present in several aspects of attentional functioning (including selective, sustained, and divided attention), speed of processing information, working memory (including executive control, storage, and manipulation), language production, visual and verbal learning and memory, and executive functions (including abstraction, conceptual shifting, disinhibition, planning). Some studies have found evidence for more severe impairment in specific areas such as executive functioning and verbal declarative memory (Reichenberg et al., 2009), but others suggest an impairment that is characterized by a general factor most closely linked to information processing speed (Dickinson et al., 2007). Data reduction techniques often support the notion of a generalized cognitive factor in schizophrenia (Dickinson et al., 2008; Keefe et al., 2006), yet some studies find evidence for separable domains (Bowie et al., 2008; Genderson et al., 2007). Czobor and colleagues (2007) used confirmatory factor analysis for a large group of individuals with bipolar disorder derived from a schizophrenia model of six underlying functions created from a large battery of tests: attention, working memory, learning, verbal knowledge, nonverbal functions, and executive functions. The results supported consistence in factor structure across the two conditions and were observed in spite of several demographic differences.

Magnitude of impairment

Consideration of a cognitive profile of mental disorders includes an evaluation of the magnitude (severity) of impairments, in addition to the specific types of domains that are affected. There has been considerable controversy regarding the degree of difference in performance in bipolar versus schizophrenia samples.

Studies that find comparable levels of impairment between schizophrenia and bipolar disorders tend to have limited breadth of cognitive assessment (Docherty et al., 1996) and/or unique sample characteristics such as older age (Depp et al., 2007), or clinical remission. The broader literature base suggests that impairments observed in bipolar disorders follow a similar pattern but with a magnitude that is intermediate to healthy controls and schizophrenia (Figure 3.2). Consistent with those studies, epidemiological data from Reichenberg and colleagues (2009) reported cognitive performance of consecutive admission patients with psychosis from 12 hospitals in Suffolk County, New York. Compared to the bipolar group, those with schizophrenia were more severely impaired on verbal memory, visual memory, executive functions, attention and processing speed, language skills, sensory motor skills, and visual processing, but not general verbal ability. The bipolar group was intermediate to the schizophrenia group and normal performance, with impairments in the mild to moderate range in verbal memory, visual memory, executive functions, attention, and processing speed.

Course of cognition

The longitudinal course of cognitive impairments, like the variability in clinical symptoms, provides a window into the differences between primary psychotic and affective disorders. Chapter 7 offers a detailed review of the course of cognition in schizophrenia, where we see impairments prior to illness onset and relative stability throughout the lifespan, with the exception of declines in late life for those with a more recalcitrant course. Although the course of cognitive functioning in schizophrenia is more dynamic than once thought, several investigators support the notion that variability of performance is typical of bipolar disorders. While not yet as thoroughly investigated as the schizophrenia literature,

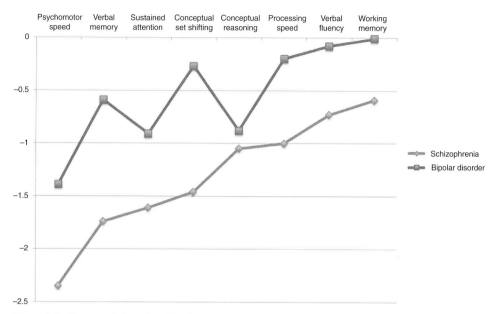

Figure 3.2. Neuropsychological profile of cognitive impairments in schizophrenia and bipolar disorder. (Adapted from data in Bowie et al., 2010.)

premorbid cognitive impairment appears to be absent or at least more limited in scope in bipolar disorders. Retrospective reviews (Uzelac et al., 2006) and epidemiological cohort studies (Reichenberg et al., 2002) using global measures of intellectual and cognitive functioning find normal performance prior to bipolar disorder onset, yet after the initial onset of the illness, intellectual abilities are closer to those with schizophrenia (Touloupoulou et al., 2006). Moving beyond global measures, it is likely that more discrete cognitive impairments are observed during the premorbid period of those who are later diagnosed with bipolar disorder. A small number of studies have found premorbid visuospatial and executive functioning impairments in bipolar disorders during prospective studies (Meyer et al., 2004; Tiihonen et al., 2005).

Changes in cognition during the prodromal period are being addressed in bipolar disorder at present and are far from answered in schizophrenia. A small study (Olvet et al., 2010) failed to differentiate a clinical high-risk psychosis group that converted to bipolar disorder or schizophrenia on a neurocognitive composite score. A number of ongoing clinical and genetic high-risk studies now include bipolar disorders along with schizophrenia, so the specific profile and possibly a distinction between the two groups are likely to be addressed in the next few years.

Following a first episode of psychosis, impairments are relatively stable in schizophrenia (Heaton et al., 2001), but in bipolar disorder several domains appear to be more dynamic even over two-year periods (an exception is stable sustained attention impairments). Interestingly, these changes are not well explained by clinical symptom changes (Arts et al., 2011). In late life, cognitive impairments worsen for schizophrenia patients who have greater institutionalization histories (Harvey et al., 2010), yet preliminary reports have found severe impairments in older individuals with bipolar disorder in spite of the sample being clinically stable (Depp et al., 2007; Schouws et al., 2007). More episodes of mania are positively associated with greater cognitive impairments, particularly in executive function-ing tasks (Elshahawi et al., 2011; Lopez-Jaramillo et al., 2010). Disentangling the long-term course of cognition in the two conditions is difficult due to differences in the stability and pseudospecificity of symptoms, but clearly the longitudinal nature of bipolar disorder is in need of further study. Work in this area will help clarify whether bipolar disorder, or certain individuals such as those with recurrent mood episodes, are associated with a neurotoxic disease process – one that would further complicate a Kraepelinian distinction based on course of illness.

Thus, cognition in schizophrenia is characterized by broad impairments with selective severe deficits in executive skills and memory. Bipolar disorder is also associated with selective impairment in those domains, but several areas of cognitive functioning, while following the profile observed in schizophrenia, are within the normal range of function-ing. Several positions have been put forward to explain the core of cognitive impairments in schizophrenia, from perceptual processing, working memory, to top-down executive control. Fewer proposals have been advanced for the core of cognitive impairment of bipolar disorders. From a qualitative perspective, the types of impairments might manifest due to differences in core cognitive impairments, test taking strategy, or behaviors. For example, substantial differences in the magnitude of impairment in more elementary cognitive functions such as processing speed and sensory–motor functioning might suggest that, in schizophrenia, dysfunction in the higher processes is a consequence of those systems that subserve higher-order skills. In contrast, intact basic functions in bipolar disorders might point to higher order skills representing the core feature of impairment. As such, executive dysfunction has been proposed as the core feature of bipolar disorder (Mur et al., 2007). Pathological mechanisms might thus be explored as we increase our understanding of the mechanisms responsible for these discrete cognitive skills and their interactions.

Social cognition

Social cognition refers to the mental operations that underlie social interactions and the skills that govern navigation of social environments. Fundamentally, social cognition allows people to understand and interact with one another effectively; its impairment in both schizophrenia and bipolar disorders appears to be partially responsible for impairments in everyday functioning. Chapter 8 reviews social cognition in schizophrenia; this section will focus on findings in bipolar disorders and contrast them to those in schizophrenia.

Emotional processing

The ability to infer the emotional state of another from observable information from their prosody and facial expression is a crucial skill for interpersonal functioning. Compara-tively, the effect size of emotion processing deficits in affective disorders (collapsed across depression and bipolar) is -0.49 compared to -0.91 in schizophrenia (Kohler et al., 2010, 2011). Impaired emotion processing in schizophrenia may be a consequence of scanning facial features that are not important in the evaluation of emotion expression (Gordon et al., 1992; Green et al., 2003). The mechanisms for impairments in bipolar disorder are not well understood. There is evidence to suggest that fear and sadness are especially challenging emotions to recognize for those with schizophrenia (Edwards et al., 2001). During mania there appears to be a mood-congruent bias, with a specific deficit in recognition of negative over positively valenced faces (Lembke & Ketter, 2002), whereas individuals in a depressed state demonstrate a mood-congruent negative bias during facial emotion processing tasks (Gur et al., 1992).

Social perception

Social perception encompasses a person's ability to judge social cues and includes awareness of the roles of others, rules, and goals that typically characterize social situations and guide social interactions (Corrigan & Green, 1993). Individuals with schizophrenia consistently demonstrate a deficit on measures of social perception (Horan et al., 2008). In bipolar disorder, social perception has not been studied directly, but inferences suggest that these individuals struggle with understanding the social expectations of situations and roles in interpersonal relationships. Spouses of those with bipolar disorder reported that their partners offer less emotional and practical support as compared to healthy control marital couples (Horesh & Fennig, 2000). In tasks of evaluating intentions of others in a social situation, manic patients performed significantly worse than healthy controls, demonstrating a deficit in understanding interpretations of social behaviors (Bazin et al., 2009). Individuals with bipolar disorder perform worse than healthy controls in tasks of social knowledge and judgment, but, similar to most other social cognitive tasks, better than those with schizophrenia (Cutting & Murphy, 1990).

Theory of mind

Theory of mind refers to the ability to ascribe mental states, such as beliefs, desires, and intentions to the self and others (Premack & Woddruff, 1978), and is generally conceptualized as having both cognitive (understanding another's perspective) and affective (emotional response to the feelings of others) components. Theory of mind deficits in schizophrenia are very large ($d=1.25$) (Sprong et al., 2007), while those in bipolar disorder range from -0.86 to -1.02 (Kerr et al., 2003; Sarfati & Harde-Bayle, 1999). It has been suggested that acute psychosis may have a significant moderating influence on theory of mind performance, indicating that mentalizing deficits may be trait-like characteristics of schizophrenia (Bora et al., 2009). Other studies demonstrate a role for negative symptoms in their maintenance of impairments in mentalizing (Frith & Corcoran, 1996) and there appear to be specific deficits (e.g., first- and second-order verbal theory of mind tasks) that are associated with paranoia (Harrington et al., 2005). In bipolar disorders, the literature suggests a gradient in theory of mind performance with lesser or no impairment on tasks requiring low cognitive demands, and a more severe deficit in more cognitively taxing tasks (Cusi et al., in press).

Mood episodes may play a role in the degree and type of theory of mind impairment. Euthymic patients perform similar to healthy controls on lower-order tasks but worse on tasks that require high levels of cognitive processing demands (Bora et al., 2005). A similar but more severe pattern emerges with subsyndromal symptoms, demonstrating a deficit on both higher- and lower-level theory of mind tasks, with a milder impairment on lower-level tasks (McKinnon et al., 2010). Among actively ill patients (manic and depressed mood states), we observe impairments on both low and high cognitive demand tasks (Kerr et al., 2003). Thus, the presence of specific symptoms in both disorders and clinical state in bipolar disorders are contributing factors to theory of mind deficits.

Attributional style

Attributional style refers to the manner by which individuals characteristically explain the causes for positive and negative events in their lives. Individuals with persecutory delusions have a higher tendency to blame others rather than situational factors for negative events – an inference style known as a "personalizing bias" (Langdon et al., 2006). Comorbid depressive symptoms in schizophrenia are related to excessive attribution of positive events to external causes and negative events to internal causes (Fraguas et al., 2008). Specific temperament and personality factors that are frequently observed in bipolar disorder, such as ruminative tendencies and neuroticism, may play a role in the style in which these individuals interpret the causal role of events in their lives (McKinnon et al., 2010). Negative attributional style for negative events interacts with subsequent negative events and predicts increases in depressive symptoms, while a positive attributional style for positive events predicts an increase in hypomanic symptoms (Alloy et al., 1999).

Empathy

Empathy refers to the ability to appraise and vicariously experience the emotional state of another. Similar in structure to theory of mind, empathy is hypothesized to encompass cognitive (understanding another's perspective) and affective (emotional response to the feeling states of others) components (Davis, 1980). Individuals with schizophrenia have difficulties with perspective taking and might also experience challenges with affective responsiveness (Derntl et al., 2009). The scarce literature on empathy in individuals with bipolar disorder suggests lower levels of cognitive empathy (i.e., perspective taking) and increased affective discomfort in response to others' distress (Davis, 1980) or elevated affective empathy (Shamay-Tsoory et al., 2009). This suggests that there is indeed an active affective empathy component in bipolar disorders, but it is dysregulated such that the experienced emotional response to the feeling states of others is inappropriate in magnitude and/or direction. There is little evidence to suggest whether the impairments demonstrated by individuals with bipolar disorder are state- or trait-like in nature, whereas these same impairments have been proposed to be a possible prodromal risk marker in schizophrenia (Bota et al., 2007).

Neurophysiological findings

Cognitive functions can be indexed at a level more proximal to neurological function through various psychophysiological methods, such as eye tracking and electroencephalogram experiments. The impairments indexed with these neurophysiological instruments are more sensitive than neuropsychological instruments to endophenotypic impairment (Thaker, 2008) and treatment-related change (Lencer et al., 2008). Perhaps more so than neuropsychological assessment methods, these measures might offer greater distinction between primary affective and psychotic disorders.

Deficits in the smooth pursuit eye movement system are observed in both disorders, with more severe impairment in schizophrenia, in the ability to predictively respond to a moving target; however, the initiation of pursuit appears disordered in schizophrenia but intact in bipolar disorders (Thaker, 2008). These impairments may be more pronounced for those with psychosis and are stable even after pharmacological treatment (Lencer et al., 2010). Similarly, negative symptoms and poor outcome are associated with mismatch negativity, which is an evoked response potential (ERP) observed in response to an auditory stimulus that is inconsistent with a series of previous auditory stimuli (Catts et al., 1995). However, this ERP is not associated with mood episode or symptom severity in bipolar disorder (Takei et al., 2010). This ERP has been found intact in large samples of those with bipolar disorder and their relatives (Hall et al., 2009), although a recent study found no difference between the two diagnostic groups at the time of first-episode psychosis (Kaur et al., 2011).

In addition to smooth pursuit initiation, positive symptoms appear to be associated with several other psychophysiological measures. Sensory and sensory–motor gating are abilities measured with repetitive (sensory gating; the P50 ERP) or sudden excessive auditory stimuli (sensory–motor gating; measured by electromyography), respectively, that filter out excessive stimuli and attenuate the organism's neurophysiological or startle responses. Impairments in gating are well replicated and stable in schizophrenia, but appear to be more specific to acute manic and/or presence or history of psychosis in bipolar disorder (Thaker, 2008). The strong relationships at the neurobiological level to dopaminergic functioning and at a conceptual level to filtering excessive information provide insights into the mechanisms underlying psychotic symptoms.

The P300 component of ERP is typically elicited by the presentation of a target stimulus that is presented less frequently than repetitive, non-target stimuli and is thought to reflect attentional engagement (P3a; observed in frontal and central regions) and working memory (P3b; observed in posterior regions). There is high heritability of the ERP response in both schizophrenia (Blackwood et al., 1991) and bipolar disorder (Hall et al., 2009), which provides support for its inclusion as a nonspecific endophenotype for both disorders. The impairment appears to be stable; following clinical remission from a first episode of psychosis, both diagnostic groups present reduced amplitude in P3a (Kaur et al., 2011). However, there is evidence for a topographical differential deficit during active illness, with a frontal reduction in amplitude in actively manic bipolar but posterior reduction in schizophrenia patients (Salisbury et al., 1999).

Moderating variables: demographics and clinical state

Most comparative studies of cognition in schizophrenia and bipolar disorders focus the distinction at the level of diagnosis. It is critical that we also consider the heterogeneous nature of symptom presentations within each diagnostic class. Several moderating variables have been identified that affect the differences that we observe at the diagnostic level. The variable symptom presentation within diagnoses and, at least in the case of bipolar disorders, the cyclical nature of symptoms interspersed with periods of euthymia, present a great challenge but exciting opportunities to further examine the overlap and discontinuities among the schizophrenia and bipolar spectra.

Gender

Although prevalence of the two disorders is consistent in men and women, several factors such as age of onset and course of illness are associated with gender differences, with women generally having a later onset and better long-term functioning. Cognitive deficits are also moderately associated with gender, with female patients functioning better than male patients on most tasks. Comparison studies that have relied heavily on recruitment from facilities where men are more prominent (e.g., veteran's affairs hospitals) are thus typically skewed toward identifying more impairment, an important factor when comparing across studies or considering differences in sample recruitment (Bora et al., 2009). Matching on gender is an important consideration in comparison studies, yet it is not always achieved in published reports.

Negative symptoms

Negative symptoms are modestly correlated with cognition in schizophrenia, although these domains are distinct (Harvey et al., 2006). Comparisons of cognitive impairments in bipolar disorders and schizophrenia have found that the differences can be partially attributed to the prevalence of individuals with high levels of negative symptoms in schizophrenia, but not in bipolar disorders (Bora et al., 2009). Negative symptoms overlap with depression (e.g., restricted behaviors and anhedonia), but examining specific items (Chemerinski et al., 2008) or utilizing scales such as the Calgary Depression Scale (Addington et al., 1992) and the Schedule for Deficit Syndrome (Kirkpatrick et al., 1989), the two symptom domains are better distinguished.

The assessment of negative symptoms is even more complicated in bipolar disorders given the increased likelihood of persistent depressive symptoms, and this is an area that needs further work. While some have argued that certain negative symptoms are specific to schizophrenia (Reddy et al., 1992), other studies find them to be present in bipolar disorder (Toomey et al., 1998), distinct from depressive symptoms, and related to functioning (Bowie et al., 2010). Whether negative symptoms are present in bipolar disorder is not well understood, although some studies have identified similar profiles with schizophrenia. Examination of comparative cognitive deficits in schizophrenia and bipolar disorders should consider the confounding effects of samples with over-representation of specific symptoms that are associated with cognition, particularly negative symptoms.

Clinical remission

Periods of clinical remission are more characteristic of bipolar disorders than schizophrenia, a point of distinction in early definitions. Here too we now recognize the overlap of this dimension, with the identification of the chronic nature of subsyndromal symptoms and functional disability in bipolar disorders (Jaeger et al., 2007) and the higher than previously presumed rates of clinical symptom remission (although this is very rarely associated with functional recovery) in schizophrenia (Robinson et al., 2004). Yet, it is in this aspect, which is related to the course of cognition (see previously), that we might find the greatest distinction between the profile of cognition in schizophrenia and bipolar disorders.

In spite of the apparent disruptive nature of clinical symptoms of schizophrenia, very small correlations are found between psychosis and cognitive functioning (Heaton et al., 2001). Impairments in cognition persist even during periods of clinical remission and do not appear to increase with repeated episodes. In contrast, there is evidence for greater cognitive impairment as the number of manic episodes increases (Martinez-Aran et al., 2004), underscoring the aforementioned need to examine a possible neurotoxic disease process in individuals who experience recurrent mood episodes. Further, concerning periods of remission, selective cognitive impairments that are observed during periods of manic and/or depressive episodes of bipolar disorder might improve during periods of euthymic mood on sustained attention (Addington & Addington, 1997), visual memory (Martinez-Aran et al., 2004), and executive functions (Ferrier et al., 1999). However, a cross-sectional study found similar performance of euthymic bipolar disorder with stable schizophrenia patients on sustained attention, visual memory and selective measures of executive functioning (disinhibition, planning or conceptual reasoning but less impairment on conceptual set shifting and verbal working memory), and verbal memory (total learning or recall but less impairment in immediate verbal recall and recognition) (Sanchez-Morla et al., 2009).

To date, very few investigations have used longitudinal within-subject designs to examine relationships of cognition with changes in affective state. Chaves and colleagues (2011) found only a linear relationship between improved depression and better verbal fluency, but no significant associations with change in information processing speed, attention, working memory, declarative memory, and executive functions. Changes in ratings of mania severity were not correlated with any cognitive measures. Studies have not directly compared performance as individuals shift from euthymia to an episode or between episodes, owing in part to the difficulty with recruitment and retention of subjects who have mood transitions that are challenging to predict.

Psychosis

Individuals with bipolar disorder and current psychotic features have cognitive impairments equivalent in magnitude to those observed in individuals with schizophrenia (Glahn et al., 2006). The distinction between the groups persists after inpatient stabilization of psychosis (Levy & Weiss, 2010), and there is evidence for more severe impairment based on history of psychotic episodes even when currently not psychotic, particularly in declarative memory, working memory, processing speed, and executive skills, but not visual memory or attention (Bora et al., 2007). This suggests that cognitive functioning depends to a large extent on the history of psychosis, and this distinction might be a more useful method than diagnostic category of classifying patients, at least from a cognitive perspective. The field appears to be heading in this direction with the consideration of cognitive impairment in the classification of at least schizophrenia spectrum disorders in the upcoming DSM-V.

The relationship of cognition with functional outcomes

Individuals with chronic mental disorders experience impairment across multiple life domains, including interpersonal relationships, independent living, academic/occupational achievement, and community involvement. These difficulties cause significant cost and burden to both the individual and society. Cognition is one of the most robust predictors of functional outcomes in schizophrenia and bipolar disorder.

Schizophrenia is among the most debilitating illnesses worldwide (Lopez et al., 2006), with significant personal costs and decreased quality of life. Historically, the role of cognition was largely over-shadowed by the perceived importance of clinical symptoms, and only recently has cognition emerged as one of the most prominent predictors of functioning in schizophrenia, independent of the contribution of positive, negative, and depressive symptoms (Green, 1996). There is substantial evidence to indicate that cognition is a prominent predictor of social, adaptive, and vocational functioning, and is a rate-limiter for the response to psychosocial treatment. Chapter 5 of this book provides an extensive review of the robust role of cognition in predicting functional abilities and outcomes in schizophrenia.

As in schizophrenia, functional disability is a major problem for many people with bipolar disorder, during both euthymic and symptomatic states (Sanchez-Moreno et al., 2009). Disability persists in many of the same domains as we see in schizophrenia, including social functioning, adaptive functioning, independent living, and occupational/academic functioning. When comparing functional outcomes between schizophrenia and bipolar disorder, clinician-rated functioning is often poorer in schizophrenia than in bipolar disorder; however, self-rated functioning is similar across both clinical groups, while still being significantly poorer than the self-reported functioning of healthy controls (Simonsen et al., 2011). This might speak to the perceived distress or quality of life in bipolar disorder that might go underappreciated in schizophrenia, where more prevalent and severe anhedonia and amotivation reduce the desire or recognition of impairments.

In the last few years, evidence has emerged to support the notion that neurocognitive performance, in addition to clinical symptoms, is strongly associated with functional disability in bipolar disorder. At one-year follow-up, independent studies have found that impairments at baseline (Martino et al., 2009) and following treatment (Tabarés-Seisdedos et al., 2008) in verbal memory, attention, and executive functions explained more than one-quarter of the variance in functional outcomes, even after considering clinical symptoms. Furthermore, at fifteen years following a manic episode, cognitive variables are associated with social and work functioning (Burdick et al., 2010).

In schizophrenia, we tend to see global cognition (Evans et al., 2003) or basic cognitive skills like information processing speed (Bowie et al., 2008) as the best predictors of everyday living skills and social outcomes, although work outcomes are best predicted by higher-order executive skills (McGurk & Meltzer, 2000). In bipolar disorders, where impairments appear to be more selective, we might expect to see differential relationships among cognitive and outcome variables. Executive functioning in particular might have a broad and robust relationship with outcomes in bipolar disorder. This domain is the strongest predictor of psychosocial functioning (Sole et al., 2011) and occupational outcomes (Altshuler et al., 2007; Bearden et al., 2011).

To date, most studies on the predictors of functioning in bipolar disorder have been conducted with euthymic patients, which complicates our understanding of the relationships, because from a statistical perspective, low levels of symptoms reduce the chances that they will be significant predictors. Indeed, very little is known about the relationship between cognition and functioning during different clinical states. A recent study by Levy et al. (2011) assessed patients with bipolar I disorder at discharge following inpatient care for acute mood disturbance. Social Security Administration disability status was related to poorer scores on visual memory, verbal memory, attention, and executive function, a relationship that was not observed with the global assessment of functioning.

Studies of functioning in bipolar disorder often rely on subjective self-report or third-party ratings of functioning, which have questionable validity in both schizophrenia and bipolar disorder (Bowie et al., 2007; Burdick et al., 2005) and may be influenced by current mood state (Dean et al., 2004). A study by Bowie and colleagues (2010) used path analyses to model the direct and indirect relationships between cognition and functioning in both schizophrenia and bipolar disorder using objective measures of functional competence, such as laboratory-based role plays, in addition to third-party ratings of observed real-world behavior on standard scales. For both diagnostic groups, neurocognition was related to real-world activities, interpersonal relationships, and work skills. However, the relationship between neurocognition and real-world functional outcomes was mediated by functional competence (skills one can demonstrate in the laboratory). For both groups, clinical symptoms were also negatively associated with real-world functional outcomes but not associated with functional competence, with the exception of depressive symptoms, which were directly related to social competence in bipolar disorder.

There are several moderating or mediating variables to consider for future work in this area. Bipolar disorder is associated with better premorbid functioning and more periods of clinical remission. As such, individuals with bipolar disorder experience a more substantial relative reduction in functioning at the onset of symptoms, but have more opportunity to acquire skills if premorbid functioning is higher. Furthermore, individuals with bipolar disorder experience fewer disruptions inter-episode with the lower rates of negative symptoms compared to the residual phase of schizophrenia.

Assessment issues
Affective saliency of tasks

The degree to which processing of information involves affective components is an important consideration in the assessment of cognition for individuals with severe mental illness (Heller, 1993; Miller, 1996). The literature presents a mixed picture of dysfunctional emotional processing of information in bipolar disorder; some find poorer performance in patients across euthymic, manic, and depressed states, relative to healthy controls (French et al., 1996), while others have found no significant differences between bipolar patients and healthy controls (Wright et al., 2005). Interestingly, patients with schizophrenia demonstrate a hypersensitivity to threatening and paranoid words (Bentall & Kaney, 1989), yet no evidence of emotional interference in response to negative, neutral, and positive stimuli (Demily et al., 2010). Of those studies that find differences in cognitive impairments as a function of affective saliency, it appears that attention and inhibition (Lyon et al., 1999; Murphy et al., 1999), and memory (Lex et al., 2011) may be affected by the presence of emotional stimuli. Evaluation of cognitive deficits should be interpreted in light of the potential emotional interference of affectively salient stimuli.

Consensus batteries

A recent large-scale effort has produced a standardized assessment battery called the Measurement and Treatment Research to Improve Cognition in Schizophrenia (MATRICS) Battery to measure treatment effects on cognition in schizophrenia (Green & Nuechterlein, 2004). This battery assesses most of the domains known to be impaired and functionally relevant in schizophrenia and includes tests with strong psychometric properties. More recent studies have examined whether the MATRICS battery is applicable to bipolar disorder. In one study, most domains, but not social cognition, reliably distinguish bipolar disorder from controls (Burdick et al., 2011); in schizophrenia in addition, the social cognition domain loads weakly with the neurocognitive domains (Eack et al., 2009). It might be that the breadth of domains and the potential for ceiling effects on the MATRICS domain make them less sensitive to treatment change in bipolar disorder. In line with this idea, a recent consensus panel recommended considering the substitution of some tests and the addition of others when examining cognitive changes in bipolar disorder (Yatham et al., 2010). For example, verbal list learning tasks with more words and components of memory, such as the California Verbal Learning Test, might be more sensitive to cognitive impairment and change scores in bipolar disorder than the Hopkins Verbal Learning Test, which contains four fewer words, two fewer learning trials, and (in the MATRICS battery) no assessment of delayed memory or recognition.

Repeated assessments

The psychometric properties of the scales and alternate forms help to minimize confounds related to repeated testing, but in bipolar disorders it is critical to also consider whether performance on measures are affected by changes in mood symptoms or even shifts in polarity to/from an episode. As of now, we have a limited understanding of the degree to which cognitive change might be pseudospecific in bipolar disorder, and this is a critical direction for future research as we continue to consider recruitment, design, instrument selection, and statistical adjustment for studying cognitive change in bipolar disorders.

Treatment of cognitive deficits

Behavioral and pharmacological treatments of cognition for schizophrenia have accelerated in the past ten years. Behavioral treatments for schizophrenia such as cognitive remediation (see Chapter 16) lead to robust changes in cognition and generalize to functional changes, particularly when implemented within a broader psychosocial rehabilitation program with multiple types of treatment. In spite of the increase in the study of cognition in bipolar disorders in the past ten years, very little information is known about the malleability of cognition. To date, only one published study, an open trial for relatively high functioning and asymptomatic bipolar patients, has examined cognitive remediation in bipolar disorder. This study found improvements in executive functioning and these cognitive changes were associated with better occupational performance, which also improved to be significant (Deckersbach et al., 2010).

Pharmacological treatments of cognition have been less successful in schizophrenia and little studied in bipolar disorder. A study of pramipexole as an adjunctive treatment of cognition in bipolar disorder found a subgroup of patients with fewer symptoms to have a greater treatment response compared to the placebo (Burdick et al., 2012).

Future studies of cognitive change in bipolar disorder might need to apply more selective recruitment and screening procedures than have been utilized in schizophrenia research, given the likelihood of already intact cognitive function for a substantial minority of the population and the dynamic nature of cognition with mood fluctuations. Recruitment of bipolar patients into cognitive treatment studies might indeed prove challenging given the possibility of poor insight into the deficits (Burdick et al., 2005).

Summary and future directions

Cognitive impairments are widely recognized as a core feature of schizophrenia and, with increasing study, an important consideration for many individuals with bipolar disorder. Compared to schizophrenia, cognitive impairments in bipolar disorder are less prevalent, manifest in fewer domains, are less severe and, at least in some domains, less persistent. We have seen more traction for the consideration of cognition in the diagnosis of schizophrenia than in bipolar disorders, although as illustrated in Figure 3.1, research on cognition in bipolar disorders is only beginning to catch up to the hefty database that exists for schizophrenia-related cognitive functions. However, the relevance of cognitive functions to both disorders is comparable, with evidence for robust relationships with everyday social and functional outcomes. With strong relationships to functioning and increasing evidence that cognition is a viable treatment target in chronic mental disorders, we will likely see an increase in treatments for cognition in both disorders. How these treatments transfer to changes in the persistent disability that is characteristic of both disorders will be an important avenue for the next several years.

References

Addington, D., Addington, J., Maticka-Tyndale, E., et al. (1992). Reliability and validity of a depression rating scale for schizophrenics. *Schizophrenia Research*, **6**, 201–208.

Addington, J. & Addington, D. (1997). Attentional vulnerability indicators in schizophrenia and bipolar disorder. *Schizophrenia Research*, **23**, 197–204.

Alloy, L. Y., Abrahamson, L. Y., Whitehouse, W. G., et al. (1999). Depressogenic cognitive styles: predictive validity, information processing and personality characteristics, and developmental origins. *Behaviour Research and Therapy*, **37**, 503–531.

Altshuler, L., Tekell, J., Biswas, K., et al. (2007). Executive function and employment status among veterans with bipolar disorder. *Psychiatric Services*, **58**, 1441–1447.

Arts, B., Jabben, N., Krabbendam, L., et al. (2011). A 2-year naturalistic study on cognitive functioning in bipolar disorder. *Acta Psychiatrica Scandinavica*, **123**, 190–205.

Bazin, N., Brunet-Gouet, E., Bourdet, C., et al. (2009). Quantitative assessment of attribution of intentions to others in schizophrenia using an ecological video-based task: a comparison with manic and depressed patients. *Psychiatry Research*, **167**, 28–35.

Bearden, C. E., Shih, V. H., Green, M. F., et al. (2011). The impact of neurocognitive impairment on occupational recovery of clinically stable patients with bipolar disorder: a prospective study. *Bipolar Disorders*, **13**, 323–333.

Bentall, R. P. & Kaney, S. (1989). Content specific information processing and persecutory delusions: an investigation using the emotional Stroop test. *British Journal of Medical Psychology*, **62**, 355–364.

Blackwood, D. H., Young, A. H., McQueen, J. K., et al. (1991). Magnetic resonance imaging in schizophrenia: altered brain morphology associated with P300 abnormalities and eye tracking dysfunction. *Biological Psychiatry*, **30**, 753–769.

Bora, E., Vahip, S., Akdeniz, F., et al. (2007). The effect of previous psychotic mood episodes on cognitive impairment in euthymic bipolar patients. *Bipolar Disorders*, **9**, 468–477.

Bora, E., Vahip, S., Gonul, A. S., et al. (2005). Evidence for theory of mind deficits in euthymic patients with bipolar disorder. *Acta Psychiatrica Scandinavica*, **112**, 110–116.

Bora, E., Yucel, M., & Pantelis, C. (2009). Theory of mind impairment in schizophrenia: meta-analysis. *Schizophrenia Research*, **109**, 1–9.

Bota, R. G. & Ricci, W. F. (2007). Empathy as method toward identification of the debut of prodome of schizophrenia. *Bulletin of the Menninger Clinic*, **71**, 312–324.

Bowie, C. R., Leung, W. W., Reichenberg, A., et al. (2008). Predicting schizophrenia patients' real-world behavior with specific neuropsychological and functional capacity measures. *Biological Psychiatry*, **63**, 505–511.

Bowie, C. R., Depp, C., McGrath, J. A., et al. (2010). Prediction of real-world functional disability in chronic mental disorders: a comparison of schizophrenia and bipolar disorder. *American Journal of Psychiatry*, **167**, 1116–1124.

Bowie, C. R., Twamley, E. W., Anderson, H., et al. (2007). Self-assessment of functional status in schizophrenia. *Journal of Psychiatric Research*, **41**, 1012–1018.

Burdick, K. E., Braga, R. J., Nnadi, C. U., et al. (2012). Placebo-controlled adjunctive trial of pramipexole in patients with bipolar disorder: targeting cognitive dysfunction. *Journal of Clinical Psychiatry*, **73**, 103–112.

Burdick, K. E., Endick, C. J., & Goldberg, J. F. (2005). Assessing cognitive deficits in bipolar disorder: are self-reports valid? *Psychiatry Research*, **136**, 43–50.

Burdick, K. E., Goldberg, T. E., Cornblatt, B. A., et al. (2011). MATRICS consensus cognitive battery in patients with bipolar disorder. *Neuropsychopharmacology*, **36**, 1587–1592.

Burdick, K. E., Goldberg, J. F., & Harrow, M. (2010). Neurocognitive dysfunction and psychosocial outcome in patients with bipolar I disorder at 15-year follow-up. *Acta Psychiatrica Scandinavica*, **122**, 499–506.

Catts, S. V., Shelley, A. M., Ward, P. B., et al. (1995). Brain potential evidence for an auditory sensory memory deficit in schizophrenia. *American Journal of Psychiatry*, **152**, 213–219.

Chaves, O. C., Lombardo, L. E., Bearden, C. E., et al. (2011). Association of clinical symptoms and neurocognitive performance in bipolar disorder: a longitudinal study. *Bipolar Disorders*, **13**, 118–123.

Chemerinski, E., Bowie, C., Anderson, H., et al. (2008). Depression in schizophrenia: methodological artifact or distinct feature of the illness? *Journal of Neuropsychiatry and Clinical Neuroscience*, **20**, 431–440.

Corrigan, P. W. & Green, M. F. (1993). Schizophrenic patients' sensitivity to social cues: the role of abstraction. *American Journal of Psychiatry*, **150**, 589–594.

Cusi, A. M., Nazarov, A., Holshausen, K., et al. (2012). A review of the neural and behavioural correlates of social cognition in mood disorders. *Journal of Psychiatry and Neuroscience* [In Press].

Cutting, J. & Murphy, D. (1990). Impaired ability of schizophrenics, relative to manics or depressives, to appreciate social knowledge about their culture. *British Journal of Psychiatry*, **157**, 355–358.

Czobor, P., Jaeger, J., Berns, S. M., et al. (2007). Neuropsychological symptom dimensions in bipolar disorder and schizophrenia. *Bipolar Disorders*, **9**, 71–92.

Davis, M. H. (1980). A multidimensional approach to individual differences in empathy. *JSAS Catalog of Selected Documents in Psychology*, **10**, 85.

Dean, B. B., Gerner, D., & Gerner, R. H. (2004). A systematic review evaluating health-related quality of life, work impairment, and healthcare costs and utilization in bipolar disorder. *Current Medical Research and Opinion*, **20**, 139–154.

Deckersbach, T., Nierenberg, A. A., Kessler R., et al. (2010). Cognitive rehabilitation for bipolar disorder: an open trial for employed patients with residual depressive symptoms. *CNS Neuroscience and Therapeutics*, **15**, 298–307.

Demily, C., Attala, N., Fouldrin, G., et al. (2010). The emotional Stroop task: a comparison between schizophrenia subjects and controls. *European Psychiatry*, **2**, 75–79.

Depp, C. A., Moore, D. J., Sitzer, D., et al. (2007). Neurocognitive impairment in middle-aged and older adults with bipolar disorder: comparison to schizophrenia and normal comparison subjects. *Journal of Affective Disorders*, **101**, 201–209.

Derntl, B., Finkelmeyer, A., Toygar, T. K., et al. (2009). Generalized deficit in all core components of empathy in schizophrenia. *Schizophrenia Research*, **108**, 197–206.

Dickinson, D., Ragland, J. D., Gold, J. M., et al. (2008). General and specific cognitive deficits in schizophrenia: Goliath defeats David? *Biological Psychiatry*, **64**, 823–827.

Dickinson, D., Ramsey, M. E., & Gold, J. M. (2007). Overlooking the obvious: a meta-analytic comparison of digit symbol coding tasks and other cognitive measures in schizophrenia. *Archives of General Psychiatry*, **64**, 532–542.

Docherty, N. M., Hawkins, K. A., Hoffman, R. E., et al. (1996). Working memory, attention, and communication disturbances in schizophrenia. *Journal of Abnormal Psychology*, **105**, 212–219.

Eack, S. M., Pogue-Geile, M. F., Greeno, C. G., et al. (2009). Evidence of factorial variance of the Mayer–Salovey–Caruso Emotional Intelligence Test across schizophrenia and normative samples. *Schizophrenia Research*, **114**, 105–109.

Edwards, J., Pattison, P. E., Jackson, H. J., et al. (2001). Facial affect and affective prosody recognition in first-episode schizophrenia. *Schizophrenia Research*, **48**, 235–253.

Elshahawi, H. H., Essawi, H., Rabie, M. A., et al. (2011). Cognitive functions among euthymic bipolar I patients after a single manic episode versus recurrent episodes. *Journal of Affective Disorders*, **130**, 180–191.

Evans, J. D., Heaton, R. K., Paulsen, J. S., et al. (2003). The relationship of neuropsychological abilities to specific domains of functional capacity in older schizophrenia patients. *Biological Psychiatry*, **53**, 422–430.

Ferrier, I. N., Stanton, B. R., Kelly, T. P., et al. (1999). Neuropsychological function in euthymic patients with bipolar disorder. *British Journal of Psychiatry*, **175**, 246–251.

Fraguas, D., Mena, A., Franco, C., et al. (2008). Attributional style, symptomatology and awareness of illness in schizophrenia. *Psychiatry Research*, **158**, 316–323.

French, C. C., Richards, A., & Scholfield, E. J. C. (1996). Hypomania, anxiety and the emotional Stroop. *British Journal of Clinical Psychology*, **35**, 617–626.

Frith, C. D. & Corcoran, R. (1996). Exploring "theory of mind" in people with schizophrenia. *Psychological Medicine*, **26**, 521–530.

Genderson, M. R., Dickinson, D., Diaz-Asper, C. M., et al. (2007). Factor analysis of neurocognitive tests in a large sample of schizophrenic probands, their siblings, and healthy controls. *Schizophrenia Research*, **94**, 231–239.

Glahn, D. C., Bearden, C. E., Cakir, S., et al. (2006). Differential working memory impairment in bipolar disorder and schizophrenia: effects of lifetime history of psychosis. *Bipolar Disorders*, **8**, 117–123.

Goldberg, T. E., Ragland, J. D., Torrey, E. F., et al. (1990). Neuropsychological assessment of monozygotic twins discordant for schizophrenia. *Archives of General Psychiatry*, **47**, 1066–1072.

Goodwin, F. K. & Jamison, K. R. (2007). *Manic Depressive Illness: Bipolar Disorders and Recurrent Depression*. (2nd edn.). New York, NY: Oxford University Press.

Gordon, E., Coyle, S., Anderson, J., et al. (1992). Eye movement response to a facial stimulus in schizophrenia. *Biological Psychiatry*, **31**, 626–629.

Green, M. F. (1996). What are the functional consequences of neurocognitive deficits in schizophrenia? *American Journal of Psychiatry*, **153**, 321–330.

Green, M. F. & Nuechterlein, K. H. (2004). The MATRICS initiative: developing a consensus cognitive battery for clinical trials. *Schizophrenia Research*, **72**, 1–3.

Green, M. J., Williams, L. M., & Davidson, D. (2003). Visual scan paths to threat-related faces in deluded schizophrenia. *Psychiatry Research*, **119**, 271–285.

Gur, R. C., Erwin, R. J., Gur, R. E., et al. (1992). Facial emotion discrimination: II. Behavioral findings in depression. *Psychiatry Research*, **42**, 241–251.

Hall, M. H., Schulze, K., Rijsdijk, F., et al. (2009). Are auditory P300 and duration MMN heritable and putative endophenotypes of psychotic bipolar disorder? A Maudsley Bipolar Twin and Family Study. *Psychological Medicine*, **39**, 1277–1287.

Harrington, L., Langdon, R., Siegert, R., et al. (2005). Schizophrenia, theory of mind and persecutory delusions. *Cognitive Neuropsychology*, **10**, 87–104.

Harvey, P. D., Koren, D., Reichenberg, A., et al. (2006). Negative symptoms and cognitive deficits: what is the nature of their relationship? *Schizophrenia Bulletin*, **32**, 250–258.

Harvey, P. D., Reichenberg, A., Bowie, C. R., et al. (2010). The course of neuropsychological performance and functional capacity in older patients with schizophrenia: influences of previous history of long-term institutional stay. *Biological Psychiatry*, **67**, 933–939.

Heaton, R. K., Gladsjo, J. A., Palmer, B. W., et al. (2001). Stability and course of neuropsychological deficits in schizophrenia. *Archives of General Psychiatry*, **58**, 24–32.

Heller, W. (1993). Neuropsychological mechanism of individual differences in emotion, personality, and arousal. *Neuropsychology*, **7**, 476–489.

Horan, W. P., Kern, R. S., Green, M. F., et al. (2008). Social cognition training for individuals with schizophrenia: emerging evidence. *American Journal of Psychiatric Rehabilitation*, **11**, 205–252.

Horesh, N. & Fennig, S. (2000). Perception of spouses and relationships: a matched control study of patients with severe affective disorder in remission and their spouses. *Journal of Nervous and Mental Disease*, **188**, 463–466.

Jaeger, J., Berns, S., Loftus, S., et al. (2007). Neurocognitive test performance predicts functional recovery from acute exacerbation leading to hospitalization in bipolar disorder. *Bipolar Disorders*, **9**, 93–102.

Kaur, M., Battisti, R. A., Ward, P. B., et al. (2011). MMN/P3a deficits in first episode psychosis: comparing schizophrenia-spectrum and affective-spectrum subgroups. *Schizophrenia Research*, **130**, 203–209.

Keefe, R. S., Bilder, R. M., Harvey, P. D., et al. (2006). Baseline neurocognitive deficits in the CATIE schizophrenia trial. *Neuropsychopharmacology*, **31**, 2033–2046.

Keefe, R. S. E. & Fenton, W. S. (2007). How should DSM-V criteria for schizophrenia include cognitive impairment? *Schizophrenia Bulletin*, **33**, 912–920.

Kerr, N., Dunbar, R. I. M., & Bentall, R. P. (2003). Theory of mind deficits in bipolar affective disorder. *Journal of Affective Disorders*, **73**, 253–259.

Kirkpatrick, B., Buchanan, R. W., McKenny, P. D., et al. (1989). The schedule for the deficit syndrome: an instrument for research in schizophrenia. *Psychiatry Research*, **30**, 119–123.

Kohler, C. G., Hoffman, L. J., Eastman, L. B., et al. (2011). Facial emotion perception in depression and bipolar disorder: a quantitative review. *Psychiatry Research*, **188**, 303–309.

Kohler, C. G., Walker, J. B., Martin, E. A., et al. (2010). Facial emotion perception in schizophrenia: a meta-analytic review. *Schizophrenia Bulletin*, **36**, 1009–1019.

Langdon, R., Corner, T., McLaren, J., et al. (2006). Externalizing and personalizing biases in persecutory delusions: the relationship with poor insight and theory-of-mind. *Behaviour Research and Therapy*, **44**, 699–713.

Lembke, A. & Ketter, T. A. (2002). Impaired recognition of facial emotion in mania. *American Journal of Psychiatry*, **159**, 302–304.

Lencer, R., Reilly, J. L., Harris, M. S., et al. (2010). Sensorimotor transformation deficits for smooth pursuit in first-episode affective psychoses and schizophrenia. *Biological Psychiatry*, **67**, 217–223.

Lencer, R., Sprenger, A., Harris, M. S., et al. (2008). Effects of second-generation antipsychotic medication on smooth pursuit performance in antipsychotic-naive schizophrenia. *Archives of General Psychiatry*, **65**, 1146–1154.

Levy, B., Medina, A. M., Hintz, K., et al. (2011). Ecologically valid support for the link between cognitive and psychosocial functioning in bipolar disorder. *Psychiatry Research*, **185**, 353–357.

Levy, B. & Weiss, R. D. (2010). Neurocognitive impairment and psychosis in bipolar I disorder during early remission from an acute episode of mood disturbance. *Journal of Clinical Psychiatry*, **71**, 201–206.

Lex, C., Hautzinger, M., & Meyer, T. D. (2011). Cognitive styles in hypomanic episodes of bipolar I disorder. *Bipolar Disorders*, **13**, 355–364.

Lopez, A. D., Mathers, C. D., Ezzati, M., et al. (2006). *Global Burden of Disease and Risk Factors*. Washington, DC: World Bank.

López-Jaramillo, C., Lopera-Vásquez, J., Gallo, A., et al. (2010). Effects of recurrence on the cognitive performance of patients with bipolar I disorder: implications for relapse prevention and treatment adherence. *Bipolar Disorders*, **12**, 557–567.

Lyon, H. M., Startup, M., & Bentall, R. P. (1999). Social cognition and the manic defense: attributions selective attention, and self-schema in bipolar affective disorder. *Journal of Abnormal Psychology*, **108**, 273–282.

Martínez-Arán, A., Vieta, E., Reinares, M., et al. (2004). Cognitive function across manic or hypomanic, depressed, and euthymic states in bipolar disorder. *American Journal of Psychiatry*, **161**, 262–270.

Martino, D. J., Marengo, E., Igoa, A., et al. (2009). Neurocognitive and symptomatic predictors of functional outcome in bipolar disorders: a prospective 1-year follow-up study. *Journal of Affective Disorders*, **116**, 37–42.

McGurk, S. R. & Meltzer, H. Y. (2000). The role of cognition in vocational functioning in schizophrenia. *Schizophrenia Research*, **45**, 175–184.

McKinnon, M. C., Cusi, A. M., & MacQueen, G. M. (2010). Impaired theory of mind performance in patients with recurrent bipolar disorder: moderating effect of cognitive load. *Psychiatry Research*, **177**, 261–262.

Meyer, S. E., Carlson, G. A., Wiggs, E. A., et al. (2004). A prospective study of the association among impaired executive functioning, childhood attentional problems, and the development of bipolar disorder. *Development and Psychopathology*, **16**, 461–476.

Miller, G. A. (1996). Presidential address: How we think about cognition, emotion, and biology in psychopathology. *Psychophysiology*, **33**, 615–628.

Mur, M., Portella, M. J., Martínez-Arán, A., et al. (2007). Persistent neuropsychological deficit in euthymic bipolar patients: executive function as a core deficit. *Journal of Clinical Psychiatry*, **68**, 1078–1086.

Murphy, F. C., Sahakian, B. J., Rubinsztein, J. S., et al. (1999). Emotional bias and inhibitory control processes in mania and depression. *Psychological Medicine*, **29**, 1307–1321.

Olvet, D. M., Stearns, W. H., McLaughlin, D., et al. (2010). Comparing clinical and neurocognitive features of the schizophrenia prodrome to the bipolar prodrome. *Schizophrenia Research*, **123**, 59–63.

Premack, D. & Woodruff, G. (1978). Does the chimpanzee have a theory of mind? *Behavioral and Brain Sciences*, **4**, 515–526.

Reddy, R., Mukherjee, S., & Schnur, D. B. (1992). Comparison of negative symptoms in schizophrenic and poor outcome bipolar patients. *Psychological Medicine*, **22**, 361–365.

Reichenberg, A., Harvey, P. D., Bowie, C. R., et al. (2009). Neuropsychological function and dysfunction in schizophrenia and psychotic affective disorders. *Schizophrenia Bulletin*, **35**, 1022–1029.

Reichenberg, A., Weiser, M., Rabinowitz, J., et al. (2002). A population-based cohort study of premorbid intellectual, language, and behavioral functioning in patients with schizophrenia, schizoaffective disorder, and nonpsychotic bipolar disorder. *American Journal of Psychiatry*, **159**, 2027–2035.

Robinson, D. G., Woerner, M. G., McMeniman, M., et al. (2004). Symptomatic and functional recovery from a first episode of schizophrenia or schizoaffective disorder. *American Journal of Psychiatry*, **161**, 473–479.

Salisbury, D. F., Shenton, M. E., & McCarley, R. W. (1999). P300 topography differs in schizophrenia and manic psychosis. *Biological Psychiatry*, **45**, 98–106.

Sanchez-Moreno, J., Martinez-Aran, A., Tabares-Seisdedos, R., et al. (2009). Functioning and disability in bipolar disorder: an extensive review. *Psychotherapy and Psychosomatics*, **78**, 285–297.

Sánchez-Morla, E. M., Barabash, A., Martínez-Vizcaíno, V., et al. (2009). Comparative study of neurocognitive function in euthymic bipolar patients and stabilized schizophrenic patients. *Psychiatry Research*, **169**, 220–228.

Sarfati, Y. & Harde-Bayle, M. C. (1999). How do people with schizophrenia explain the behaviour of others? A study of theory of mind and its relationship to thought and speech disorganization in schizophrenia. *Psychological Medicine*, **29**, 613–620.

Schouws, S. N., Zoeteman, J. B., Comijs, H. C., et al. (2007). Cognitive functioning in elderly patients with early onset bipolar disorder. *International Journal of Geriatric Psychiatry*, **22**, 856–861.

Shamay-Tsoory, S., Harari, H., Szepsenwol, O., et al. (2009). Neuropsychological evidence of impaired cognitive empathy in euthymic bipolar disorder. *Journal of Neuropsychiatry and Clinical Neurosciences*, **21**, 59–67.

Simonsen, C., Sundet, K., Vaskinn, A., et al. (2011). Neurocognitive dysfunction in bipolar and schizophrenia spectrum disorders depends on history of psychosis rather than diagnostic group. *Schizophrenia Bulletin*, **37**, 73–83.

Sole, B., Bonnin, C. M., Torrent, C., et al. (2011). Neurocognitive impairment and psychosocial functioning in bipolar II disorder. *Acta Psychiatrica Scandinavica*, **125**, 1–9.

Sprong, M., Schothorst, P., Vos, E., et al. (2007). Theory of mind in schizophrenia: meta-analysis. *British Journal of Psychiatry*, **191**, 5–13.

Tabarés-Seisdedos, R., Balanzá-Martínez, V., Sánchez-Moreno, J., et al. (2008). Neurocognitive and clinical predictors of functional outcome in patients with schizophrenia and bipolar I disorder at one-year follow-up. *Journal of Affective Disorders*, **109**, 286–299.

Takei, Y., Kumano, S., Maki, Y., et al. (2010). Preattentive dysfunction in bipolar disorder: an MEG study using auditory mismatch negativity. *Progress in Neuro-psychopharmacology and Biological Psychiatry*, **34**, 903–912.

Thaker, G. K. (2008). Neurophysiological endophenotypes across bipolar and schizophrenia psychosis. *Schizophrenia Bulletin*, **34**, 760–773.

Tiihonen, J., Haukka, J., Henriksson, M., et al. (2005). Premorbid intellectual functioning in bipolar disorder and schizophrenia: results from a cohort study of male conscripts. *American Journal of Psychiatry*, **162**, 1904–1910.

Toomey, R., Faraone, S. V., Simpson, J. C., et al. (1998). Negative, positive, and disorganized symptom dimensions in schizophrenia, major depression, and bipolar disorder. *Journal of Nervous and Mental Disease*, **186**, 470–476.

Toulopoulou, T., Quraishi, S., McDonald, C., et al. (2006). The Maudsley Family Study: premorbid and current general intellectual function levels in familial bipolar I disorder and schizophrenia. *Journal of Clinical and Experimental Neuropsychology*, **28**, 243–259.

Uzelac, S., Jaeger, J., Berns, S., et al. (2006). Premorbid adjustment in bipolar disorder: comparison with schizophrenia. *Journal of Nervous and Mental Disease*, **194**, 654–658.

Wilk, C. M., Gold, J. M., McMahon, R. P., et al. (2005). No, it is not possible to be schizophrenic yet neuropsychologically normal. *Neuropsychology*, **19**, 778–786.

Wright, K., Lam, D., & Newsom-Davis, I. (2005). Induced mood change and dysfunctional attitudes in remitted bipolar I affective disorder. *Journal of Abnormal Psychology*, **114**, 689–696.

Yatham, L. N., Torres, I. J., Malhi, G. S., et al. (2010). The International Society for Bipolar Disorders–Battery for Assessment of Neurocognition (ISBD-BANC). *Bipolar Disorders*, **12**, 351–363.

Chapter

Cognitive impairment and symptom dimensions in psychosis

Manuela Russo, Robin Murray, and Abraham Reichenberg

Introduction

The aim of this chapter is to present the relationship between symptom dimensions and neuropsychological functioning in psychosis. In the first part of the chapter, we present a short overview on neuropsychological functioning in schizophrenia and in other psychotic disorders. In the second part, studies investigating the association between symptom dimensions and neuropsychological functioning in both schizophrenia and other psychoses are described. Finally, an integrated model based on current evidence on the relationship between symptom dimensions and neuropsychological functioning is presented and discussed.

Neuropsychological functioning in schizophrenia and other psychoses

It is well established that schizophrenia patients show deficits on a wide range of cognitive domains including verbal memory, working memory, executive functions, attention, and processing speed on a background of general intellectual impairment (Reichenberg & Harvey, 2007; Seidman et al., 2002). It is also acknowledged that cognitive impairments are not just a consequence of symptoms, treatment, or the course of the disease. Cognitive deficits are core features of many patients with schizophrenia as they are present already at the onset of the illness (Addington & Addington, 2002; Elvevag & Goldberg, 2000; Heinrichs & Zakzanis, 1998; MacCabe, 2008; Woodberry et al., 2008). It has also been demonstrated that there is likely a genetic susceptibility to cognitive impairment in schizophrenia as evident by the presence of cognitive deficits, although not prominent, in nonaffected relatives of schizophrenia patients (Dickinson et al., 2007, Keefe et al., 1994, Toulopoulou et al., 2007).

Meta-analytic studies have shown that across cognitive domains the average impairment is of approximately one standard deviation below the mean (Dickinson et al., 2007; Fioravanti et al., 2005; Knowles et al., 2010; Mesholam-Gately et al., 2009; Reichenberg & Harvey, 2007). Some individuals who later develop schizophrenia present cognitive impairment during their childhood and adolescence (Jones et al., 1994; Reichenberg et al., 2010, 2002) and are more likely to have impairments in childhood educational scores (MacCabe et al., 2008). It has been demonstrated that there is a linear relationship between decreased

Cognitive Impairment in Schizophrenia, ed. Philip D. Harvey. Published by Cambridge University Press. © Cambridge University Press 2013.

IQ at the age of 18 years old and a greater risk to develop the disorder, and that deficits on specific cognitive skills may confer an additional risk (David et al., 1997).

The cognitive impairment seen in bipolar disorder patients is persistent (Bearden et al., 2001) and present at the onset of the illness (Albus et al., 1996) and in unaffected first-degree relatives (Ferrier et al., 2004; Gourovitch et al., 1999). Yet some of the neuropsychological impairments are mild, transitory, and mainly due to the affective state (Malhi et al., 2008). In a review by Quraishi & Frangou (2002) that examined the neuropsychological profile of impairment in bipolar patients during different stages of illness it was concluded that general intellectual functioning is usually preserved, that cognitive abnormalities in attention and executive functions are present in symptomatic bipolar patients, while verbal memory was impaired even in euthymic phases. Results from a meta-analysis of cognitive deficits during the euthymic phase found evidence for a trait-related neuropsychological impairment in bipolar patients involving attention, processing speed, memory, and executive functions (Torres et al., 2007). Another meta-analysis reported that euthymic patients showed varying degrees of impairment, from relatively marked impairment in executive functions and verbal memory to less severe impairment in verbal fluency and sustained attention (Robinson et al., 2006). Lower IQ in adolescence was associated with increased risk for developing psychotic depression and bipolar disorder in some (Zammit et al., 2004) but not all studies (Reichenberg et al., 2002).

Studies that examined differences in cognitive functioning between schizophrenia and affective psychoses reported an increasing gradient of severity of cognitive impairment, from less severe deficits in bipolar disorder to most severe deficits in schizophrenia-like disorders (Krabbendam et al., 2005b; Reichenberg et al., 2009). It has been suggested that profiles of neuropsychological impairment vary only minimally between psychotic disorders and that differences are largely quantitative (Reichenberg et al., 2009; Stefanopoulou et al., 2009).

Reichenberg et al. (2009), using the Suffolk County Mental Health Project study, examined neuropsychological performance profiles in three distinct diagnostic groups: schizophrenia, psychotic major depressive disorder, and psychotic bipolar disorder 24 months after the first admission (see Figure 4.1). The authors concluded that the profiles of neuropsychological impairment vary only minimally and differences are largely quantitative. In order to provide an individual-level assessment of impairment, the authors calculated the level of impairment based on the Clinically Significant Cognitive Impairment (CSGI) criteria. According to the CSGI criteria, an impairment is present in an individual when a performance of at least one standard deviation below the mean is shown in two or more neuropsychological domains. The authors found that a clinically significant cognitive impairment was present in 84% of the schizophrenia patients, 58.3% of the psychotic major depression patients, and 57.7% of the psychotic bipolar patients.

Similar patterns of dysfunction were evident in another first episode psychosis study (Zanelli et al., 2010). In this study, neuropsychological performance was assessed within six months after first admission. Schizophrenia patients performed worse than healthy subjects on all neuropsychological tasks. Patients with depressive psychosis also showed widespread impairments in comparison to healthy controls. In contrast, bipolar patients performed significantly worse than controls only on specific neuropsychological tasks measuring verbal memory and language abilities. Neuropsychological performance profiles by domain are presented in Figure 4.2.

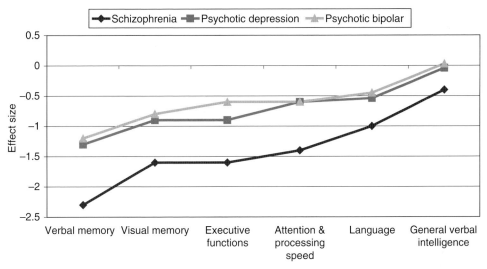

Figure 4.1. Neuropsychological performance profiles of schizophrenia, psychotic major depressive disorder, and psychotic bipolar disorder patients 24 months after first admission. (See color plate section for colored image.)

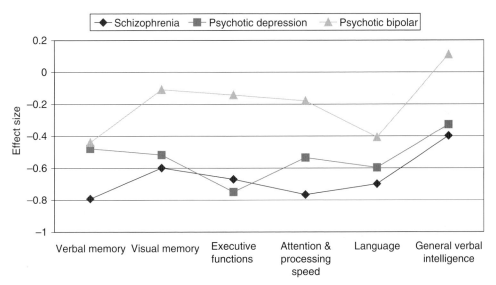

Figure 4.2. Neuropsychological performance profiles of schizophrenia, psychotic major depressive disorder, and psychotic bipolar disorder patients six months after first admission. (See color plate section for colored image.)

From the cognitive heterogeneity of schizophrenia to symptom dimensions: the heterogeneity of the cognitive impairment in schizophrenia

Although the cognitive deficit is considered a core feature of schizophrenia, there is considerable heterogeneity among patients. Individual patients differ in the extent of the overall impairment and the specific neuropsychological functions that are severely impaired. Furthermore, at least a proportion of patients with normal cognitive functioning exists (Reichenberg et al., 2009). Some studies suggest that there are groups of patients with a specific pattern of impairment on executive functions and/or memory at all stages of the illness (Joyce and Roiser, 2007; Weickert et al., 2000). Joyce et al. (2005) identified three cognitive subgroups of patients: one with IQ decline from higher premorbid values, another with low premorbid IQ, and the last one with specific deficits on executive functions. Furthermore, a percentage of schizophrenia patients without cognitive abnormalities emerged in different studies. Estimates of the proportion of schizophrenia patients without neuropsychological impairment are around 20%, varying from 16% (Reichenberg et al., 2009) to 19% (Holthausen et al., 2002) and 23% (Kremen et al., 2000). Among depressive psychosis and psychotic bipolar patients, rates of non-impaired patients were even higher (around 42%) (Reichenberg et al., 2009).

Potential explanations for cognitively intact schizophrenia

Several explanations have been put forward in order to explain the cognitive hetero-geneity and the presence of this "isolated" group of cognitively intact schizophrenia patients.

The neurodevelopmental hypothesis (Murray & Lewis, 1987) suggested prominent neurodevelopmental causes of schizophrenia originating from genetic defects and occur-rence of environmental risk factors early in life (such as obstetric complications). According to this view, schizophrenia subjects whose cognitive profile remains within the normal range had fewer neurodevelopmental adversities, and compared to patients with cognitive impairment, should show fewer premorbid symptoms and motor and behavioral problems, have a later age of onset, and have a lower severity of negative symptoms. Overall, patients who present within the normal range of cognitive functioning are likely to have a less severe disease. On the basis of this explanation, the cognitively intact schizophrenia patients lie on a continuum of severity along with the group of patients presenting cognitive deficits. This would imply that specific illness symptoms can affect neuropsychological functioning differently. Indeed, it is well established that nega-tive symptoms are significantly associated with poorer cognitive performance from the onset of the disease (Heinrichs and Zakzanis, 1998). Some studies (Kremen et al., 2000; Palmer et al., 1997) found that schizophrenia patients without cognitive impairment presented more positive symptomatology and specifically more paranoid symptoms. Furthermore, being cognitively intact does not mean that patients necessarily have normal cognitive functioning. Performance could still be worse than that of normal controls, thus attesting that their impairment is subclinical (Kremen et al., 2000).

Another explanation for the presence of schizophrenia patients without cognitive impairment applies the brain reserve capacity theory (Satz, 1993), a theory more com-monly applied to dementia. According to this theory, individuals develop a set of cognitive reserves (due to genetic predisposition and environmental factors such as level of educa-tion) that, acting as a protective factor, are able to compensate for brain dysfunctions. Holthausen et al. (2002) found that although there are schizophrenia patients without a clinically significant cognitive impairment, the profile of performance they show (i.e., relative strengths and weaknesses) is very similar to that of patients with a cognitive impairment. The authors concluded that patients performing below normal controls only at subclinical levels could represent a difference in cognitive compensation capacity in this group of patients.

Summary

Three main conclusions can be drawn from the review presented in the first part of this chapter. First, differences in neuropsychological functioning between schizophrenia patients and patients with other psychotic disorders are mainly quantitative (Reichenberg et al., 2009; Stefanopoulou et al., 2009; Zanelli et al., 2010) with an increased severity of impairment seen across the schizophrenia spectrum (Krabbendam et al., 2005a). Second, a heterogeneity in cognitive impairment is evident in schizophrenia as well as other psychotic disorders, characterized by different levels of impairment between cognitive domains and among individual patients, ranging from within normal range levels of performance to moderate impairment to severe deficits (one or more standard deviations below the mean), especially in verbal and visual memory, executive functions, working memory, and processing speed (Reichenberg et al., 2009). Third, a minority of schizophrenia patients, characterized by exposure to fewer early risk factors, later onset and lower severity of negative symptoms, and predominant positive symptomatology (Kremen et al., 2000), perform within the normal range; however, the pattern of performance is similar to that of those patients with cognitive deficits (Holthausen et al., 2002).

Taken together it can be hypothesized that the overall severity of the illness and severity and presence of specific symptoms (negative, positive/paranoid symptoms and occurrence of frank symptomatology as in the acute phases of bipolar disorder) can be related to neuropsychological functioning. Studying the relationship between cognition and groups of symptoms (i.e., symptom dimensions) instead of categorical diagnosis could therefore be a more promising way for unveiling different brain mechanisms responsible for biological and phenomenological differences among psychotic disorders.

Symptom dimensions

With a background of general criticism of categorical classification of psychotic disorders within the current classification systems (DSM-IV and ICD-10), due to evidence from interdiagnostic biological overlapping (Kaymaz & Van Os, 2009; Squires & Saederup, 1991; van Os & Kapur, 2009) and evidence for clinical heterogeneity within diagnoses of psychotic disorders (Jablensky, 2006; Joyce & Roiser, 2007; Stroup, 2007), the use of symptom dimensions as a valid alternative construct to categorical diagnosis is obtaining increasing consensus.

Validity of symptom dimensions as neurobiological constructs has been supported by several genetic and neurobiological studies. A twin study in psychotic disorders provided evidence for heritability of some psychotic symptom dimensions (disorganization) but not all (positive and negative symptoms) (Rijsdijk et al., 2011). Brain imaging studies suggested the existence of a cognitive neuropsychiatric basis of specific symptoms (i.e., auditory hallucination) (McGuire et al., 1993; Shergill et al., 2000). It has been suggested that rather than using the traditional binary classification of psychosis, a more meaningful formulation might be to conceptualize alternative categories or clinical symptoms with susceptibility conferred by sets of genes (Craddock et al., 2006).

Research on symptom dimensions in psychosis focuses predominantly on schizophrenia. The first model proposed was one of a dichotomy that differentiated the disorder into two subtypes: Type I and Type II (Crow, 1980). Type I described the acute phase of schizophrenia, defined by positive symptoms (Schneiderian classification), while Type II was characterized by negative symptoms (Kraepelian classification). In the late 1980s,

Carpenter and colleagues proposed to use the term "deficit syndrome" to describe a condition of enduring traits the symptomatology of which (mainly characterized by blunted affect, social withdrawal) was not secondary to other symptoms (Carpenter et al., 1988). Deficit symptoms could therefore be present even between episodes of positive symptom exacerbation and regardless of medication status (Carpenter et al., 1988). However, because the dichotomy model was considered too reductive to account for the entire phenomenology of schizophrenia, factor analytical studies were carried out in order to identify more comprehensive models empirically. A three-factor model was proposed by Liddle et al. (1989). This model was composed of symptoms of reality distortion (namely, positive symptoms such as hallucinations and delusions), psychomotor poverty (poverty of speech, flat affect, and decreased voluntary movement), and disorganization (formal thought disorder, inappropriate affect, and bizarre behavior) (Andreasen et al., 1995a, 1995b; Johnstone & Frith, 1996). Inclusion of the entire spectrum of psychotic disorders (i.e., affective and nonaffective psychoses) frequently resulted in a wider range of symptom dimensions. Overall, when ignoring semantic differences between the various labels that have been given to symptom dimensions, manic and depressive symptoms were the factors that, together with positive and negative symptoms and disorganization, emerged in most of the studies (Allardyce et al., 2007; Demjaha et al., 2009; Dikeos et al., 2006; Lindenmayer et al., 1995).

Neuropsychological functioning and symptom dimensions of schizophrenia

Early investigations into correlates of symptom dimensions provided evidence for an association between the dimensions and intraindividual differences in cognitive functioning. Andreasen and Olsen (1982) showed that the negative subtype was characterized by poorer premorbid functioning and more cognitive deficits compared to the positive subtype. Overall negative and disorganized symptoms have been found to be associated with poor performance on a variety of measures of executive functions (Cuesta & Peralta, 1995; Heinrichs & Zakzanis, 1998; O'Leary et al., 2000). In a study comparing cognitive profiles across psychotic disorders, severe negative symptoms accounted for some of the differences in neuropsychological functioning between groups of patients (Bora et al., 2009).

Basso et al. (1998), in a study analyzing the relationship between neuropsychological functioning and three symptom dimensions of schizophrenia (positive, negative, and disorganization), found that negative and disorganized symptom dimensions were significantly associated with cognitive measures and positive symptoms were only negatively associated with the Trial Making Test-Part A, a test of visual processing and motor speed (semipartial correlation of -0.34). Both negative symptoms and disorganization were negatively associated with IQ (semipartial correlation was -0.49 and -0.36, respectively). Severity of negative symptoms was characterized by a modest to large association with measures of executive functions (highest partial correlation was -0.62) and memory and attention (highest partial correlation -0.58). Additionally, disorganization reached a moderate negative association with memory and attention span, and visual memory performance (Basso et al., 1998).

Nieuwenstein et al. (2001) carried out a meta-analysis of the relationship between negative symptoms, positive symptoms, and disorganization, and executive functions and sustained attention. Only studies that used the Wisconsin Card Sorting Test (WCST) and the Continuous Performance Test (CPT) were considered in the analysis. Results showed that more severe negative symptoms were significantly associated with worse performance in both cognitive domains; more severe symptoms of disorganization were associated with worse performance in WCST, but not with CPT performance; in contrast, positive symptoms did not significantly correlate with either measure (Nieuwenstein et al., 2001). Although statistically significant, the effect sizes of these associations were moderate (highest correlation was 0.31), thus accounting for no more than 10% of the individual differences in cognitive functioning. Another, more recent, meta-analytic study (Dibben et al., 2009) reported similar results. Negative and disorganized symptoms showed correlations of -0.20 and -0.28 (respectively) with executive functions, while the association with positive symptoms was negligible ($r = 0.01$).

Another meta-analytic study, focusing on the positive and disorganized dimensions, confirmed that while positive symptoms have a very weak association with cognition (meta-analysis pooled correlation $r = -0.04$), disorganization showed a modest association (meta-analysis pooled correlation $r = -0.23$). The authors used composite measures of neurocognition accounting for measures from six individual cognitive domains. Moreover, findings showed that positive symptoms were significantly associated with only two individual cognitive domains (meta-analysis pooled correlation for attention/vigilance, $r = -0.12$ and reasoning and problem solving $r = 0.06$). In contrast, disorganization was significantly associated with all individual measures (meta-analysis pooled correlation range between $r = -20$ for verbal/visual/working memory and $r = -0.26$ for processing speed) (Ventura et al., 2010).

The dimension of depressive symptoms has been much less frequently investigated in schizophrenia, possibly because it emerged as a symptom dimension mainly when affective psychoses are also considered in factor analytical studies. Depressive symptoms were associated with attention and psychomotor functions in one study (Holthausen et al., 1999) while no correlation was found in other studies (Bozikas et al., 2004; Lucas et al., 2004).

A recent large systematic review was carried out to investigate the associations between symptom dimensions and cognitive domains in nonaffective psychoses (Dominguez et al., 2009). A total of 5009 individuals (from 58 studies) were included in the analysis. The authors considered four symptom dimensions: positive, negative, depressive, and disorganized. Nine cognitive domains were examined. These included the six domains identified by the Measurement and Treatment Research to Improve Cognition in Schizophrenia (MATRICS) consensus (Nuechterlein et al., 2008): reasoning and problem solving, speed of processing, attention, verbal working memory, verbal learning and memory, and visual learning and memory; as well as three additional cognitive domains: IQ, verbal fluency, and executive control. Although effect sizes were small (from -0.29 to -0.12), significant correlations emerged between the negative and disorganized symptoms and the majority of cognitive domains. Negative symptoms were most strongly correlated with verbal fluency (effect size, -0.29), verbal learning and memory (effect size, -0.21), and IQ (effect size, -0.24). Disorganization symptoms were most strongly correlated with attention (effect size, -0.28), visual learning and memory (effect size, -0.21), and IQ (effect size, -0.21). Apart from a very small negative correlation (effect size, -0.09) between positive symptoms and processing speed, no associations were found between positive and depressive symptoms and cognitive domains (Figure 4.3). All associations were independent of age, gender, and chronicity of illness. The authors argued that the implications of the findings were that two different pathophysiological processes account for the heterogeneity of schizophrenia and are

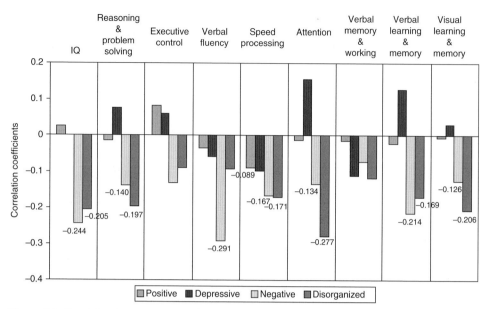

Figure 4.3. Correlations between cognitive domains and four symptom dimensions in schizophrenia (statistically significant relationships are those with reported values). (See color plate section for colored image.)

the clinical expression of differential patterns of cerebral dysfunctions: negative symptoms along with disorganization on one end, and positive and depressive symptoms on the other end.

It should be noted, however, that the association between negative symptoms and cognitive impairment can be explained by some common features of negative symptomatology and cognitive functioning, such as onset, stability over time, and presence of more adverse outcomes (Harvey et al., 2006). It has also been argued that while negative symptoms may be related to deficits involving higher cognitive functions such as concept formation, attention, and intellect, disorganized symptoms may be related prominently with deficits involving motor and sensory functions (Basso et al., 1998). The severity of disorganization symptoms was found to be related to working memory and specifically to both reduced ability to suppress distraction and reduced access to representations in semantic memory (Cameron et al., 2002).

Neuropsychological functioning and symptom dimensions of psychoses

The findings reported in the previous section are schizophrenia specific. The relationship between a broader range of psychotic symptomatology and cognitive performance has not been thoroughly investigated.

One such effort to characterize the relationship between the broader range of psychotic symptomatology and cognition has been the focus of an investigation in a cohort of first-episode psychotic patients, which included both affective and nonaffective cases (Demjaha et al., 2009). Using patients soon after their first episode of psychotic illness has several methodological advantages; importantly, measurement of symptomatology and cognitive functioning in patients not affected by either prolonged hospitalization or long-term

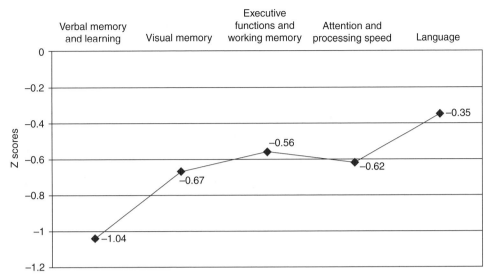

Figure 4.4. Performance of patients across five cognitive domains.

antipsychotic treatment. Data were collected on 100 first-episode psychosis (FEP) patients, recruited in South East London, and were used to examine the relationship between symptom dimensions and cognitive functioning in FEP. In order to compare results from this study with those that emerged from the meta-analysis by Dominguez et al. (2009) (presented in the previous section), findings were restricted to equivalent symptom dimensions with the exception of positive symptoms, which were divided into hallucinations and delusions (in accordance with the DSM-IV conceptualization). Therefore, the symptom dimensions that were taken into account were: negative symptoms, disorganization, depressive symptoms, and positive symptoms. Cognitive measures were slightly different from those used in the meta-analysis (Dominguez et al., 2009); however, they covered the range of cognitive domains known to be affected in schizophrenia and included: general intelligence (IQ) (obtained from the Wechsler Adult Intelligence Scale (WAIS, version III)) and five specific cognitive domains, including verbal memory and learning, visual memory, attention-concentration and processing speed, executive functions and working memory, and language.

Patients showed a typical pattern of cognitive impairment (Figure 4.4). Full-scale IQ (mean, 92.74±13.22) and all individual cognitive domains were significantly lower in patients than in healthy controls. Verbal memory emerged as the most affected cognitive domain with patients performing one standard deviation below the mean (z score, −1.04), followed by visual memory (z score, −0.67), attention and processing speed (z score, −0.62), executive functions and working memory (z score, −0.56), and language (z score, −0.35).

All symptom dimensions, except for positive symptoms, had statistically significant correlations with at least one cognitive domain. The statistically significant correlations were of moderate effect size. Negative symptoms showed a negative linear relationship with the verbal memory and learning domain (r = −0.261, P = 0.014). Disorganized

Table 4.1. Associations between symptom dimensions and cognitive domains

Symptom dimensions	Negative symptoms	Disorganization	Depressive symptoms	Positive symptoms	Variance explained
Cognitive domains					
IQ	P = 0.216 r = −0.126	P = 0.136 r = −0.151	P = 0.104 r = 0.164	P = 0.564 r = −0.061	7.4%
Verbal memory and learning	P = 0.014 r = −0.261	P = 0.031 r = −0.230	P = 0.033 r = 0.228	P = 0.581 r = 0.057	18.1%
Visual memory	P = 0.633 r = 0.055	P = 0.274 r = −0.118	P = 0.759 r = −0.032	P = 0.930 r = 0.000	1.8%
Executive functions and working memory	P = 0.641 r = 0.045	P = 0.491 r = 0.071	P = 0.001* r = 0.338	P = 0.546 r = 0.004	13%
Attention and processing speed	P = 0.834 r = 0.000	P = 0.239 r = −0.126	P = 0.001* r = 0.336	P = 0.505 r = 0.079	14.6%
Verbal fluency	P = 0.065 r = −0.214	P = 0.606 r = 0.063	P = 0.401 r = 0.100	P = 0.691 r = −0.004	13.6%

*Statistically significant after Bonferroni correction for multiple testing (P≤0.05/6=0.008).

symptoms negatively correlated with the verbal memory and learning domain (r = −0.230, P = 0.031). The depressive symptoms dimension had a positive relationship with the verbal memory and learning domain (r = 0.228, P = 0.033), executive functions and working memory domain (r = 0.337, P = 0.001), and attention, concentration, and processing speed domain (r = 0.336, P = 0.001). The relationship between depressive symptoms and both the domain of executive functions and working memory and the domain of attention-concentration and processing speed withheld correction for multiple comparisons set to P = 0.008. Variance in cognitive domains accounted for by symptoms ranged from 1.8% in the visual memory domain and up to 18.1% in the verbal memory and learning domain (Table 4.1).

In order to compare the relationships between symptom dimensions and cognitive domains in psychotic disorders to those reported for schizophrenia, associations between symptom dimensions and cognitive domains in our study are presented in Figure 4.5. The pattern that emerged was contrasted with the one reported by Dominguez et al. (2009) in a meta-analysis of schizophrenia. Negative symptoms and disorganization were associated only with verbal memory and learning (r = −0.261 and −0.230, respectively). In the meta-analysis (see Figure 4.3 for comparison), these symptom dimensions had much broader associations with a range of cognitive domains. In psychotic disorders, depressive symptoms showed a broad relationship with cognitive domains. Correlations ranged from 0.228 to 0.338 for depressive symptoms and verbal memory and learning, executive functions and working memory, and attention and processing speed domains. Similar to the meta-analysis, positive symptoms were not associated with cognitive functions, confirming the independence between positive symptomatology and cognition.

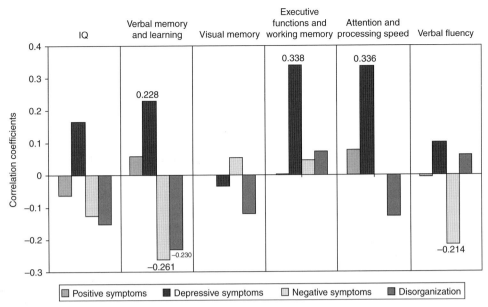

Figure 4.5. Pearson's correlations between symptom dimensions of psychoses and cognitive domains. (See color plate section for colored image.)

Summary

The relationship between symptom dimensions and cognitive domains varies across groups of symptoms. Studies have demonstrated that negative symptoms and disorganization are associated with cognitive functions, with more severe symptoms related to poorer cognitive performance. In contrast, positive symptoms are not associated with the severity of cognitive impairment. Dimensions of mood symptoms such as mania and depression have been investigated less frequently compared to other psychotic symptomatology, and findings are therefore less conclusive. Results reviewed here, however, suggest that mood symptom dimensions (e.g., depressive symptoms) might be associated with better cognitive functioning.

Schizophrenia patients are generally characterized by more severe negative and disorganized symptoms, and show more impaired cognitive functioning compared with bipolar disorder patients (Zanelli et al., 2010). Overall results might indicate some important contrasts between different psychopathological signs and neuropsychological functioning (Bozikas et al., 2004; Dominguez et al., 2009). Specific patterns of association between cognitive functions and symptom dimensions are detectable. Variations within the same symptom dimensions (e.g., according to severity of symptoms) and across symptom dimensions can explain differences in neuropsychological functioning in psychotic disorders. Overall, symptoms explained up to 18% of variance in cognitive functioning (Table 4.1). Taken together these results suggest that negative symptoms along with disorganization and positive and depressive symptoms can be the clinical expression of different cerebral patterns of dysfunctions.

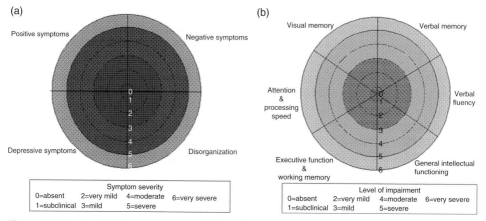

Figure 4.6. Scoring wheel for symptom severity (a) and cognitive impairment (b).

Conclusion

The results discussed in this chapter may also be considered in relation to future typology of psychotic disorders. It has recently been proposed (van Os & Kapur, 2009) to include cognitive impairment among five dimensions of psychosis. Applying this model to the symptom dimensions we used in this chapter, patients are characterized based on the combination of individual symptom dimension scores. For example, if the four symptom dimensions (positive, negative, depressive symptoms, and disorganization) are used to rate psychopathology and considering a gradient of severity from 0 (absent) to 6 (very severe), scoring would go from 0 (none) to 24 (maximum score on each symptom dimension). Two patients with the same categorical diagnosis of schizophrenia and with an identical total score of severity of psychopathology of 12, nevertheless, may have different scores on different dimensions of psychopathology (e.g., Patient A: positive symptoms = 5, disorganization = 4, depression = 0; mania = 3; Patient B: psychosis = 5, disorganization = 3, depression = 4; mania = 0) (Figure 4.6a). The cognitive heterogeneity across and within psychosis and the findings described in this chapter, however, suggest that cognitive functioning should perhaps be better viewed as a transversal component, intersecting with the psychopathological components of psychosis, and requiring multiple dimensions of classification by itself. Thus, the same two patients described here will also be similarly classified based on the severity of their impairment on different cognitive domains. Their overall cognitive profile might therefore look different according to the level of impairment in terms of standard deviations from the mean of the general population across cognitive domains (Figure 4.6b).

References

Addington, J. & Addington, D. (2002). Cognitive functioning in first-episode schizophrenia. *Journal of Psychiatry and Neuroscience* **27**, 188–192.

Albus, M., Hubmann, W., Wahlheim, C., et al. (1996). Contrasts in neuropsychological test profile between patients with first-episode schizophrenia and first-episode affective disorders. *Acta Psychiatrica Scandinavica* **94**, 87–93.

Allardyce, J., McCreadie, R. G., Morrison, G., et al. (2007). Do symptom dimensions or categorical diagnoses best discriminate between known risk factors for psychosis? *Social Psychiatry and Psychiatric Epidemiology* **42**, 429–437.

Andreasen, N. C., Arndt, S., Alliger, R., et al. (1995a). Symptoms of schizophrenia. Methods, meanings, and mechanisms. *Archives of General Psychiatry* **52**, 341–351.

Andreasen, N. C. & Olsen, S. (1982). Negative v. positive schizophrenia. Definition and validation. *Archives of General Psychiatry* **39**, 789–794.

Basso, M. R., Nasrallah, H. A., Olson, S. C., et al. (1998). Neuropsychological correlates of negative, disorganized and psychotic symptoms in schizophrenia. *Schizophrenia Research* **31**, 99–111.

Bearden, C. E., Hoffman, K. M., & Cannon, T. D. (2001). The neuropsychology and neuroanatomy of bipolar affective disorder: a critical review. *Bipolar Disorders* **3**, 106–150.

Bora, E., Yucel, M., & Pantelis, C. (2009). Cognitive functioning in schizophrenia, schizoaffective disorder and affective psychoses: meta-analytic study. *British Journal of Psychiatry* **195**, 475–482.

Bozikas, V. P., Kosmidis, M. H., Kioperlidou, K., et al. (2004). Relationship between psychopathology and cognitive functioning in schizophrenia. *Comprehensive Psychiatry* **45**, 392–400.

Cameron, A. M., Oram, J., Geffen, G. M., et al. (2002). Working memory correlates of three symptom clusters in schizophrenia. *Psychiatry Research* **110**, 49–61.

Carpenter, W. T. Jr., Heinrichs, D. W., & Wagman, A. M. (1988). Deficit and nondeficit forms of schizophrenia: the concept. *American Journal of Psychiatry* **145**, 578–583.

Craddock, N., O'Donovan, M. C., & Owen, M. J. (2006). Genes for schizophrenia and bipolar disorder? Implications for psychiatric nosology. *Schizophrenia Bulletin* **32**, 9–16.

Crow, T. J. (1980). Positive and negative schizophrenic symptoms and the role of dopamine. *British Journal of Psychiatry* **137**, 383–386.

Cuesta, M. J. & Peralta, V. (1995). Cognitive disorders in the positive, negative, and disorganization syndromes of schizophrenia. *Psychiatry Research* **58**, 227–235.

David, A. S., Malmberg, A., Brandt, L., et al. (1997). IQ and risk for schizophrenia: a population-based cohort study. *Psychological Medicine* **27**, 1311–1323.

Demjaha, A., Morgan, K., Morgan, C., et al. (2009). Combining dimensional and categorical representation of psychosis: the way forward for DSM-V and ICD-11? *Psychological Medicine* **39**, 1943–1955.

Dibben, C. R. M., Rice, C., Laws, K., et al. (2009). Is executive impairment associated with schizophrenic syndromes? A meta-analysis. *Psychological Medicine* **39**, 381–392.

Dickinson, D., Ramsey, M. E., & Gold, J. M. (2007). Overlooking the obvious: a meta-analytic comparison of digit symbol coding tasks and other cognitive measures in schizophrenia. *Archives of General Psychiatry* **64**, 532–542.

Dikeos, D. G., Wickham, H., McDonald, C., et al. (2006). Distribution of symptom dimensions across Kraepelinian divisions. *British Journal of Psychiatry* **189**, 346–353.

Dominguez, G., Viechtbauer, W., Simons, C. J., et al. (2009). Are psychotic psychopathology and neurocognition orthogonal? A systematic review of their associations. *Psychological Bulletin* **135**, 157–171.

Elvevag, B. & Goldberg, T. E. (2000). Cognitive impairment in schizophrenia is the core of the disorder. *Critical Reviews in Neurobiology* **14**, 1–21.

Ferrier, I. N., Chowdhury, R., Thompson, J. M., et al. (2004). Neurocognitive function in unaffected first-degree relatives of patients with bipolar disorder: a preliminary report. *Bipolar Disorders* **6**, 319–322.

Fioravanti, M., Carlone, O., Vitale, B., et al. (2005). A meta-analysis of cognitive deficits in adults with a diagnosis of schizophrenia. *Neuropsychology Review* **15**, 73–95.

Gourovitch, M. L., Torrey, E. F., Gold, J. M., et al. (1999). Neuropsychological performance of monozygotic twins discordant for bipolar disorder. *Biological Psychiatry* 45, 639–646.

Harvey, P. D., Koren, D., Reichenberg, A., et al. (2006). Negative symptoms and cognitive deficits: what is the nature of their relationship? *Schizophrenia Bulletin* 32, 250–258.

Heinrichs, R. W. & Zakzanis, K. K. (1998). Neurocognitive deficit in schizophrenia: a quantitative review of the evidence. *Neuropsychology* 12, 426–445.

Holthausen, E. A. E., Wiersma, D., Knegtering, R. H., et al. (1999). Psychopathology and cognition in schizophrenia spectrum disorders: the role of depressive symptoms. *Schizophrenia Research* 39, 65–71.

Holthausen, E. A. E., Wiersma, D., Sitskoorn, M. M., et al. (2002). Schizophrenic patients without neuropsychological deficits: subgroup, disease severity or cognitive compensation? *Psychiatry Research* 112, 1–11.

Jablensky, A. (2006). Subtyping schizophrenia: implications for genetic research. *Molecular Psychiatry* 11, 815–836.

Johnstone, E. C. & Frith, C. D. (1996). Validation of three dimensions of schizophrenic symptoms in a large unselected sample of patients. *Psychological Medicine* 26, 669–679.

Jones, P., Rodgers, B., Murray, R., et al. (1994). Child development risk factors for adult schizophrenia in the British 1946 birth cohort. *Lancet* 344, 1398–1402.

Joyce, E. M., Hutton, S. B., Mutsatsa, S. H., et al. (2005). Cognitive heterogeneity in first-episode schizophrenia. *British Journal of Psychiatry* 187, 516–522.

Joyce, E. M. & Roiser, J. P. (2007). Cognitive heterogeneity in schizophrenia. *Current Opinion in Psychiatry* 20, 268–272.

Kaymaz, N. & Van Os, J. (2009). Murray et al. (2004) revisited: is bipolar disorder identical to schizophrenia without developmental impairment? *Acta Psychiatrica Scandinavica* 120, 249–252.

Keefe, R. S., Silverman, J. M., Roitman, S. E., et al. (1994). Performance of nonpsychotic relatives of schizophrenic patients on cognitive tests. *Psychiatry Research* 53, 1–12.

Knowles, E. E., David, A. S., & Reichenberg, A. (2010). Processing speed deficits in schizophrenia: reexamining the evidence. *American Journal of Psychiatry* 167, 828–835.

Krabbendam, L., Arts, B., van Os, J., et al. (2005a). Cognitive functioning in patients with schizophrenia and bipolar disorder: a quantitative review. *Schizophrenia Research* 80, 137–149.

Krabbendam, L., Myin-Germeys, I., Bak, M., et al. (2005b). Explaining transitions over the hypothesized psychosis continuum. *Australian and New Zealand Journal of Psychiatry* 39, 180–186.

Kremen, W. S., Seidman, L. J., Faraone, S. V., et al. (2000). The paradox of normal neuropsychological function in schizophrenia. *Journal of Abnormal Psychology* 109, 743–752.

Liddle, P. F., Barnes, T. R., Morris, D., et al. (1989). Three syndromes in chronic schizophrenia. *British Journal of Psychiatry*, S119–122.

Lindenmayer, J. P., Grochowski, S., & Hyman, R. B. (1995). Five factor model of schizophrenia: replication across samples. *Schizophrenia Research* 14, 229–234.

Lucas, S., Fitzgerald, D., Redoblado-Hodge, M. A., et al. (2004). Neuropsychological correlates of symptom profiles in first episode schizophrenia. *Schizophrenia Research* 71, 323–330.

Maccabe, J. H. (2008). Population-based cohort studies on premorbid cognitive function in schizophrenia. *Epidemiol Rev* 30, 77–83.

MacCabe, J. H., Lambe, M. P., Cnattingius, S., et al. (2008). Scholastic achievement at age 16 and risk of schizophrenia and other psychoses: a national cohort study. *Psychological Medicine* 38, 1133–1140.

Malhi, G. S., Green, M., Fagiolini, A., et al. (2008). Schizoaffective disorder: diagnostic issues and future recommendations. *Bipolar Disorders* 10, 215–230.

McGuire, P. K., Shah, G. M., & Murray, R. M. (1993). Increased blood flow in Broca's area during auditory hallucinations in schizophrenia. *Lancet* **342**, 703–706.

Mesholam-Gately, R. I., Giuliano, A. J., Goff, K. P., et al. (2009). Neurocognition in first-episode schizophrenia: a meta-analytic review. *Neuropsychology* **23**, 315–336.

Murray, R. M. & Lewis, S. W. (1987). Is schizophrenia a neurodevelopmental disorder? *British Medical Journal (Clinical Research Ed.)* **295**, 681–682.

Nieuwenstein, M. R., Aleman, A., & de Haan, E. H. (2001). Relationship between symptom dimensions and neurocognitive functioning in schizophrenia: a meta-analysis of WCST and CPT studies. Wisconsin Card Sorting Test. Continuous Performance Test. *Journal of Psychiatric Research* **35**, 119–125.

Nuechterlein, K. H., Green, M. F., Kern, R. S., et al. (2008). The MATRICS consensus cognitive battery, part 1: test selection, reliability, and validity. *American Journal of Psychiatry* **165**, 203–213.

O'Leary, D. S., Flaum, M., Kesler, M. L., et al. (2000). Cognitive correlates of the negative, disorganized, and psychotic symptom dimensions of schizophrenia. *Journal of Neuropsychiatry and Clinical Neurosciences* **12**, 4–15.

Palmer, B. W., Heaton, R. K., Paulsen, J. S., et al. (1997). Is it possible to be schizophrenic yet neuropsychologically normal? *Neuropsychology* **11**, 437–446.

Quraishi, S. & Frangou, S. (2002). Neuropsychology of bipolar disorder: a review. *Journal of Affective Disorders* **72**, 209–226.

Reichenberg, A., Caspi, A., Harrington, H., et al. (2010). Static and dynamic cognitive deficits in childhood preceding adult schizophrenia: a 30-year study. *American Journal of Psychiatry* **167**, 160–169.

Reichenberg, A. & Harvey, P. D. (2007). Neuropsychological impairments in schizophrenia: integration of performance-based and brain imaging findings. *Psychological Bulletin* **133**, 833–858.

Reichenberg, A., Harvey, P. D., Bowie, C. R., et al. (2009). Neuropsychological function and dysfunction in schizophrenia and psychotic affective disorders. *Schizophrenia Bulletin* **35**, 1022–1029.

Reichenberg, A., Weiser, M., Rabinowitz, J., et al. (2002). A population-based cohort study of premorbid intellectual, language, and behavioral functioning in patients with schizophrenia, schizoaffective disorder, and nonpsychotic bipolar disorder. *American Journal of Psychiatry* **159**, 2027–2035.

Rijsdijk, F. V., Gottesman, I. I., McGuffin, P., et al. (2011). Heritability estimates for psychotic symptom dimensions in twins with psychotic disorders. *American Journal of Medical Genetics. Part B, Neuropsychiatric Genetics* **156**B, 89–98.

Robinson, L. J., Thompson, J. M., Gallagher, P., et al. (2006). A meta-analysis of cognitive deficits in euthymic patients with bipolar disorder. *Journal of Affective Disorders* **93**, 105–115.

Satz, P. (1993). Brain reserve capacity on symptom onset after brain injury: a formulation and review of evidence for threshold theory. *Neuropsychology* **7**, 273–295.

Seidman, L. J., Kremen, W. S., Koren, D., et al. (2002). A comparative profile analysis of neuropsychological functioning in patients with schizophrenia and bipolar psychoses. *Schizophrenia Research* **53**, 31–44.

Shergill, S. S., Brammer, M. J., Williams, S. C., et al. (2000). Mapping auditory hallucinations in schizophrenia using functional magnetic resonance imaging. *Archives of General Psychiatry* **57**, 1033–1038.

Squires, R. F. & Saederup, E. (1991). A review of evidence for GABergic predominance/ glutamatergic deficit as a common etiological factor in both schizophrenia and affective psychoses: more support for a continuum hypothesis of "functional" psychosis. *Neurochemical Research* **16**, 1099–1111.

Stefanopoulou, E., Manoharan, A., Landau, S., et al. (2009). Cognitive functioning in patients with affective disorders and schizophrenia: a meta-analysis. *International Review of Psychiatry* **21**, 336–356.

Stroup, T. S. (2007). Heterogeneity of treatment effects in schizophrenia. *American Journal of Medicine* **120**, S26–31.

Torres, I. J., Boudreau, V. G., & Yatham, L. N. (2007). Neuropsychological functioning in euthymic bipolar disorder: a meta-analysis. *Acta Psychiatrica Scandinavica*, S17–26.

Toulopoulou, T., Picchioni, M., Rijsdijk, F., et al. (2007). Substantial genetic overlap between neurocognition and schizophrenia: genetic modeling in twin samples. *Archives of General Psychiatry* 64, 1348–1355.

van Os, J. & Kapur, S. (2009). Schizophrenia. *Lancet* 374, 635–645.

Ventura, J., Thames, A. D., Wood, R. C., et al. (2010). Disorganization and reality distortion in schizophrenia: a meta-analysis of the relationship between positive symptoms and neurocognitive deficits. *Schizophrenia Research* 121, 1–14.

Weickert, T. W., Goldberg, T. E., Gold, J. M., et al. (2000). Cognitive impairments in patients with schizophrenia displaying preserved and compromised intellect. *Archives of General Psychiatry* 57, 907–913.

Woodberry, K. A., Giuliano, A. J., & Seidman, L. J. (2008). Premorbid IQ in schizophrenia: a meta-analytic review. *American Journal of Psychiatry* 165, 579–587.

Zammit, S., Allebeck, P., David, A. S., et al. (2004). A longitudinal study of premorbid IQ score and risk of developing schizophrenia, bipolar disorder, severe depression, and other nonaffective psychoses. *Archives of General Psychiatry* 61, 354–360.

Zanelli, J., Reichenberg, A., Morgan, K., et al. (2010). Specific and generalized neuropsychological deficits: a comparison of patients with various first-episode psychosis presentations. *American Journal of Psychiatry* 167, 78–85.

Neurocognition and functional outcome in schizophrenia: filling in the gaps

Michael F. Green, William P. Horan, Kristopher I. Mathis, and Jonathan K. Wynn

Acknowledgments

Funding for this project came from NIH grant MH043292 (to MFG).

Introduction and overview

The goal of treatments for schizophrenia has moved beyond management of psychotic symptoms to the goal of "recovery." Recovery refers to achieving independent living, vocational or educational activities, and satisfying interpersonal relationships (Kopelowicz et al., 2005; Liberman & Kopelowicz, 2005). This goal remains elusive for many patients with schizophrenia, as evidenced by the disappointing statistics on the worldwide level of disability associated with the illness (Murray & Lopez, 1996; WHO, 2008). An important step for public health improvement is to identify the determinants of poor functioning that interfere with successful community adaptation. One of the most consistent correlates and determinants of functional outcome for individuals with schizophrenia has been neurocognition (i.e., episodic memory, attention, working memory, reasoning and problem solving abilities, and speed of processing).

Relationships between neurocognition and functional outcome have been well documented in several reviews of this literature (Green, 1996; Green et al., 2000; Green et al., 2004). The relationships are present in cross-sectional studies, as well as in prospective studies in which neurocognition is assessed at baseline and outcome is assessed one or two years later (Green et al., 2004). The specific types of functional outcome vary across studies, but they usually include aspects of role functioning (work, housekeeping, school), independent living, and/or social functioning with friends and family. Associations between neurocognition and functional outcome are typically stronger than those found between psychotic symptoms and functional outcome, and sometimes even stronger than those between negative symptoms and outcome. Most of the studies in the reviews examined patients with chronic illness, but the linkages are also present in first-episode and prodromal (high-risk) samples (Carrion et al., 2011; Nuechterlein et al., 2011). While the magnitude of these relationships is often modest at the level of individual cognitive domains, a substantial amount of variance in outcome can be explained when summary scores that combine multiple domains are examined (Green et al., 2000).

Given the well-established nature of this literature, this chapter will not conduct a new review. Instead, it will attempt to place this literature in a larger context. Although the connections between neurocognition and outcome are well established, the mechanisms through which neurocognition measured in the laboratory ultimately relate to real-world functioning are not well understood. Over the last decade, investigators have switched from asking *if* neurocognition is related to outcome to asking *how* neurocognition is related to outcome. In doing so, research has started to identify the intervening steps between neurocognition and daily living, and also to look to perceptual factors earlier in the processing stream.

The purpose of the chapter is to sketch out a preliminary integrative model of outcome that incorporates factors that run from basic perception to functional outcome, with neurocognition as a lynchpin. We will first consider a close cousin of neurocognition, namely, social cognition. This area is also considered in Chapter 8 in this book; our focus here is on how social cognition relates to outcome beyond neurocognition. Neurocognition and social cognition can collectively be considered types of "ability." Second, we will move earlier in the processing stream to examine how early auditory and visual perception help to explain pathways from brain-based processes to ability measures and subsequently to community outcome. Third, we will examine motivational factors as promising intervening steps between ability and daily functioning. Finally, we conclude with recent efforts to evaluate how these domains (perception, ability, and motivation) can be integrated in a single model of outcome.

Social cognition and functional outcome in schizophrenia

Although some aspects of social cognition in schizophrenia have been studied for decades (e.g., facial affect perception), interest in this area has increased substantially in the last decade. Social cognition refers to the mental operations underlying social interactions, including perceiving, interpreting, and generating responses to the intentions, dispositions, and behaviors of others (Fiske & Taylor, 1991; Kunda, 1999). It includes processing a range of social information from how we identify an emotion on a face to how we draw inferences about another person's intentions. At the most basic level, social cognition is what enables us to understand and effectively interact with other people. Based on a rapidly expanding data-based literature, we know that schizophrenia is characterized by substantial wide-ranging social cognitive impairments (Bora et al., 2009; Green et al., 2008; Kohler et al., 2010). Intuitively, problems with social cognition, such as misperceiving the actions of other people and reacting in a manner confusing to others, are likely to have an adverse effect on functioning for patients.

Research in social cognition in schizophrenia has tended to cluster around four types of social cognitive processes: emotion processing, social perception, attributional style, and mental state attribution (i.e., theory of mind). **Emotion processing** includes perceiving and using emotion to facilitate adaptive functioning. One influential model of emotional processing (also called emotional intelligence) includes four components: identifying emotions, using emotions to facilitate cognition, understanding emotions, and managing emotions (Mayer et al., 2002; Mayer et al., 2003). Of these components, perceiving emotions (e.g., identifying emotions in faces) has been the most extensively studied social cognitive process in schizophrenia. **Social perception** refers to the ability to judge social cues from contextual information and communicative gestures (Corrigan & Green, 1993; Sergi & Green, 2002). In social perception tasks, participants typically process nonverbal, paraverbal, and/or verbal cues to make inferences about the social situations that contained such cues. **Attributional style** refers to how individuals characteristically explain the causes for positive and negative events in their lives (Bentall et al., 2001). Key distinctions are typically made between external personal attributions (i.e., causes attributed to other people), external situational attributions (i.e., causes attributed to situational factors), and internal attributions (i.e., causes attributed to oneself). In schizophrenia research, attributional style has been studied primarily to understand psychological mechanisms of persecutory delusions and paranoid beliefs in which there is a bias for patients with these symptoms to perceive malicious intent in other people. **Mental state attribution** (also called theory of mind, or mentalizing) involves inferring the intentions, dispositions, and beliefs of others (Baron-Cohen et al., 2001; Brune, 2005; Frith and Corcoran, 1996). This process includes the ability to understand false beliefs, hints, intentions, humor, deceptions, metaphor, and irony. This process requires one to "stand in someone's shoes." Mental state attribution studies in schizophrenia have relied heavily on measurements that were borrowed from the developmental literature, such as those used with autism spectrum disorders. The use of tests that were developed for children and adolescents means that the psychometric characteristics of mental state attribution measures used in schizophrenia are often problematic, but some newer measures have better psychometric properties in this population (Kern et al., 2009).

A growing literature has examined relationships between the domains of social cognition described earlier and various aspects of community functioning in schizophrenia (e.g., work, social, independent living). A previous review of this literature concluded that there were consistent functional correlates of social perception and emotion perception (Couture et al., 2006). A recent meta-analysis examined the amount of variance in functioning explained by neurocognition and social cognition in 52 studies that included 2692 subjects (Fett et al., 2011). The associations across studies between outcome and key social cognitive domains were all relatively strong: mental state attribution/theory of mind, 0.48; social perception, 0.41; emotion processing, 0.31. When the explanatory value of neurocognition and of social cognition were compared, the neurocognitive factor accounted for 6% of variance in community functioning, whereas the average of social cognitive domains explained 16%. Hence, social cognition is not only related to functional outcome–the strength of that relationship appears to be greater than for neurocognition.

The distinction between neurocognitive and social cognitive tasks depends mainly on the types of stimuli (e.g., people/faces vs. objects) and the types of responses (e.g., judgments about mental states of other people vs. simple speed and accuracy). Neurocognitive and social cognitive tasks often share cognitive demands, such as working memory and perception. Hence, one might question whether neurocognition and social cognition are truly different constructs. However, several data sets have shown that neurocognitive tests and social cognitive tests are only partially interrelated. Studies using confirmatory factor analysis with schizophrenia patients (Allen et al., 2007; Bell et al., 2009; Sergi et al., 2007) or exploratory factor analysis in participants with psychosis or heightened vulnerability to psychosis (van Hooren et al., 2008; Williams et al., 2008) indicate that models fit better when the two domains are separated compared to when they are combined. The general conclusion from these studies is that social cognition in schizophrenia is associated with neurocognition, but is not redundant to it. The relative distinctiveness of neurocognition and social cognition supported by the schizophrenia literature has also been found using healthy samples.

The conclusion that there is both partial overlap and relative distinctiveness between neurocognition and social cognition is consistent with studies from the social neuroscience literature that reveal partially overlapping and partially distinct patterns of neural activation associated with nonsocial and social cognitive activation tasks (van Overwalle, 2009).

The observation that neurocognition and social cognition are separable raises the question of how these domains work together to determine outcome. We previously found social cognition to be a mediator between neurocognition and functioning (Brekke et al., 2005). Being a mediator means that social cognition is associated with neurocognition, social cognition is related to functional outcome after controlling for its relationship to neurocognition, and the direct pathway between neurocognition and functional outcome becomes significantly smaller when social cognition is included in the model. This role of social cognition as a mediator is supported by a large number of data sets: out of 15 studies that considered whether social cognition was a significant mediator between neurocognition and functional outcome, 14 studies supported that role (Schmidt et al., 2011). The fact that social cognition is a mediator between neurocognition and functional outcome is additional evidence that the two domains are not redundant. If they were, it would not be possible for social cognition to have a significant relationship with outcome while controlling for its relationship to neurocognition.

Overall, social cognition appears to be a consistent correlate of functional outcome. In addition, it helps to provide a mechanism through which problems in neurocognition lead to problems in functional outcome. Social cognition acts as a mediator between the two; variance from neurocognition "flows through" social cognition to impact functional outcome. Consistent with this view, social cognition explains unique variance in functional outcome (Brekke et al., 2005; Poole et al., 2000; Vauth et al., 2004). That is, it has incremental validity that accounts for variance in outcome above and beyond that provided by neurocognition. Both neurocognition and social cognition can be considered reflections of integrative cognitive processes and are both reflections of the general category of ability. The next section covers what happens if we move earlier in processing and consider perceptual processes.

Perception as a correlate and predictor of social cognition and outcome

As opposed to later (more integrative) stages, such as neurocognition or social cognition, many studies of functional outcome have moved earlier in the processing stream to examine the effects of visual and auditory perception. Individuals with schizophrenia have abnormalities in both of these modalities and starting with perceptual measures in mechanistic models of outcome has some interpretive advantages for two reasons (Javitt, 2009). First, perceptual variables have rather direct and established ties to neural processes. Neural models of perception are better specified than they are for many of the neurocognitive domains that depend on integrating information from different sources. Second, perceptual variables are relatively less influenced by later-stage processes. Although top-down processes influence some early perceptual variables, their effects tend to be relatively small. Hence, early perceptual variables, in a model of outcome, are much more likely to influence later variables than later-stage variables (e.g., neurocognition, social cognition, motivation, etc.) are to influence perception.

Several studies in schizophrenia have found associations between lower-level perceptual processing and higher-level variables. In previous publications from our laboratory we found that early visual perception is a contributor in models of functional outcome (Rassovsky et al., 2011; Sergi et al., 2006). Perceptual variables can contribute to outcome either directly, or indirectly via social cognition. Our studies used versions of visual masking in which the processing of a visual target is disrupted by a visual mask that is briefly presented shortly before (forward masking) or after (backward masking) the target. The visual masking paradigm provides excellent temporal resolution by manipulating the interval between the target and mask, and can be used to assess the first 100 ms of visual processing. Other early visual processing measures, including visual evoked potentials assessed using electroencephalography, have shown similar connections to functional outcome (Butler et al., 2005). In addition, more integrative visual tasks have been used to examine visual integration. In these tasks, subjects are asked to detect a contour in an array of separate small visual elements. This ability to integrate visual elements into contours is related to higher-level social cognitive processes, such as mental state attribution (Schenkel et al., 2005; Uhlhaas et al., 2006).

In addition to the role played by visual processing impairments in leading to social cognitive deficits, impaired early auditory processing leads to problems in emotion detection from the prosody of voices (Javitt, 2009; Leitman et al., 2005, 2010). Basic auditory processing in schizophrenia, assessed with tasks such as simple tone matching, was correlated with poor prosody detection (Leitman et al., 2005). In a follow-up study, poor early auditory processing was associated with poorer ability to detect complex pitch changes inherent in prosodic speech (Leitman et al., 2010).

In addition to behavioral measures, early auditory processing can be assessed with specific event-related potentials (ERPs). Mismatch negativity (MMN) is one ERP index of early auditory discrimination that reflects the difference in neural response to an expected (standard) tone and an unexpected (rare) tone. Mismatch negativity can be evoked even when stimuli are not directly or fully attended, making it an ideal measure of early auditory processing without any cognitive or effortful processing by the participant. Reduced MMN (meaning less of a difference between standard and rare tones) is indicative of dysfunctional early auditory processing. Mismatch negativity is related to lower levels of functioning and independent living in schizophrenia patients (Light & Braff, 2005). In addition, MMN has been shown to be related to an aspect of social cognition, namely, social perception that is heavily reliant on processing brief perceptual cues (Wynn et al., 2010).

The connections between auditory and visual perceptual processes and later processes (e.g., social cognition, and eventually community outcome) are typically viewed within a "cascade" model. In such models, early impairments produce perceptual information that is eroded, partial, or unstable in some way. This poorly formed perceptual information is fed forward to higher-level processing stages. However, because the perceptual information is imperfect initially, subsequent processing of this information is impaired as well (Javitt, 2009).

Overall, support for starting outcome models very early in the processing stream has become increasingly persuasive, because perceptual factors are seen to relate to higher-level ability factors (neurocognition and social cognition). Further, there are benefits to constructing models that begin at a perceptual level due to the well-established links to neural substrates. The following section addresses the question of how the perception-to-ability linkages eventually lead to community functioning.

Role of negative symptoms with cognition and functional outcome

A key unresolved question in this area is how motivation and negative symptoms fit with ability factors to lead to functional outcome. Negative symptoms reflect a decrease or absence of normal functions within two broad domains: (1) internal experience-related impairments, including diminished emotional experience (anhedonia), motivation to engage in productive activities (avolition), and desire for social affiliation (asociality); (2) expressive or communicative impairments, including diminished facial expressivity, gestures, prosody, and speech production (Blanchard et al., 2011; Kirkpatrick et al., 2006). In general, motivation and negative symptoms are highly overlapping and can be considered reflections of the same underlying avolitional state (Nakagami et al., 2008, 2010). It has been known for a long time that, like neurocognition, negative symptoms are consistent predictors of daily functioning (Breier et al., 1991; Fenton & McGlashan, 1994). What is less clear is how neurocognition and negative symptoms interact so that they are both determinants of outcome. There is surprisingly little theoretical discussion about this issue in the literature (see Harvey et al., 2006, for an example).

There are two general possibilities. One is that two independent paths to functional outcome exist: one that flows through neurocognition and a separate one that is based on motivation. Such a model is depicted in Figure 5.1. In this model, problems start with impaired perception, as in the cascade models mentioned earlier. Next, a variety of performance-based skills, including neurocognition, social cognition, and functional capacity that can be collectively called measures of ability are diminished (Harvey et al., 2011). We have already discussed neurocognition and social cognition. Functional capacity (also called competence) refers to the ability to demonstrate activities of daily living or social communications in a simulated setting (Green et al., 2011; McKibbin et al., 2004). Measures of functional capacity are performance-based simulations in which a participant demonstrates how he/she would conduct daily activities such as paying a bill, taking their medication, or planning an outing to a local recreational site (Patterson et al., 2001, 2002). Similar to social cognition, functional capacity can act as a mediator between

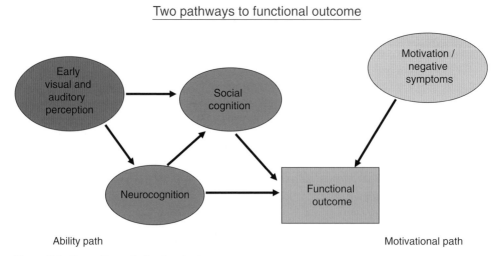

Two pathways to functional outcome

Ability path | Motivational path

Figure 5.1. Two pathways to functional outcome.

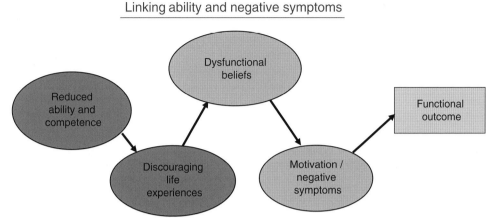

Figure 5.2. Linking of ability and negative symptoms.

neurocognition and functional outcome (Bowie et al., 2006, 2010). These three types of measures, neurocognition, social cognition, and functional capacity, are distinctive but typically they are intercorrelated. Hence, they are shown as part of the same category of ability.

Alternative models can be formally tested with statistical techniques such as structural equation modeling or path analysis. In this two pathway model (Figure 5.1), the ability path reflects what one *can* do, whereas the motivational path reflects what one *wants* to do. The two pathway model is reflected in everyday speech; people commonly describe others (e.g., their family members, or even themselves) as being fully capable of accomplishing tasks, but not having enough motivation to give it a try. A clinical example would be a patient who appears to have the skills and competence to function at work or college, but does not get out of bed early enough to catch the bus on a regular basis. We might attribute that problem to decreased motivation in the presence of good ability.

Instead of two pathways, there could be a single path in which ability helps to determine motivation. An example of a single path model that includes both cognitive (i.e., ability) variables and negative symptoms comes from the work of Beck and colleagues (Beck & Rector, 2005). This theory proposes that ability (e.g., neurocognition and functional capacity) and functional outcome are related via intervening variables in a causal pathway involving dysfunctional beliefs (Figure 5.2). According to this model, reduced ability leads to discouraging life circumstances as individuals find themselves repeatedly failing at basic life tasks. These discouraging experiences engender negative attitudes and beliefs about one's self. For example, patients may start to feel that they are likely to fail before they even undertake daily activities. These dysfunctional attitudes, in turn, contribute to decreased motivation, energy, and interest; which manifest clinically as negative symptoms. The theory by Beck and colleagues proposes a single indirect pathway that runs from impaired ability (and its resulting discouraging experiences) to dysfunctional attitudes to negative symptoms to functional outcome.

This provocative theory regarding the connection between dysfunctional beliefs and negative symptoms has received some empirical support. Studies have shown connections between ability and dysfunctional beliefs (Horan et al., 2010), dysfunctional beliefs and negative symptoms (Grant & Beck, 2009), and dysfunctional beliefs and social functioning

(Grant & Beck, 2010). A study from our laboratory found that one type of dysfunctional attitudes, "defeatist beliefs," was connected to a measure of functional capacity and to negative symptoms (Horan et al., 2010). Defeatist beliefs refer to overgeneralized conclusions about one's ability to perform tasks (e.g., "If you cannot do something well, there is little point in doing it at all." "Taking even a small risk is foolish because the loss is likely to be a disaster."). A variety of dysfunctional beliefs exist, such as maladaptive beliefs about one's ability to communicate effectively (Beck et al., 2009), but defeatist beliefs has been a focus of research in schizophrenia.

The published data are inconclusive on the question of one versus two pathways. Some studies suggest that negative symptoms lie on a separate pathway from ability (Bowie et al., 2006, 2008), whereas other studies suggest it lies on the same pathway as perceptual or ability measures (Couture et al., 2011; Grant & Beck, 2009; Rassovsky et al., 2011). Most studies have not had enough variables and subjects to formally test one versus two causal pathways, so there is little way to arbitrate between the possibilities.

From perception to community functioning: trying to put it all together

The final section of this chapter is more speculative and it includes our best guess for a useful integrative model of outcome that incorporates perception, ability, and motivation. In describing this model, we will rely on the published data mentioned earlier, and unpublished data from our laboratory. Our findings are generally supportive of a single pathway model, similar to that proposed by Beck and colleagues. The data suggest that functional outcome in schizophrenia can be considered the result of a relatively linear and streamlined series of steps from perception to ability to beliefs/motivation to functional outcome (see Figure 5.3). This figure has several connections that are largely expected based on previous data and theories. For example, there are considerable data to support the linkages between perception and ability, and between negative symptoms and daily functioning. Less data exist on the idea that ability leads to motivation (via dysfunctional attitudes), although that is predicated by the theoretical framework of Beck and colleagues.

Single pathway to functional outcome

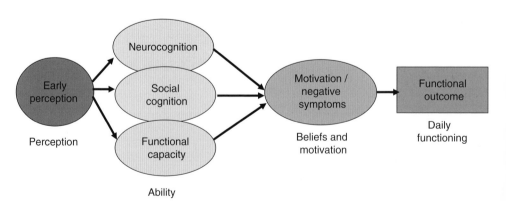

Figure 5.3. Single pathway to functional outcome.

The model shown in Figure 5.3 is relatively parsimonious compared to the two pathway model, but it also raises some questions. For example, negative symptoms are a multi-faceted construct composed of two separable subdomains: diminished *expression* (affective flattening and alogia) and diminished *experience* (avolition/apathy and anhedonia/asociality) (Blanchard & Cohen, 2006). Experiential negative symptoms are particularly close to concepts of motivation; they refer to a reduction in internal drive and emotion, as opposed to a reduction in outward expressions and communication. Additionally, experiential negative symptoms appear to be more closely related to outcome than expressive symptoms (Horan et al., 2006; Orsel et al., 2004; Rassovsky et al., 2011). It will be important to determine whether negative symptoms in general or experiential negative symptoms in particular are relevant for models of functional outcome in schizophrenia. The initial findings suggest the functional implications of experiential symptoms are greater.

A second consideration is that the association between experiential negative symptoms and functional outcome might be influenced by the degree of overlap in how the two are assessed. Interviews for functional outcome and those for negative symptoms ask similar types of questions regarding the extent to which a patient is engaged in activities in daily life. This issue of measurement overlap has provided a rationale for the development of new scales that assess experiential negative symptoms independently from current community functioning (Blanchard et al., 2010). Such a scale, the Clinical Assessment Interview for Negative Symptoms (CAINS), was recently developed through an NIMH-sponsored consortium (Blanchard et al., 2011) and will be a valuable addition for future studies of outcome.

Conclusions

In summary, research on outcome in schizophrenia has moved beyond the question of whether neurocognition is related to outcome and has started asking how the relationship works. Although the pathway(s) through which neurocognition leads to outcome are complex, we are beginning to understand how ability variables (including neurocognition, social cognition, and functional capacity) interface with more fundamental processes (perception) on the one hand, and motivational factors on the other, to impact functioning. These models emphasize the importance of considering both what a person can do and what the person wants to do, as both can limit one's successful adaptation. Models of outcome will become more complex as additional relevant factors are considered. Such factors would include additional within-person factors (e.g., insight, metacognition, premorbid history), as well as external factors (e.g., social and family support, opportunities for supported employment). In addition, future research will consider factors that influence outcome at a particular phase of illness (prodromal, first-episode, and chronic).

A better understanding of the mechanisms and intervening steps through which neurocognition ultimately impacts outcome is critical for the development of new recovery-oriented treatments. It is notable that all of the components of the final model in Figure 5.3 are also targets for interventions. Recovery-oriented treatments are showing promise on several fronts, including neurocognitive and social cognitive remediation, cognitive behavioral therapy for negative symptoms, and drug development for both neurocognition and negative symptoms. A greater understanding of how neurocognition and other factors contribute to outcome can help guide the implementation of these promising treatment approaches.

References

Allen, D. N., Strauss, G. P., Donohue, B., et al. (2007). Factor analytic support for social cognition as a separable cognitive domain in schizophrenia. *Schizophrenia Research*, **93**, 325–333.

Baron-Cohen, S., Wheelwright, S., Hill, J., et al. (2001). The "Reading the Mind in the Eyes" Test, revised version: a study with normal adults, and adults with Asperger syndrome or high-functioning autism. *Journal of Child Psychology and Psychiatry*, **42**, 241–251.

Beck, A. T. & Rector, N. A. (2005). Cognitive approaches to schizophrenia: theory and therapy. *Annual Review of Clinical Psycholology*, **1**, 577–606.

Beck, A. T., Rector, N. A., Stolar, N., et al. (2009). *Schizophrenia: cognitive theory, research, and therapy*. New York, NY: Guilford Press.

Bell, M., Tsang, H. W., Greig, T. C., et al. (2009). Neurocognition, social cognition, perceived social discomfort, and vocational outcomes in schizophrenia. *Schizophrenia Bulletin*, **35**, 738–747.

Bentall, R. P., Corcoran, R., Howard, R., et al. (2001). Persecutory delusions: a review and theoretical integration. *Clinical Psychology Review*, **21**, 1143–1192.

Blanchard, J. J. & Cohen, A. S. (2006). The structure of negative symptoms within schizophrenia: implications for assessment. *Schizophrenia Bulletin*, **32**, 238–245.

Blanchard, J. J., Forbes, C., Bennett, M., et al. (2010). Initial development and preliminary validation of a new negative symptom measure: the clinical assessment inventory for negative symptoms. *Schizophrenia Research*, **124**, 36–42.

Blanchard, J. J., Kring, A. M., Horan, W. P., et al. (2011). Toward the next generation of negative symptom assessments: the collaboration to advance negative symptom assessment in schizophrenia. *Schizophrenia Bulletin*, **37**, 291–299.

Bora, E., Yucel, M., & Pantelis, C. (2009). Theory of mind impairment in schizophrenia: meta-analysis. *Schizophrenia Research*, **109**, 1–9.

Bowie, C. R., Depp, C., McGrath, J. A., et al. (2010). Prediction of real-world functional disability in chronic mental disorders: a comparison of schizophrenia and bipolar disorder. *American Journal of Psychiatry*, **167**, 1116–1124.

Bowie, C. R., Leung, W. W., Reichenberg, A., et al. (2008). Predicting schizophrenia patients' real-world behavior with specific neuropsychological and functional capacity measures. *Biological Psychiatry*, **63**, 505–511.

Bowie, C. R., Reichenberg, A., Patterson, T. L., et al. (2006). Determinants of real-world functional performance in schizophrenia subjects: correlations with cognition, functional capacity, and symptoms. *American Journal of Psychiatry*, **163**, 418–425.

Breier, A., Schreiber, J. L., Dyer, J., et al. (1991). National Institutes of Mental Health longitudinal study of chronic schizophrenia: prognosis and predictors of outcome. *Archives of General Psychiatry*, **48**, 239–246.

Brekke, J. S., Kay, D. D., Kee, K. S., et al. (2005). Biosocial pathways to functional outcome in schizophrenia. *Schizophrenia Research*, **80**, 213–225.

Brune, M. (2005). "Theory of mind" in schizophrenia: a review of the literature. *Schizophrenia Bulletin*, **31**, 21–42.

Butler, P. D., Zemon, V., Schechter, I., et al. (2005). Early-stage visual processing and cortical amplification deficits in schizophrenia. *Archives of General Psychiatry*, **62**, 495–504.

Carrion, R. E., Goldberg, T. E., Mclaughlin, D., et al. (2011). Impact of neurocognition on social and role functioning in individuals at clinical high risk for psychosis. *American Journal of Psychiatry*, **168**, 806–813.

Corrigan, P. W. & Green, M. F. (1993). Schizophrenic patients' sensitivity to social cues: the role of abstraction. *American Journal of Psychiatry*, **150**, 589–594.

Couture, S. M., Granholm, E. L., & Fish, S. C. (2011). A path model investigation of neurocognition, theory of mind, social competence, negative symptoms and real-world functioning in schizophrenia. *Schizophrenia Research*, **125**, 152–160.

Couture, S. M., Penn, D. L., & Roberts, D. L. (2006). The functional significance of social cognition in schizophrenia: a review. *Schizophrenia Bulletin*, **32**, S44–63.

Fenton, W. S. & McGlashan, T. H. (1994). Antecedents, symptom progression, and long-term outcome of the deficit syndrome in schizophrenia. *American Journal of Psychiatry*, **151**, 351–356.

Fett, A. K., Viechtbauer, W., Dominguez, M. D., et al. (2011). The relationship between neurocognition and social cognition with functional outcomes in schizophrenia: a meta-analysis. *Neuroscience and Biobehavioral Reviews*, **35**, 573–588.

Fiske, S. T. & Taylor, S. E. (1991). *Social Cognition*. New York, NY: McGraw-Hill.

Frith, C. D. & Corcoran, R. (1996). Exploring 'theory of mind' in people with schizophrenia. *Psychological Medicine*, **26**, 521–530.

Grant, P. M. & Beck, A. T. (2009). Defeatist beliefs as a mediator of cognitive impairment, negative symptoms, and functioning in schizophrenia. *Schizophrenia Bulletin*, **35**, 798–806.

Grant, P. M. & Beck, A. T. (2010). Asocial beliefs as predictors of asocial behavior in schizophrenia. *Psychiatry Research*, **177**, 65–70.

Green, M. F. (1996). What are the functional consequences of neurocognitive deficits in schizophrenia? *American Journal of Psychiatry*, **153**, 321–330.

Green, M. F., Kern, R. S., Braff, D. L., et al. (2000). Neurocognitive deficits and functional outcome in schizophrenia: Are we measuring the "right stuff"? *Schizophrenia Bulletin*, **26**, 119–136.

Green, M. F., Kern, R. S., & Heaton, R. K. (2004). Longitudinal studies of cognition and functional outcome in schizophrenia: implications for MATRICS. *Schizophrenia Research*, **72**, 41–51.

Green, M. F., Penn, D. L., Bentall, R., et al. (2008). Social cognition in schizophrenia: an NIMH workshop on definitions, assessment, and research opportunities. *Schizophrenia Bulletin*, **34**, 1211–1220.

Green, M. F., Schooler, N. R., Kern, R. S., et al. (2011). Evaluation of functionally meaningful measures for clinical trials of cognition enhancement in schizophrenia. *American Journal of Psychiatry*, **168**, 400–407.

Harvey, P. D., Koren, D., Reichenberg, A., et al. (2006). Negative symptoms and cognitive deficits: what is the nature of their relationship? *Schizophrenia Bulletin*, **32**, 250–258.

Harvey, P. D., Raykov, T., Twamley, E. W., et al. (2011). Validating the measurement of real-world functional outcomes: Phase I results of the VALERO study. *American Journal of Psychiatry*, **168**, 1195–1201.

Horan, W. P., Kring, A. M., & Blanchard, J. J. (2006). Anhedonia in schizophrenia: a review of assessment strategies. *Schizophrenia Bulletin*, **32**, 259–273.

Horan, W. P., Rassovsky, Y., Kern, R. S., et al. (2010). Further support for the role of dysfunctional attitudes in models of real-world functioning in schizophrenia. *Journal of Psychiatric Research*, **44**, 499–505.

Javitt, D. C. (2009). When doors of perception close: bottom-up models of disrupted cognition in schizophrenia. *Annual Review of Clinical Psychology*, **5**, 249–275.

Kern, R. S., Green, M. F., Fiske, A. P., et al. (2009). Theory of mind deficits for processing counterfactual information in persons with chronic schizophrenia. *Psychological Medicine*, **39**, 645–654.

Kirkpatrick, B., Fenton, W., Carpenter, W. T., et al. (2006). The NIMH-MATRICS Consensus Statement on Negative Symptoms. *Schizophrenia Bulletin*, **32**, 296–303.

Kohler, C. G., Walker, J. B., Martin, E. A., et al. (2010). Facial emotion perception in schizophrenia: a meta-analytic review. *Schizophrenia Bulletin*, **36**, 1009–1019.

Kopelowicz, A., Liberman, R. P., Ventura, J., et al. (2005). Neurocognitive correlates of recovery from schizophrenia. *Psychological Medicine*, **35**, 1165–1173.

Kunda, Z. (1999). *Social Cognition: Making Sense of People*. Cambridge, MA: MIT Press.

Leitman, D. I., Foxe, J. J., Butler, P. D., et al. (2005). Sensory contributions to impaired prosodic processing in schizophrenia. *Biological Psychiatry*, **58**, 56–61.

Leitman, D. I., Laukka, P., Juslin, P. N., et al. (2010). Getting the cue: sensory contributions to auditory emotion recognition impairments in schizophrenia. *Schizophrenia Bulletin*, **36**, 545–556.

Liberman, R. P. & Kopelowicz, A. (2005). Recovery from schizophrenia: a concept in search of research. *Psychiatric Services*, **56**, 735–742.

Light, G. A. & Braff, D. L. (2005). Mismatch negativity deficits are associated with poor functioning in schizophrenia patients. *Archives of General Psychiatry*, **62**, 127–136.

Mayer, J. D., Salovey, P., & Caruso, D. R. (2002). *Mayer–Salovey–Caruso Emotional Intelligence Test (MSCEIT) User's Manual*. Toronto: MHS Publishers.

Mayer, J. D., Salovey, P., Caruso, D. R., et al. (2003). Measuring emotional intelligence with the MSCEIT V2.0. *Emotion*, **3**, 97–105.

McKibbin, C. L., Brekke, J. S., Sires, D., et al. (2004). Direct assessment of functional abilities: relevance to persons with schizophrenia. *Schizophrenia Research*, **72**, 53–67.

Murray, C. J. L. & Lopez, A. D. (eds.). (1996). *The Global Burden of Disease*. Boston, MA: Harvard School of Public Health.

Nakagami, E., Hoe, M., & Brekke, J. S. (2010). The prospective relationships among intrinsic motivation, neurocognition, and psychosocial functioning in schizophrenia. *Schizophrenia Bulletin*, **36**, 935–948.

Nakagami, E., Xie, B., Hoe, M., et al. (2008). Intrinsic motivation, neurocognition and psychosocial functioning in schizophrenia: testing mediator and moderator effects. *Schizophrenia Research*, **105**, 95–104.

Nuechterlein, K. H., Subotnik, K. L., Green, M. F., et al. (2011). Neurocognitive predictors of work outcome in recent-onset schizophrenia. *Schizophrenia Bulletin*, **37**, S33–40.

Orsel, S., Akdemir, A., & Dag, I. (2004). The sensitivity of quality-of-life scale

WHOQOL-100 to psychopathological measures in schizophrenia. *Comprehensive Psychiatry*, **45**, 57–61.

Patterson, T. L., Goldman, S., McKibbin, C. L., et al. (2001). UCSD performance-based skills assessment: development of a new measure of everyday functioning for severely mentally ill adults. *Schizophrenia Bulletin*, **27**, 235–245.

Patterson, T. L., Lacro, J., McKibbin, C. L., et al. (2002). Medication management ability assessment: results from a performance-based measure in older outpatients with schizophrenia. *Journal of Clinical Psychopharmacology*, **22**, 11–19.

Poole, J. H., Tobias, F. C., & Vinogradov, S. (2000). The functional relevance of affect recognition errors in schizophrenia. *Journal of the International Neuropsychological Society*, **6**, 649–658.

Rassovsky, Y., Horan, W. P., Lee, J., et al. (2011). Pathways between early visual processing and functional outcome in schizophrenia. *Psychological Medicine*, **41**, 487–497.

Schenkel, L. S., Spaulding, W. D., & Silverstein, S. M. (2005). Poor premorbid social functioning and theory of mind deficit in schizophrenia: evidence of reduced context processing? *Journal of Psychiatric Research*, **39**, 499–508.

Schmidt, S. J., Mueller, D. R., & Roder, V. (2011). Social cognition as a mediator variable between neurocognition and functional outcome in schizophrenia: empirical review and new results by structural equation modeling. *Schizophrenia Bulletin*, **37**, S41–54.

Sergi, M. J. & Green, M. F. (2002). Social perception and early visual processing in schizophrenia. *Schizophrenia Research*, **59**, 233–241.

Sergi, M. J., Rassovsky, Y., Nuechterlein, K. H., et al. (2006). Social perception as a mediator of the influence of early visual processing on functional status in schizophrenia. *American Journal of Psychiatry*, **163**, 448–454.

Sergi, M. J., Rassovsky, Y., Widmark, C., et al. (2007). Social cognition in schizophrenia: relationships with neurocognition and negative symptoms. *Schizophrenia Research*, **90**, 316–324.

Uhlhaas, P. J., Phillips, W. A., Schenkel, L. S., et al. (2006). Theory of mind and perceptual context-processing in schizophrenia. *Cognitive Neuropsychiatry*, **11**, 416–436.

Van Hooren, S., Versmissen, D., Janssen, I., et al. (2008). Social cognition and neurocognition as independent domains in psychosis. *Schizophrenia Research*, **103**, 257–265.

Van Overwalle, F. (2009). Social cognition and the brain: a meta-analysis. *Human Brain Mapping*, **30**, 829–858.

Vauth, R., Rusch, N., Wirtz, M., et al. (2004). Does social cognition influence the relation between neurocognitive deficits and vocational functioning in schizophrenia? *Psychiatry Research*, **128**, 155–165.

World Health Organization (WHO). (2008). *The Global Burden of Disease: 2004 update.* Geneva: WHO Press.

Williams, L. M., Whitford, T. J., Flynn, G., et al. (2008). General and social cognition in first episode schizophrenia: identification of separable factors and prediction of functional outcome using the IntegNeuro test battery. *Schizophrenia Research*, **99**, 182–191.

Wynn, J. K., Sugar, C., Horan, W. P., et al. (2010). Mismatch negativity, social cognition, and functioning in schizophrenia patients. *Biological Psychiatry*, **67**, 940–947.

Chapter

6

Cognition and work functioning in schizophrenia

Susan R. McGurk and Kim T. Mueser

Introduction

Schizophrenia has a profound effect on reducing the capacity of individuals to engage in and sustain productive employment (American Psychiatric Association, 1994). Impaired work functioning has important implications for both the overall quality of life for people with the disorder, and for the costs to their families and society. We begin this chapter with a brief review of the magnitude of the problem of poor vocational functioning in schizophrenia, as well as the benefits of work for this population. We next consider important factors related to schizophrenia that contribute to the poor work outcomes, first focusing on impaired premorbid functioning and reduced educational attainment, followed by the impact of symptoms and social impairments. We then address the impact of impaired cognitive functioning on work capacity in schizophrenia and response to vocational rehabilitation. As impaired cognitive ability is the most important clinical correlate of vocational functioning and response to vocational rehabilitation, we briefly review cognitive remediation approaches aimed at improving cognitive performance and employment outcomes.

Work functioning in schizophrenia

Rates of employment in schizophrenia are typically low, with usually fewer than 15%–20% of people with the illness working either part- or full-time (Lindamer et al., 2003; Marwaha et al., 2007; Salkever et al., 2007). Even when people with schizophrenia obtain jobs, they often have difficulties maintaining their employment due to problems such as poor work performance or relapses and hospitalizations (Suslow et al., 2000; Tsang et al., 2010). As a result of this impairment in work functioning, many people with schizophrenia live in poverty (Draine et al., 2002), and are dependent upon family members and disability benefits for having their basic needs met. Because of the early onset of the disorder, combined with its long-term effects on impaired ability to work and to care for oneself, schizophrenia is ranked as one of the ten most globally burdensome illnesses to individuals and societies throughout the world, including in developing nations as well as industrialized ones (Murray & Lopez, 1996).

Work for people with schizophrenia is associated with a range of benefits, including meaningful daily activity, social contact, community integration, self-esteem, modest reductions in symptoms, and a better quality of life (Bond et al., 2001; Burns et al., 2007). For

Cognitive Impairment in Schizophrenia, ed. Philip D. Harvey. Published by Cambridge University Press. © Cambridge University Press 2013.

these reasons, work is a common goal endorsed by the majority of people with schizophrenia (Brekke et al., 1993; Mueser et al., 2001b; Rogers et al., 1991). Numerous first-person accounts attest to the importance of work as a central part of the recovery process (Bailey et al., 1998; Provencher et al., 2002).

Premorbid functioning and educational attainment

Poor vocational functioning in schizophrenia is the result of a host of different factors related to the illness, some of which antedate the onset of the disorder itself. Two of the most important of these factors are poor premorbid adjustment and curtailed level of educational attainment. Problems in childhood and adolescent premorbid social and academic functioning are a well-established antecedent of schizophrenia (Hans et al., 1992; Malmberg et al., 1998; Robins, 1966). Furthermore, impaired premorbid functioning is predictive of a worse course of illness, both symptomatically and in terms of psychosocial functioning including work (MacBeth &Gumley, 2008; Malla & Payne, 2005; Strauss & Carpenter, 1977; Zigler & Glick, 1986). Thus, reduced social competence prior to the onset of schizophrenia may persist or worsen after the illness develops, thereby contributing to difficulties obtaining jobs and performing well at work (Mueser et al., 1990).

The florid psychotic symptoms that define the onset of schizophrenia and that characterize episodes of the illness usually begin in early adulthood. However, it is now well established that this first break is preceded by a pattern of other problems that on average last two to three years, including depression, social difficulties, and reduced cognitive abilities (Häfner & an der Heiden, 2008). A common consequence of this gradual deterioration in functioning is that people who develop schizophrenia are often unable to complete important sociocultural educational milestones, such as finishing high school or college (Kessler et al., 1995). The interruption of individuals' educational striving can be demoralizing for someone with schizophrenia (Lewine, 2005). In addition, lower levels of education put people at a disadvantage in the labor market, both in the general population (Jencks, 1979) and among people with schizophrenia (Mueser et al., 2001b; Tsang et al., 2010). Thus, both impaired premorbid functioning and lower education are an impediment to vocational success in people who develop schizophrenia, even before they experience their first episode of psychosis.

Symptoms, social competence, and work

Both the psychotic and negative symptoms of schizophrenia can interfere with the ability to work. Between 25% and 40% of people with schizophrenia have persistent psychotic symptoms (Mueser et al., 1991b; Tarrier, 1987), which are associated with worse vocational functioning (Racenstein et al., 2002). Psychotic symptoms most often include hallucinations and delusions, but may also include bizarre behavior, and formal thought disorder (e.g., neologisms, disordered syntax).

Hallucinations such as hearing voices can interfere with obtaining a job or adequately performing work tasks by distracting the individual, reducing his/her ability to focus attention on relevant work-related stimuli (e.g., the interviewer, a customer or co-worker, or a job task). Hallucinations are often distressing and contribute to anxiety or depression (Chadwick & Birchwood, 1994), which can reduce job performance independent of their effects on attention. Delusions or false beliefs, which are tenaciously held despite overwhelming evidence against them, take a variety of forms in schizophrenia, most often including paranoia, delusions of control (e.g., thought insertion, thought withdrawal), or religious or grandiose delusions. Delusions can interfere with work when they lead to strange or inexplicable behaviors at the workplace, either compromising work performance directly, or having a negative effect on the social milieu at work by frightening or annoying other people.

The negative symptoms of schizophrenia include blunted affect (reduced facial and vocal expressiveness), alogia (reduced verbal output or content), apathy (difficulty initiating or following through on plans of action), and anhedonia (reduced pleasure). Negative symptoms tend to be relatively stable over time, and can interfere with the ability to work in a variety of ways. Blunted affect during social interactions can inadvertently convey to the conversational partner that the person is not interested in what they are saying, or suggest lack of enthusiasm or motivation, which can have damaging effects at the workplace. In truth, when blunted affect is present it does not accurately convey the person's internal feelings, which have generally been found to be intact rather than muted (Berenbaum & Oltmanns, 1992), and therefore the person must learn to communicate his or her feelings verbally.

Apathy and anhedonia are closely related to each other as a diminished capacity for pleasure, including the ability to anticipate and reflect back on rewarding experiences (Burbridge & Barch, 2007), can naturally reduce the individual's motivation to initiate and pursue presumably reinforcing activities. Not surprisingly, apathy and anhedonia can be reflected in reduced effort to seek and maintain employment, as the individual perceives (and potentially experiences) less reinforcement from work. Negative symptoms are well established predictors of psychosocial impairment in schizophrenia, including work (McGurk & Mueser, 2004; Pogue-Geile, 1989), with apathy–anhedonia most strongly associated with impaired functioning (Sayers et al., 1996).

Social competence, or the ability to be effective in interpersonal situations, requires a combination of social skills and social cognition. Social skills are the specific verbal, nonverbal, and paralinguistic (e.g., voice tone and loudness) behaviors that are used in social situations to communicate with others. Social cognition is the broad set of cognitive skills and knowledge necessary to accurately understand and perceive social information that has relevance to effective and appropriate behaviors during an encounter, such as recognizing the other person's emotions through facial expressions and voice tone, under-standing what the other person might be thinking based on clues and the nature of the situation (i.e., theory of mind), awareness of the relationship between the two individuals (e.g., friend, co-worker, case manager), and familiarity with "unwritten social rules" (e.g., the "rules" of the workplace). People with schizophrenia have significant impairments in both social skills and social cognition (Bellack et al., 1990, 1992; Penn et al., 1997). Some evidence suggests that impaired social cognition mediates the association between impaired cognitive functioning and functional outcomes (Brekke et al., 2005).

Poor social skills and social cognition can have a prominent impact on getting and keeping a job. Problems accurately tracking another person's feelings during an interaction, and being able to recognize hints or someone's intentions, can render people less sensitive to interpersonal nuances that are critical to effective interactions with co-workers, super-visors, and customers. Suboptimal social skills can interfere with accurately communicating appropriate interest, understanding, concern, or empathy during interactions at the work-place. For these reasons, impaired social skills and social communication have been linked to worse vocational functioning in schizophrenia (Bae et al., 2010; Bellack et al., 1990; Mueller, 1988; Mueser, 2002).

Cognitive functioning and work

Cognitive impairments frequently precede the onset of schizophrenia, worsen during the prodrome, and are a prominent feature over the long-term course of the disorder (Lewandowski et al., 2011). Impairments occur across a wide range of cognitive domains, including attention and vigilance, working memory, processing speed, learning and memory, and executive functions (Heaton et al., 1994). Poor cognitive functioning is an important correlate of the broad range of psychosocial adjustment in schizophrenia (Green, 1996; Harvey et al., 2004), including work (Kaneda et al., 2010; McGurk & Mueser, 2004). The relationship between cognition and work outcomes has been evaluated in cross-sectional comparisons of employed versus unemployed clients (McGurk & Meltzer, 2000; McGurk & Mueser, 2004; Meltzer, 1999), retrospectively in clients with good versus poor vocational outcomes (Bellack et al., 1999), and prospectively (Gold et al., 2002; McGurk & Mueser, 2004; Mueser et al., 2001b; Tsang et al., 2010). Despite differences in methods across these studies, a consistent pattern has emerged from this literature: better cognitive functioning is associated with better work outcomes (McGurk & Mueser, 2004). One recent study found that self-reports of impaired cognitive functioning in schizophrenia were also linked to worse occupational functioning (Verdoux et al., 2010).

Poor cognitive functioning is also related to an attenuated response to vocational rehabilitation. People with serious mental illness who have more compromised cognitive functioning have more difficulty engaging in vocational rehabilitation services (O'Connor et al., 2011). Once they are receiving vocational rehabilitation, clients with impaired cognitive functioning have worse employment outcomes (Bell & Bryson, 2001; Bryson et al., 1998; Lysaker et al., 1995), including when receiving supported employment (McGurk et al., 2003; Mueser, 2002), an evidence-based practice for improving work outcomes in schizophrenia and other serious mental illnesses.

Supported employment

The Individual Placement and Support (IPS) model of supported employment was developed and standardized to improve competitive work in people with a serious mental illness. Supported employment is defined by the inclusion of all clients who want to work, rapid job search and no prevocational training, focus on competitive jobs in integrated community settings, attention to consumer preferences regarding types of jobs and services received, follow-along supports after job acquisition, and benefits counseling (Becker & Drake, 2003). Numerous quasi-experimental (Bailey et al., 1998; Becker et al., 2001; Drake et al., 1994, 1996a; Torrey et al., 1995, 1997) and randomized controlled trials (Bond et al., 2008) have demonstrated the superiority of supported employment over other vocational rehabilitation models for improving work outcomes.

Although supported employment is the only evidence-based vocational rehabilitation model for schizophrenia, there is still much room for improvement. Research on supported employment indicates that 30%–60% of clients do not get competitive jobs or work very little, and when work is obtained clients often hold jobs for relatively brief periods of time (Drake et al., 1996b, 1999; Gervey & Bedell, 1994; Lehman et al., 2002; McGurk et al., 2003; Mueser et al., 2004; Shafer & Huang, 1995; Wong et al., 2004). Furthermore, competitive jobs often end unsuccessfully, with the client being fired or walking off the job (Becker et al., 1998; Mueser et al., 2001a). While a variety of reasons for unsuccessful job endings have been identified, problems with poor job performance due to impaired cognitive functioning are common, a finding that has led to research on the effects of providing cognitive remediation or enhancement to clients participating in vocational rehabilitation programs.

Cognitive remediation and vocational rehabilitation

The recognition of the importance of cognitive impairment in schizophrenia to community functioning, including work, has led to the proliferation of cognitive remediation programs (Kurzban et al., 2010). Cognitive remediation interventions differ along a broad range of dimensions, including the methods and technology used to improve cognitive functioning (e.g., computer-based vs. paper-and-pencil practice), the cognitive domains targeted for enhancement (one or two specific cognitive domains vs. a broad range of cognitive functions), the use and specific activities of a program facilitator to guide the cognitive remediation exercises (e.g., directions for independent use of software, teaching of meta-cognitive and compensatory strategies), the use of ancillary group processes (e.g., discussion or practice groups), duration and intensity of training sessions, and the relationship of the cognitive remediation intervention to other psychiatric rehabilitation services (stand-alone cognitive programs vs. programs that are parallel or fully integrated with psychosocial rehabilitation). Despite these programmatic differences, there is a core element included in most programs, which is the provision of drill-and-practice exercises designed to engage various cognitive areas in focused, repeated practice or "exercise" (Fisher et al., 2009; Greig et al., 2007) in order to improve them.

Over the past several decades numerous randomized controlled trials have been conducted evaluating the effects of cognitive remediation programs for serious mental illness. Recently, two meta-analyses of controlled research on cognitive remediation for schizophrenia have been published, including 26 and 40 studies, respectively (McGurk et al., 2007b; Wykes et al., 2011). The findings of the two meta-analyses were remarkably similar, with both reporting significant moderate effects for improved cognitive remediation on cognitive functioning (effect sizes, 0.41 and 0.45, respectively) and psychosocial functioning (effect sizes, 0.36 and 0.43, respectively), and small effects on reducing symptoms (effect sizes, 0.28 and 0.18, respectively). Most importantly, both meta-analyses found that the effect of cognitive remediation on psychosocial functioning was moderated by the provision of adjunctive psychiatric rehabilitation (e.g., social skills training, vocational rehabilitation). Specifically, studies that provided cognitive remediation in addition to psychiatric rehabilitation (compared to psychiatric rehabilitation alone) demonstrated even stronger effects of remediation on psychosocial outcomes, whereas significantly weaker effects on psychosocial functioning were found in studies comparing cognitive remediation and usual services to usual services alone. The results of these meta-analyses suggest that improved cognitive functioning facilitates the ability of people with schizophrenia to learn and benefit more from psychiatric rehabilitation, and that it is the psychiatric rehabilitation, not the cognitive remediation, that has the most direct impact on improving psychosocial functioning. This interpretation is consistent with the well-established association between cognitive impairment and diminished response to rehabilitation approaches such as vocational rehabilitation (Evans et al., 2004; McGurk et al., 2003) and social skills training (Mueser et al., 1991a; Silverstein et al., 1998; Smith et al., 1999).

The results of seven randomized controlled trials comparing cognitive remediation and vocational rehabilitation to vocational rehabilitation alone for clients with schizophrenia or other serious mental illnesses have all demonstrated significant effects on work outcomes favoring the addition of cognitive remediation (Bell et al., 2001, 2004, 2005, 2007, 2008; Greig et al., 2007; Lindenmayer et al., 2008; McGurk et al., 2005, 2007a, 2009; Vauth et al., 2005; Wexler & Bell, 2005). Despite the positive effects of cognitive remediation in these studies, as can be seen from Table 6.1, they were quite disparate in important methodological aspects, such as the client population, the vocational rehabilitation model, the work outcomes reported, the nature of the cognitive intervention and the intensity of the training program, and the methods of combining the cognitive remediation and vocational programs. While the mechanisms underlying the beneficial effects of cognitive remediation on the outcomes of vocational rehabilitation programs remain to be determined, improved capacity for learning and skills for managing persistent cognitive impairments that can interfere with work are leading candidates (McGurk & Wykes, 2008).

Another important question raised by research on the effects of adding cognitive remediation to vocational rehabilitation is the most effective combination of the two treatment approaches. Current methods are quite varied. For example, some approaches involve staging the cognitive remediation by providing it first, followed by vocational rehabilitation (Vauth et al., 2005). Another approach is to provide the two programs in a parallel fashion (Bell et al., 2005, 2007), and yet another approach is to integrate the cognitive remediation with the vocational rehabilitation (McGurk et al., 2005, 2007a, 2009). It is possible that the optimal approach depends on the vocational rehabilitation and/or cognitive remediation model employed, or pertinent characteristics of the client, such as the nature of his/her cognitive impairment, educational level, and prior work experience.

Summary and conclusions

Poor vocational functioning is a hallmark of schizophrenia that contributes to the high global burden of the disease on individuals, their families, and society. A wide range of disadvantages and impairments contribute to the low rates of competitive work in schizophrenia, including poor premorbid functioning, low levels of educational attainment, positive and negative symptoms, social skill deficits, and impaired cognitive functioning. Difficulties with cognitive functioning in schizophrenia are associated with worse vocational outcomes in the competitive labor market, and with reduced benefit from vocational rehabilitation programs, including evidence-based supported employment.

The strong association between impaired cognitive functioning and poor psychosocial adjustment in schizophrenia, especially work, has led to efforts to improve cognitive abilities through systematic training efforts, or cognitive remediation. Meta-analyses of multiple randomized controlled trials of cognitive remediation in schizophrenia have demonstrated positive effects on cognitive functioning and psychosocial adjustment, and small improvements in symptoms. However, this research also shows that the beneficial effects of cognitive remediation on psychosocial functioning are contingent upon the provision of adjunctive psychiatric rehabilitation; thus, whereas cognitive remediation has negligible effects on psychosocial functioning (including work) when provided alone, it has substantial effects on improving psychosocial functioning when added to a psychiatric rehabilitation program, such as supported employment. Seven randomized controlled trials have demonstrated the positive effects of cognitive remediation on work outcomes when provided in addition to vocational rehabilitation for schizophrenia, compared to vocational rehabilitation alone. While the mechanisms underlying the effects of these cognitive

Table 6.1. Summary of studies of cognitive remediation and psychiatric rehabilitation

Studies	Subject population	Cognitive remediation program	Psychiatric rehabilitation program	Timing of cognitive remediation and psychosocial rehabilitation	Functional outcomes/ follow-up period
Bell et al., 2001, Bell et al., 2005	Unemployed VA patients	Neurocognitive enhancement therapy (NET): 36 hours of computerized drill-and-practice (Odie Bracie) over 26 weeks, and weekly social and work processing groups	Inpatient compensated work therapy	Parallel	Paid work in VA work therapy program/ 12 months
Wexler & Bell, 2005	Unemployed outpatients with interest in work	NET: 72 hours of computerized drill-and-practice (Odie Bracie) over 52 weeks and weekly social and work processing groups	Vocational rehabilitation	Parallel	Subsidized and competitive work/ 12 months
Vauth et al., 2005	Unemployed inpatients	Cognitive enhancement program: 24 hours over 8 weeks of teaching coping strategies, computerized drill-and-practice and environmental modifications in simulated work environments	Vocational rehabilitation	Sequential: cognitive remediation program followed by vocational rehabilitation	All paid work/ 12 months
McGurk et al., 2007a, McGurk et al., 2005	54 outpatients enroled in supported employment with history of job loss	The thinking skills for work program: 24 hours of computerized practice (Cogpack) with strategy coaching over 12 weeks; consultation of cognitive specialist with employment specialist regarding the use of compensatory strategies during job search and job performance	Supported employment	Integrated	Competitive work/ 24–36 months
Bell et al., 2007, Greig et al., 2007	Outpatients	NET: 126 hours of computerized drill-and-practice over 34 weeks and weekly social and work processing groups	Vocational rehabilitation	Parallel	Work/12 months
Lindenmayer et al., 2008	Inpatients	24 hours of computerized cognitive remediation over 12 weeks drill-and-practice	Inpatient work program	Parallel	Compensated work/12 months
McGurk et al., 2009	34 outpatients enroled in a work-oriented day treatment program	The thinking skills for work program (see McGurk et al., 2005)	Vocational rehabilitation	Integrated	Competitive and non competitive work/12 months

remediation programs remain unknown, as does the optimal approach to combining cognitive remediation with vocational rehabilitation, these recent findings provide hope that targeting impaired cognitive functioning may facilitate learning and response to these programs, leading to improved employment outcomes, economic standing, and quality of life.

References

American Psychiatric Association. (1994). *Diagnostic and Statistical Manual of Mental Disorders (DSM-IV)*. Washington, DC: American Psychiatric Association.

Bae, S.-M., Lee, S.-H., Park, Y.-M., et al. (2010). Predictive factors of social functioning in patients with schizophrenia: exploration for the best combination of variables using data mining. *Psychiatry Investigation*, **7**, 93–101.

Bailey, E. L., Ricketts, S. K., Becker, D. R., et al. (1998). Do long-term day treatment clients benefit from supported employment? *Psychiatric Rehabilitation Journal*, **22**, 24–29.

Becker, D. R., Bond, G. R., McCarthy, D., et al. (2001). Converting day treatment centers to supported employment programs in Rhode Island. *Psychiatric Services*, **52**, 351–357.

Becker, D. R. & Drake, R. E. (2003). *A Working Life for People with Severe Mental Illness*. New York, NY: Oxford University Press.

Becker, D. R., Drake, R. E., Bond, G. R., et al. (1998). Job terminations among persons with severe mental illness participating in supported employment. *Community Mental Health Journal*, **34**, 71–82.

Bell, M. D. & Bryson, G. (2001). Work rehabilitation in schizophrenia: does cognitive impairment limit improvement? *Schizophrenia Bulletin*, **27**, 269–279.

Bell, M. D., Bryson, G., Greig, T., et al. (2001). Neurocognitive enhancement therapy with work therapy. *Archives of General Psychiatry*, **58**, 763–768.

Bell, M. D., Bryson, G. J., Greig, T. C., et al. (2005). Neurocognitive enhancement therapy with work therapy: productivity outcomes at 6- and 12-month follow-ups. *Journal of Rehabilitation Research and Development*, **42**, 829–838.

Bell, M. D., Fiszdon, J., Bryson, G. J., et al. (2004). Effects of neurocognitive enhancement therapy in schizophrenia: normalisation of memory performance. *Cognitive Neuropsychiatry*, **9**, 199–211.

Bell, M. D., Fiszdon, J., Greig, T., et al. (2007). Neurocognitive enhancement therapy with work therapy in schizophrenia: 6-month followup of neuropsychological performance. *Journal of Rehabilitation Research and Development*, **44**, 761–770.

Bell, M. D., Zito, W., Greig, T., et al. (2008). Neurocognitive enhancement therapy with vocational services: work outcomes at two-year follow-up. *Schizophrenia Research*, **105**, 18–29.

Bellack, A. S., Gold, J. M., & Buchanan, R. W. (1999). Cognitive rehabilitation for schizophrenia: problems, prospects, and strategies. *Schizophrenia Bulletin*, **25**, 257–274.

Bellack, A. S., Morrison, R. L., Wixted, J. T., et al. (1990). An analysis of social competence in schizophrenia. *British Journal of Psychiatry*, **156**, 809–818.

Bellack, A. S., Mueser, K. T., Wade, J. H., et al. (1992). The ability of schizophrenics to perceive and cope with negative affect. *British Journal of Psychiatry*, **160**, 473–480.

Berenbaum, H. & Oltmanns, T. F. (1992). Emotional experience and expression in schizophrenia and depression. *Journal of Abnormal Psychology*, **101**, 37–44.

Bond, G. R., Drake, R. E., & Becker, D. R. (2008). An update on randomized controlled trials of evidence-based supported employment. *Psychiatric Rehabilitation Journal*, **31**, 280–290.

Bond, G. R., Resnick, S. G., Drake, R. E., et al. (2001). Does competitive employment improve nonvocational outcomes for people with severe mental illness? *Journal of Consulting and Clinical Psychology*, **69**, 489–501.

Brekke, J. S., Kay, D. D., Lee, K. S., et al. (2005). Biosocial pathways to functional outcome in schizophrenia. *Schizophrenia Research*, **80**, 213–225.

Brekke, J. S., Levin, S., Wolkon, G. H., et al. (1993). Psychosocial functioning and subjective experience in schizophrenia. *Schizophrenia Bulletin*, **19**, 600–608.

Bryson, G., Bell, M. D., Kaplan, E., et al. (1998). The functional consequences of memory impairments on initial work performance in people with schizophrenia. *Journal of Nervous and Mental Disease*, **186**, 610–615.

Burbridge, J. A. & Barch, D. M. (2007). Anhedonia and the experience of emotion in individuals with schizophrenia. *Journal of Abnormal Psychology*, **116**, 30–42.

Burns, T., Catty, J., Becker, T., et al. (2007). The effectiveness of supported employment for people with severe mental illness: a randomized controlled trial. *Lancet*, **370**, 1146–1152.

Chadwick, P. & Birchwood, M. (1994). The omnipotence of voices: a cognitive approach to auditory hallucinations. *British Journal of Psychiatry*, **164**, 190–201.

Draine, J., Salzer, M. S., Culhane, D. P., et al. (2002). Role of social disadvantage in crime, joblessness, and homelessness among persons with serious mental illness. *Psychiatric Services*, **53**, 565–573.

Drake, R. E., Becker, D. R., Biesanz, B. A., et al. (1996a). Day treatment versus supported employment for persons with severe mental illness: a replication study. *Psychiatric Services*, **47**, 1125–1127.

Drake, R. E., Becker, D. R., Biesanz, J. C., et al. (1994). Rehabilitative day treatment vs. supported employment: I. Vocational outcomes. *Community Mental Health Journal*, **30**, 519–532.

Drake, R. E., Mchugo, G. J., Bebout, R. R., et al. (1999). A randomized clinical trial of supported employment for inner-city patients with severe mental illness. *Archives of General Psychiatry*, **56**, 627–633.

Drake, R. E., McHugo, G. J., Becker, D. R., et al. (1996b). The New Hampshire study of supported employment for people with severe mental illness: vocational outcomes. *Journal of Consulting and Clinical Psychology*, **64**, 391–399.

Evans, J. D., Bond, G. R., Meyer, P. S., et al. (2004). Cognitive and clinical predictors of success in vocational rehabilitation in schizophrenia. *Schizophrenia Research*, **70**, 331–342.

Fisher, M., Holland, C., Merzenich, M. M., et al. (2009). Using neuroplasticity-based auditory training to improve verbal memory in schizophrenia. *American Journal of Psychiatry*, **166**, 805–811.

Gervey, R. & Bedell, J. R. (1994). Supported employment in vocational rehabilitation. In J. R. Bedell (ed.), *Psychological Assessment and Treatment of Persons with Severe Mental Disorders*. Washington, DC: Taylor & Francis.

Gold, J. M., Goldberg, R. W., McNary, S. W., et al. (2002). Cognitive correlates of job tenure among patients with severe mental illness. *American Journal of Psychiatry*, **159**, 1395–1402.

Green, M. F. (1996). What are the functional consequences of neurocognitive deficits in schizophrenia? *American Journal of Psychiatry*, **153**, 321–330.

Greig, T. C., Zito, W., Wexler, B. E., et al. (2007). Improved cognitive function in schizophrenia after one year of cognitive training and vocational services. *Schizophrenia Research*, **96**, 156–161.

Häfner, H. & an der Heiden, W. (2008). Course and outcome. In K. T. Mueser & D. V. Jeste (eds.), *Clinical Handbook of Schizophrenia*. New York, NY: Guilford Press.

Hans, S. L., Marcus, J., Henson, L., et al. (1992). Interpersonal behavior of children at risk for schizophrenia. *Psychiatry*, **55**, 314–335.

Harvey, P. D., Green, M. F., Keefe, R. S., et al. (2004). Cognitive functioning in schizophrenia: a consensus statement on its role in the definition and evaluation of effective treatments for the illness. *Journal of Clinical Psychiatry*, **65**, 361–372.

Heaton, R., Paulsen, J. S., McAdams, L. A., et al. (1994). Neuropsychological deficits in schizophrenics: relationship to age, chronicity, and dementia. *Archives of General Psychiatry*, **51**, 469–476.

Jencks, C. (1979). *Who Gets Ahead? The Determinants of Economic Success in America*. New York, NY: Basic Books.

Kaneda, Y., Jayathilak, K., & Meltzer, H. (2010). Determinants of work outcome in neuroleptic-resistant schizophrenia and schizoaffective disorder: cognitive impairment and clozapine treatment. *Psychiatry Research*, **178**, 57–62.

Kessler, R. C., Foster, C. L., Saunders, W. B., et al. (1995). Social consequences of psychiatric disorders, I. Educational attainment. *American Journal of Psychiatry*, **152**, 1026–1032.

Kurzban, S., Davis, L., & Brekke, J. S. (2010). Vocational, social, and cognitive rehabilitation for individuals diagnosed with schizophrenia: a review of recent research and trends. *Current Psychiatry Reports*, **12**, 345–355.

Lehman, A. F., Goldberg, R., Dixon, L. B., et al. (2002). Improving employment outcomes for persons with severe mental illnesses. *Archives of General Psychiatry*, **59**, 165–172.

Lewandowski, K. E., Cohen, B. M., & Öngur, D. (2011). Evolution of neuropsychological dysfunction during the course of schizophrenia and bipolar disorder. *Psychological Medicine*, **41**, 225–241.

Lewine, R. R. J. (2005). Social class of origin, lost potential, and hopelessness in schizophrenia. *Schizophrenia Research*, **76**, 329–335.

Lindamer, L. A., Buse, D. C., Auslander, L., et al. (2003). A comparison of gynecological variables and service use among older women with and without schizophrenia. *Psychiatric Services*, **54**, 902–904.

Lindenmayer, J. P., McGurk, S. R., Mueser, K. T., et al. (2008). Cognitive remediation in persistently mentally ill inpatients: a randomized controlled trial. *Psychiatric Services*, **59**, 241–247.

Lysaker, P. H., Bell, M. D., Zito, W. S., et al. (1995). Social skills at work: deficits and predictors of improvement in schizophrenia. *Journal of Nervous and Mental Disease*, **183**, 688–692.

MacBeth, A. & Gumley, A. (2008). Premorbid adjustment, symptom development and quality of life in first episode psychosis: a systematic review and critical reappraisal. *Acta Psychiatrica Scandinavica*, **117**, 85–99.

Malla, A. & Payne, J. (2005). First-episode psychosis: psychopathology, quality of life, and functional outcome. *Schizophrenia Bulletin*, **31**, 650–671.

Malmberg, A., Lewis, G., David, A., et al. (1998). Premorbid adjustment and personality in people with schizophrenia. *British Journal of Psychiatry*, **172**, 308–313.

Marwaha, S., Johnson, S., Bebbington, P., et al. (2007). Rates and correlates of employment in people with schizophrenia in the UK, France and Germany. *British Journal of Psychiatry*, **191**, 30–37.

McGurk, S. R. & Meltzer, H. Y. (2000). The role of cognition in vocational functioning in schizophrenia. *Schizophrenia Research*, **45**, 175–184.

McGurk, S. R. & Mueser, K. T. (2004). Cognitive functioning, symptoms, and work in supported employment: a review and heuristic model. *Schizophrenia Research*, **70**, 147–174.

McGurk, S. R., Mueser, K. T., Derosa, T., et al. (2009). Work, recovery, and comorbidity in schizophrenia: a randomized controlled trial of cognitive remediation. *Schizophrenia Bulletin*, **35**, 319–335.

McGurk, S. R., Mueser, K. T., Feldman, K., et al. (2007a). Cognitive training for supported employment: 2–3 year outcomes of a randomized controlled trial. *American Journal of Psychiatry*, **164**, 437–441.

McGurk, S. R., Mueser, K. T., Harvey, P. D., et al. (2003). Cognitive and clinical predictors of work outcomes in clients with schizophrenia. *Psychiatric Services*, **54**, 1129–1135.

McGurk, S. R., Mueser, K. T., & Pascaris, A. (2005). Cognitive training and supported employment for persons with severe mental illness: one year results from a randomized controlled trial. *Schizophrenia Bulletin*, **31**, 898–909.

McGurk, S. R., Twamley, E. W., Sitzer, D. I., et al. (2007b). A meta-analysis of cognitive remediation in schizophrenia. *American Journal of Psychiatry*, **164**, 1791–1802.

McGurk, S. R. & Wykes, T. (2008). Cognitive remediation and vocational rehabilitation. *Psychiatric Rehabilitation Journal*, **31**, 350–359.

Meltzer, H. Y. (1999). Outcome in schizophrenia: beyond symptom reduction. *Journal of Clinical Psychiatry*, **60**, 3–7.

Mueller, H. H. (1988). Employers' reasons for terminating the employment of workers in entry-level jobs: implications for workers with mental disabilities. *Canadian Journal of Rehabilitation*, **1**, 233–240.

Mueser, K. T. (2002). Cognitive impairment, symptoms, social functioning, and vocational rehabilitation in schizophrenia. In H. Kashima, I. R. H. Falloon, M. Mizuno, et al. (eds.), *Comprehensive Treatment of Schizophrenia: Linking Neurobehavioral Findings to Psychosocial Approaches*. Tokyo: Springer-Verlag.

Mueser, K. T., Becker, D. R., & Wolfe, R. (2001a). Supported employment, job preferences, and job tenure and satisfaction. *Journal of Mental Health*, **10**, 411–417.

Mueser, K. T., Bellack, A. S., Douglas, M. S., et al. (1991a). Prediction of social skill acquisition in schizophrenic and major affective disorder patients from memory and symptomatology. *Psychiatry Research*, **37**, 281–296.

Mueser, K. T., Bellack, A. S., Morrison, R. L., et al. (1990). Social competence in schizophrenia: premorbid adjustment, social skill, and domains of functioning. *Journal of Psychiatric Research*, **24**, 51–63.

Mueser, K. T., Clark, R. E., Haines, M., et al. (2004). The Hartford study of supported employment for severe mental illness. *Journal of Consulting and Clinical Psychology*, **72**, 479–490.

Mueser, K. T., Douglas, M. S., Bellack, A. S., et al. (1991b). Assessment of enduring deficit and negative symptom subtypes in schizophrenia. *Schizophrenia Bulletin*, **17**, 565–582.

Mueser, K. T., Salyers, M. P., & Mueser, P. R. (2001b). A prospective analysis of work in schizophrenia. *Schizophrenia Bulletin*, **27**, 281–296.

Murray, C. J. L. & Lopez, A. D. (eds.). (1996). *The Global Burden of Disease: A Comprehensive Assessment of Mortality and Disability from Diseases, Injuries, and Risk Factors in 1990 and Projected to 2020*. Harvard School of Public Health on behalf of the World Health Organization and the World Bank, Cambridge, MA: Harvard University Press.

O'Connor, M. J., Mueller, L., Van Ormer, A., et al. (2011). Cognitive impairment as barrier to engagement in vocational services among veterans with severe mental illness. *Journal of Rehabilitation Research & Development*, **48**, 597–608.

Penn, D. L., Corrigan, P. W., Bentall, R. P., et al. (1997). Social cognition in schizophrenia. *Psychological Bulletin*, **121**, 114–132.

Pogue-Geile, M. F. (1989). The prognostic significance of negative symptoms in schizophrenia. *British Journal of Psychiatry Suppl*, **7**, 123–127.

Provencher, H. P., Gregg, R., Mead, S. et al. (2002). The role of work in recovery of persons with psychiatric disabilities. *Psychiatric Rehabilitation Journal*, **26**, 132–144.

Racenstein, J. M., Harrow, M., Reed, R., et al. (2002). The relationship between positive symptoms and instrumental work functioning in schizophrenia: a 10-year follow-up study. *Schizophrenia Research*, **56**, 95–103.

Robins, L. N. (1966). *Deviant Children Grown Up*. Huntington, NY: Robert E. Krieger Publishing.

Rogers, E. S., Walsh, D., Masotta, L., et al. (1991). *Massachusetts Survey of Client Preferences for Community Support Services (Final Report)*. Boston, MA, Center for Psychiatric Rehabilitation.

Salkever, D. S., Karakus, M. C., Slade, E. P., et al. (2007). Measures and predictors of community-based employment and earnings of persons with schizophrenia in a multi-site study. *Psychiatric Services*, **58**, 315–324.

Sayers, S. L., Curran, P. J., & Mueser, K. T. (1996). Factor structure and construct validity of the Scale for the Assessment of

Negative Symptoms. *Psychological Assessment*, **8**, 269–280.

Shafer, M. S. & Huang, H. W. (1995). The utilization of survival analysis to evaluate supported employment services. *Journal of Vocational Rehabilitation*, **5**, 103–113.

Silverstein, S. M., Schenkel, L. S., Valone, C., et al. (1998). Cognitive deficits and psychiatric rehabilitation outcomes in schizophrenia. *Psychiatric Quarterly*, **69**, 169–191.

Smith, T. E., Hull, J. W., Romanelli, S., et al. (1999). Symptoms and neurocognition as rate limiters in skills training for psychotic patients. *American Journal of Psychiatry*, **156**, 1817–1818.

Strauss, J. S. & Carpenter, W. T. (1977). Prediction of outcome in schizophrenia III. Five-year outcome and its predictors. *Archives of General Psychiatry*, **34**, 159–163.

Suslow, T., Schonauer, K., Ohrmann, P., et al. (2000). Prediction of work performance by clinical symptoms and cognitive skills in schizophrenic outpatients. *Journal of Nervous and Mental Disease*, **188**, 116–118.

Tarrier, N. (1987). An investigation of residual psychotic symptoms in discharged schizophrenic patients. *British Journal of Clinical Psychology*, **26**, 141–143.

Torrey, W. C., Becker, D. R., & Drake, R. E. (1995). Rehabilitative day treatment vs. supported employment: II. Consumer, family and staff reactions to a program change. *Psychosocial Rehabilitation Journal*, **18**, 67–75.

Torrey, W. C., Clark, R. E., Becker, D. R., et al. (1997). Switching from rehabilitative day treatment to supported employment.

In L. L. Kennedy (ed.), *Continuum, Developments in Ambulatory Mental Health Care*. San Francisco, CA: Jossey-Bass.

Tsang, H. W., Leung, A. Y., Chung, R. C., et al. (2010). Review on vocational predictors: a systematic review of predictors of vocational outcomes among individuals with schizophrenia: an update since 1998. *Australian and New Zealand Journal of Psychiatry*, **44**, 495–504.

Vauth, R., Corrigan, P. W., Clauss, M., et al. (2005). Cognitive strategies versus self-management skills as adjunct to vocational rehabilitation. *Schizophrenia Bulletin*, **31**, 55–66.

Verdoux, H., Monello, F., Goumilloux, R., et al. (2010). Self-perceived cognitive deficits and occupational outcome in persons with schizophrenia. *Psychiatry Research*, **178**, 437–439.

Wexler, B. E. & Bell, M. D. (2005). Cognitive remediation and vocational rehabilitation for schizophrenia. *Schizophrenia Bulletin*, **31**, 931–941.

Wong, K. K., Chiu, L.-P., Tang, S-W., et al. (2004). A supported employment program for people with mental illness in Hong Kong. *American Journal of Psychiatric Rehabilitation*, **7**, 83–96.

Wykes, T., Huddy, V., Cellard, C., et al. (2011). A meta-analysis of cognitive remediation for schizophrenia: methodology and effect sizes. *American Journal of Psychiatry*, **168**, 472–485.

Zigler, E. & Glick, M. (1986). *A Developmental Approach to Adult Psychopathology*. New York, NY: John Wiley & Sons.

Chapter

7

Cognition and functional status in adult and older patients with schizophrenia

Sara J. Czaja and David Loewenstein

Introduction

Schizophrenia is a severely disabling illness characterized by a low rate of recovery that affects about 24 million people worldwide and ranks among the top 10 causes of disability. In the United States alone, over two million people are afflicted with schizophrenia (World Health Organization, 2011). Furthermore, about three in 10 000 people worldwide are newly diagnosed with schizophrenia each year. Although the symptom profile of schizophrenia is diverse across patients and over the course of the illness, most patients experience cognitive and functional decline and impairments in everyday living skills and social functioning. Thus, the illness is not only devastating to the patient (the risk of suicide is high among schizophrenic patients) but also to families and society as a whole. Current treatments for the disorder include: antipsychotic medications, psychosocial treatments such as cognitive behavioral therapy, and functional skills training. Although these treatments have been shown to be efficacious in terms of improvements in social and functional skills, overall recovery rates for patients with schizophrenia are relatively low. Thus, as discussed in other chapters in this book, efforts continue to be directed toward the development of effective treatments for this disorder.

Successful interventions for adults with schizophrenia are predicated on understanding the characteristics of the disease across the life course. This is critically important given the current demographic trends. In 2009, in the United States, people aged 65 years and over accounted for about 13% of the population and are estimated to represent about 20% of the population by 2030, and the number of those aged 85 years and over was about 5.7 million in 2009 and is expected to increase to about 6.6 million by 2020 (Administration on Aging, 2010) (Figure 7.1). These trends are paralleled worldwide. In 2006, almost 500 million people worldwide were 65 years and older and will increase to about one billion by 2030 (National Institute on Aging, 2007). Coupled with population aging is the projected increase in the number of older adults with schizophrenia in the upcoming decades (Bartels & Pratt, 2009; Jeste et al., 1999). Moreover, with the end of large-scale institutional care for non-forensic cases, many older individuals with a long-term history of serious mental illness are being forced to function in various community settings, with a notable lack of success (Harvey et al., 1998). Mental illnesses make a substantial independent contribution to the burden of disease and significantly increase the greater risk for impairments in self-care and everyday living skills, depression, poorer health outcomes and falls, compromised quality of life, repeated inpatient treatment, institutionalization, mortality from a variety of causes, and higher healthcare costs (Bartels & Pratt, 2009; Prince et al., 2007).

Cognitive Impairment in Schizophrenia, ed. Philip D. Harvey. Published by Cambridge University Press. © Cambridge University Press 2013.

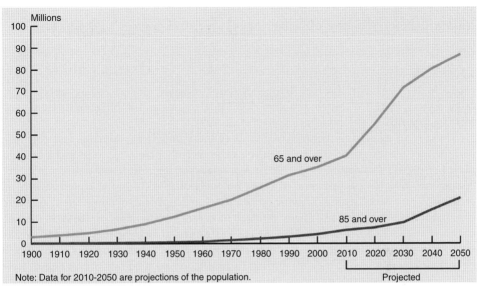

Figure 7.1. Number of people aged 65+ years of age, years 1900–2000 and projected years 2010–2050. (Source: U.S. Census Bureau, Decennial Census and Projections.)

Compared to the rather large body of research focusing on mental illness in younger people, mental illnesses such as schizophrenia have been studied only to a limited degree among older adults. An interesting and important issue is understanding to what extent the patterns of cognitive and functional impairments associated with schizophrenia are diminished, maintained, or exacerbated in later life given normative age-related declines in abilities and the greater propensity among older adults to memory impairments such as dementia. Other important issues are identifying extrinsic (e.g., education) and intrinsic (e.g., changes in brain functioning or structure) factors that impact cognitive and functional deficits over the life course in schizophrenic patients and how the effectiveness of intervention strategies varies as a function of patient age. In this chapter, we attempt to address these issues. We also discuss current techniques for assessing neurocognition and functioning and present some new potential assessment strategies. To provide a context for the remainder of the chapter, we begin by discussing normative age-related changes in cognition followed by a short discussion of memory impairments, dementia, and aging.

Normative age-related changes in sensation/perception and cognition
Visual and auditory acuity

There are a number of normative changes in visual abilities that occur with aging. The incidence of visual impairments such as cataracts and macular degeneration also increases with age. Although most older people do not experience severe visual impairments, they typically experience declines in vision sufficient to make it more difficult to perceive and comprehend visual information. Age-related changes in vision include: declines in static and dynamic visual acuity, a reduction in the range of accommodation, a loss of contrast sensitivity, decreases in dark adaptation, declines in color sensitivity (especially in the blue region), and heightened susceptibility to problems with glare. Visual search skills and the ability to detect targets against a background also decline with age (Kline & Schieber, 1985). Additionally, aging is associated with declines in auditory acuity. Many older adults experience a loss of sensitivity for high frequency tones; difficulty understanding speech, especially if the speech is distorted; problems localizing sounds and in binaural listening; and increased sensitivity to loudness (Schieber et al., 1991).

There is an association between acuity in auditory and visual domains and cognitive performance measures and this has been shown from both a cross-sectional and a longitudinal perspective (Valentijn et al., 2005). Age-related changes in sensory/perceptual processing can also have a pronounced effect on functional skills and the performance of everyday living tasks such as driving, medication management, finding one's way, and communication/socialization. These changes in sensory processing can also exacerbate cognitive declines. For example, if someone has difficulty hearing they may incorrectly interpret medication instructions presented to them by their physician. This problem will be further compounded if they are unable to read labels on medication bottles and have problems with prospective memory. Thus, it is important to recognize these changes when assessing the functional and social skills of older adults and to screen older individuals for sensory functioning so that changes in visual or auditory acuity are not interpreted as changes in cognitive or functional performance. Furthermore, these changes in abilities need to be considered in the design of remediation and intervention programs. For example, one might consider using an online multimedia training program to teach patients basic vocational skills. However, these programs will have limited utility if it is difficult for older patients to read the text on the screen or hear the narrative aspect of the program.

Cognitive processing

Aging is also associated with changes in cognitive abilities. A typical distinction when discussing aging and cognition is between crystallized abilities or abilities that reflect knowledge, such as language skills or knowledge about a particular topical area, and fluid abilities or abilities that are involved in active processing of current or new information. Fluid abilities are very important to new learning and skill acquisition and to active processing of information such as recalling medication instructions or remembering the route to a clinic. It is well established that crystallized abilities tend to remain stable until the very latter decades whereas fluid abilities tend to decline with age (Czaja et al., 2010; Park & Schwartz, 2000).

In terms of specific abilities, working memory – our ability to temporarily "hold" information while it is being processed or used – declines with age. Working memory plays an important role in learning, for example a bus route, or carrying out procedural tasks such as how to use an ATM machine to access cash. Long-term memory is a more permanent memory storage system and the memory store for knowledge. There are different types of long-term memory. Semantic long-term memory refers to the storage system for factual information that we have acquired over our lifetime. Generally, this aspect of memory shows little decline with age. Older adults may experience some problems with retrieval of semantic information if the information has not been used or activated for a while, but generally the information is not lost if appropriate cues are provided. Prospective memory or remembering to do something in the future is another type of long-term memory.

Basically there are two types of prospective memory: time-based prospective memory and event-based prospective memory. Time-based prospective memory is remembering to do something at a later time, such as show up for a clinic appointment the next day at 2 PM. Event-based prospective memory is remembering to do something after some event, such as meeting with a career counselor after the clinic appointment. There are age-related declines in both types of prospective memory but declines are typically greater for time-based prospective memory. Finally, there is procedural long-term memory or remembering how to perform some activity such as driving or using a piece of equipment or some work procedure. The degree of age-related declines in procedural memory depends on how well learned the procedure is or level of automaticity. Older adults do not typically have difficulty remembering procedures that are "automatic" or well learned and they can learn new procedures with sufficient amounts of practice.

Another well-established finding in the cognitive aging literature is that it takes older people longer to process information than younger people. Age differences in processing speed are especially pronounced in the older decades. They also increase with task complexity. Attention, our capacity for processing information, also shows age-related declines. In addition, there are age-related differences in reasoning abilities or the ability to draw inferences from newly presented information and in spatial abilities such as finding one's way or interpreting location- or route-finding information.

Our work (Czaja & Sharit, 2003; Czaja et al., 2001, 2010; Sharit et al., 2009) and that of others (Diehl et al., 1995; Hultsch et al., 1990) has shown that these normative age-related changes in cognitive abilities are important predictors of the performance of everyday living tasks such as work tasks, money management, medication management, and use of everyday technologies. When discussing age-related changes in cognition or other aspects of functioning, there are some important caveats, however. An important distinction is between the younger of the older adults, those aged 65–80 years, and those aged 80+ years. Someone in their 60s and 70s is typically vastly different from someone in their 80s. There are also important differences in characteristics between those who are 80–89 years old and those aged 90+ years. Another important caveat is that aging is associated with tremendous heterogeneity and all older people are not alike due to differences in genetics and experiences over the life course. Aging is also associated with plasticity. As will be discussed later in this chapter and other chapters in this book, older adults can experience improvements and gains in physical, cognitive, and functional performance and can learn new skills. For many tasks, especially those that are well learned, older adults can also employ strategies to compensate for ability declines. In the next section we present some general information on aging and memory impairments and dementia. We include this discussion as it has been postulated that schizophrenia is a variant of dementia. Having a clear understanding of the long-term impact of schizophrenia on cognition and functioning requires discriminating changes associated with the illness from normal age-related changes and also from changes that occur from dementia.

Aging, memory impairment, and dementia

As previously discussed, acquired knowledge and crystallized intelligence seem to be intact in neurologically healthy individuals in their 70s and beyond and there are well-known declines in cognitive processes, such as processing and psychomotor speed, working and episodic memory, and spatial abilities, as well as reductions in abilities to solve novel complex tasks dependent on executive function (Park & Schwartz, 2000; Schaie, 1996).

Fortunately, among those without underlying cerebral impairment, these changes are frequently offset by the continuing acquisition of experience and wisdom derived from life experiences. Therefore, for many individuals, the cognitive effects of aging do not have to cause deterioration in adaptive living skills or quality of life.

On the other hand, age is the greatest risk factor for pathological neurological conditions such as Alzheimer's disease (AD) and other neurodegenerative disorders. Older adults are also susceptible to an increase in other conditions such as diabetes and cardiovascular diseases that may increase the risk of cerebral infarctions secondary to stroke. An increasing number of medications and their potential interactions may also affect cognition, as do manifestations of neuropsychiatric disorders such as depression. When cognitive declines become so disruptive that they start to interfere with one's ability to perform independent activities of daily living successfully, the possibility of dementia must be considered.

Dementia is defined by DSM-IV (American Psychiatric Association, 1994) as impairment in memory and other cognitive domains (i.e., language, visuospatial function, executive abilities), which represent deterioration in premorbid function and are of sufficient severity to interfere with social and/or occupational function. This cannot occur in the presence of alterations in mental function or fluctuating consciousness ascribed to a delirium. Dementia is therefore a diagnosis based on an impaired cognition that is of sufficient severity to impair the ability to perform activities of daily living. Dementia can be caused by many potential etiologies such as AD, cerebrovascular disease, frontotemporal neurodegenerative disorders, diffuse Lewy body disease/Parkinson's disease, or Huntington's disease.

Mild cognitive impairment (MCI) (Petersen, 2003) refers to changes in memory or other cognitive domains that are reported by the patient or collateral informant, and it is confirmed by neuropsychological testing. The typical threshold for neuropsychological impairment is 1.5 SD or more below expected levels, although some groups have lower thresholds of 1.0 SD or more below expected levels (Schinka et al., 2010). The importance of the concept of MCI is that it is a risk factor for decline to a dementia state. In clinical memory disorders clinics, the rate of progression of MCI to dementia is typically 12%–15% per year (Peterson et al., 2003). While there is a greater risk factor for dementia among MCI patients diagnosed in community-based epidemiological studies, significant numbers also revert to a normal state over time, likely reflecting the greater base-rate of Alzheimer's pathology in selected clinical samples (Brooks & Loewenstein, 2010).

Dementia praecox was the term first used by Kraepelin to describe individuals with schizophrenia who were thought to have developed dementia early in life. In this regard, schizophrenia was regarded as a variant of dementia, which was progressive. In our review of the literature, we have determined that both cross-sectional and longitudinal studies have been mixed as to whether cognitive decline is a feature of schizophrenia (Loewenstein et al., 2012). However, there is evidence that those who are continuously hospitalized after the age of 65 years are at much greater risk for decline than those who are younger (Friedman et al., 2001; Harvey et al., 1999). In a recent cross-sectional study, we found that there were greater age-related effects in cognitive processes in nondemented community-dwelling schizophrenia patients relative to psychiatrically unimpaired controls (Loewenstein et al., 2012). This raises the issue of whether there is a particular neurobiological susceptibility of schizophrenic subjects to cognitive impairment that places them at higher risk for dementia. Indeed, Ortiz-Gil et al. (2011) carried out structural MRI and voxel-based morphometry studies of 23 schizophrenia patients who were cognitively preserved versus 26 schizophrenia subjects who were cognitively impaired and 39 matched controls. A subset of these subjects received functional MRI (fMRI). Results indicated the lack of differences in structural abnormalities among the impaired and non-impaired schizophrenic groups with regards to whole brain volume, white and gray matter volumes, or lateral ventricular volume. In contrast, impaired schizophrenic patients showed hypoactivation of the prefrontal cortex and other structures during activation tasks using the N-back test. This supports the notion that altered brain function rather than structural abnormalities per se underlie working memory deficits in schizophrenia. Unfortunately, this does not address the issue of the potential synergy between these functional abnormalities related to schizophrenia and the loss of synaptic connectivity and neurons in the hippocampus and cortical areas that occur as a result of normal aging. If schizophrenia patients indeed have a greater neurobiological susceptibility to structures that affect cognition in normal aging, it would stand to reason that already significant cognitive deficits associated with the disorders could become notably worse in the 70s and beyond.

Jellinger (2001) observed that over half of geriatric schizophrenia patients meet criteria for dementia although it is unknown whether this totally reflects the underlying illness or may also reflect a lifetime accumulation of different medications that affect the brain. With greater understanding of the pathological effects of abnormal beta-amyloid and disorders of tau protein in AD and other disorders, there needs to be more work focused on how pathological processes in schizophrenia interact with pathological processes for which age is a risk factor (Brooks & Loewenstein, 2010). We discuss the issue of cognition in older adults with schizophrenia in the next section.

Cognition and functional performance in older schizophrenic patients

Although there is a substantial body of literature regarding aging, cognition, and functional performance in non-mentally impaired older adults, what is less well known is how age-related changes in cognition and functional activities are manifest in older adults with persistent mental illnesses such as schizophrenia. It is generally well established in the literature that cognitive impairment is a hallmark feature of schizophrenia. The cognitive abilities that show decline with age such as episodic memory, processing speed, and working memory are also those that show impairment in younger schizophrenic patients (Harvey et al., 2006). However, it is not well known whether these impairments are exacerbated in older adults given normative age-related changes in cognitive abilities. In other words, is there an age-related "double whammy" that occurs in older adults with schizophrenia?

Available evidence regarding this question is mixed. The results of cross-sectional studies have suggested that cognition in older people with schizophrenia is either no more impaired than that seen in similarly aged psychiatrically healthy individuals controlling for education (Eyler-Zorrilla et al., 2000; Hijman et al., 2003; Mockler et al., 1997) or is considerably more impaired in comparison to normative standards and not samples of healthy controls (Bowie et al., 2008b; Fucetola et al., 2000). We (Loewenstein et al., 2012) recently examined the association between age and cognitive performance in patients with schizophrenia and psychiatrically healthy older adult controls. The performance of psychiatrically healthy adults aged 70 years and older was superior to the performance of the youngest patients with schizophrenia (aged 40–49 years) on measures of working and episodic memory, executive function, and psychomotor speed. We also found that age effects on cognition were significantly greater for schizophrenia patients on measures of verbal learning and speed of processing. Within both the schizophrenia group and the

(a)

Seconds

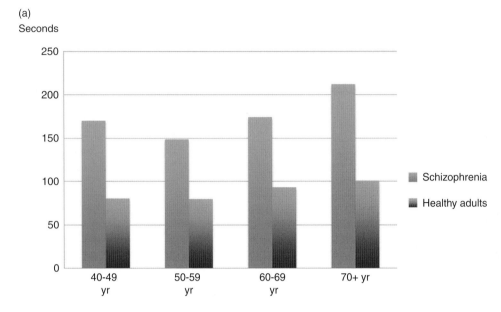

(b)

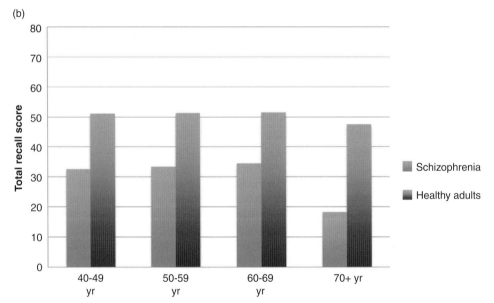

Figure 7.2. (a) Comparative performance for different age groups on Trails B: schizophrenia and healthy adults. (b) Comparative performance for different age groups on CVLT-II: schizophrenia and healthy adults.

psychiatrically healthy adults, the greatest age-related differences in performance occurred in individuals aged 70+ years (Figure 7.2A, B). However, the challenge in all cross-sectional comparisons is the potential of co-founding cohort effects such as differences in available educational programs, assessment instruments, and treatment strategies.

Unfortunately a clear picture also fails to emerge from available longitudinal studies of people with schizophrenia. Savla and colleagues (Savla et al., 2006) evaluated the trajectory of neuropsychological performance among middle-aged and older schizophrenic patients using hierarchical linear modeling. They found that age did not affect the trajectories in patients or the healthy comparison sample. However, the mean age of the patient sample was 53 years and that of the healthy comparison sample about 60 years. The results of other studies have also shown that the trajectory pattern for cognition as a function of age is fairly stable (Granholm et al., 2010; Heaton et al., 2001). Yet, the results from other longitudinal studies suggest generalized worsening in cognition with age (Friedman et al., 2001; Harvey et al., 1999). Generally, from both cross-sectional and longitudinal studies it appears, similar to normative aging, that there is a great deal of variability in the prevalence and extent of cognitive and functional decline in later life among schizophrenic patients. Certain subgroups of patients, such as those who are less educated, or have greater positive symptoms or a history of hospitalization, are more vulnerable to cognitive and functional decline with age (Bowie et al., 2004; Harvey et al., 2006). Differences are also found as a function of onset of the disease. It appears that the cognitive impairments in these populations are discriminable from normal age-related changes and from the changes associated with AD. In neurodegenerative conditions such as AD, there is typically a gradual decline in memory function representing neuronal loss and loss of synaptic function in the hippocampus, entorhinal cortex, and other parts of the medial temporal lobes. However, AD may also present with initial executive, language, and visuospatial deficits. In contrast, there are cognitive deficits in schizophrenia that appear to be most sensitive to or most resemble frontotemporal dementia with predominant executive deficits and minimal parietal lobe involvement (De Vries, 2001). In fact, many of the negative symptoms of schizophrenia including apathy are related to deficits in the dorsolateral regions of the prefrontal cortex (Salgado-Pineda, 2007). Kazui et al. (2011) found that the differences between early AD in the MCI stage and schizophrenia in older adults were that the former group displayed more difficulties with delayed recall and forgetfulness while those with schizophrenia tended to have more difficulties in working memory, attention, and executive function.

Findings regarding age, schizophrenia, and performance on functional tasks important to everyday living are highly similar to those for cognitive functioning. This is not surprising given the generally strong correlation between cognitive abilities and functional performance. For example, numerous studies using varying cognitive assessment strategies have yielded significant correlations between total scores on three versions of the University of California at San Diego (UCSD) performance-based skills assessment (UPSA) and composite neuropsychological test performance (see Leifker et al., 2011, for a review). Further, studies examining the relationship between individual neuropsychological test scores and the UPSA have also yielded significant correlations (McClure et al., 2007). Based on the findings that these measures are highly and consistently related to cognitive functioning on the one hand and everyday real-world functioning on the other, these measures and the skills they assess have been proposed to be an important mediator of the influence of cognitive functioning on everyday outcomes (Bowie et al., 2006, 2008a; McClure et al., 2007). In both schizophrenia and bipolar illness, performance on a measure of everyday functional skills, the UPSA (Patterson et al., 2001), was the best predictor of real-world outcomes in vocational and residential domains, even when the influences of cognition and symptoms were considered (Bowie et al., 2010; Mausbach et al., 2010).

Overall, the controversy surrounding the issue of aging, cognition, functional performance, and schizophrenia may be due to the fact that until recently patients with this disability did not live into the older decades. Thus as noted, the research examining this issue is rather limited. Additionally, as discussed later in this chapter, a variety of techniques are used to assess cognition and functional abilities. Functional capacity is typically rated with a variety of methods including informant reports, self-report by the patient, and performance-based assessment protocols such as the UPSA. Thus part of the discrepancy in findings may be due to differences in assessment strategies. Furthermore, there are differences in the demographics of patient populations included in these studies and other factors such as exposure to treatment strategies. Clearly, this is an important area of further research.

Impact of hospitalization and current treatments on cognitive and functional outcomes

Today, hospital stays for individuals with schizophrenia are relatively brief and involve stabilization and symptom reduction. Hospital stays often range from five to seven days with shorter stays associated with emergency room visits. This is in contrast with several generations ago, when long-term institutional care was the norm and longer hospital stays were associated with poorer outcomes (Harvey et al., in press). However, it should be noted that those individuals who remained hospitalized following the deinstitutionalization movement were more severely impaired, had higher numbers of positive and negative symptoms of schizophrenia, and had more aggressive and unpredictable patterns of behavior. Thus, it is difficult to conclude that hospitalization itself contributed to the poorer outcomes but that people with more severe symptoms remained in hospitals.

Nevertheless, what is evident is that those persons who remained continuously psychotic and treatment unresponsive were more prone to enlargement of the ventricles (preeminently left sided) relative to schizophrenia patients who were successfully treated and did not evidence such enlargement over time (Davis et al., 1998). DeLisi (1999) argues that brain volumes decrease progressively, starting at the time of the first episode or even before a formal diagnosis is made. Indeed, it has been suggested that more severe psychotic symptoms have been associated with greater decline over time (Friedman et al., 2001; Harvey et al., 2003). Thus, persistent psychosis seems associated with progressive brain volume loss as well as with cognitive and functional declines, and losses in critical brain regions may be the substrate for these changes. If persistent psychosis is associated with poorer outcomes, it would seem important to treat these symptoms as effectively as possible through appropriate interventions.

Assessment of cognitive and functional skills in patients with schizophrenia

There has been a broad array of neuropsychological measures, which have been developed to assess the core cognitive features of schizophrenia. The problem has been the many different measures that have been used to assess such areas as memory, attention, processing speed, and aspects of executive function. There have also been a variety of normative databases employed and different cut-offs resulting in the lack of a uniform standard for establishing cognitive impairment versus nonimpairment. This has made it difficult to directly compare the results of various studies conducted in many different sites throughout the world.

The Measurement and Treatment Research to Improve Cognition in Schizophrenia (MATRICS) cognitive battery was developed with the recognition that neurocognitive deficits are a core feature of the illness and should be a legitimate target for the development of pharmacological agents (Green et al., 2004). The MATRICS cognitive battery consists of seven cognitive domains, which include brief and standardized measures of: (1) speed of processing, (2) attention/vigilance, (3) verbal and nonverbal working memory, (4) verbal learning, (5) nonverbal learning, (6) reasoning and problem solving, and (7) social cognition, and has been shown to have high reliability and validity (Nuechterlein et al., 2008). Given that neurocognitive impairments are significant core features of schizophrenia and have been related to functional outcomes, it is understandable that this would be a primary target of specific interventions.

On the other hand, it is often difficulties with real-world functioning that cause the most disruption in the lives of schizophrenia patients. Nuechterlein et al. (2011) found that three principal components of cognition: attention/working memory, verbal memory, and processing speed accounted for 52% of the variance in return to work or school among those with recent-onset schizophrenia. Unfortunately, a significant amount of variance is unaccounted for, which has made it difficult to classify persons at an individual level to determine which neurocognitively impaired persons will exhibit the most impaired functional outcomes. This has led to efforts to identify measures that will capture important aspects of independent daily living. This is extremely important because longitudinal outcomes of first-episode schizophrenic subjects may be less related to initial neurocognitive status rather than what has been suggested by cross-sectional studies that have focused on chronic schizophrenia.

Informant-based reports of functional performance

It is a well-accepted practice to assess functional abilities of schizophrenia patients based upon reports from collateral informants such as a relative or friend or the patient themselves. Unfortunately, there is growing recognition that patients with severe mental illness tend to greatly overestimate their functional abilities while other informants may have positive or negative biases in their perceptions of different aspects of functional performance. This may result in informants being inaccurate in their judgments regarding a schizophrenia patient's functional capacity, and real-world functioning (Bowie et al., 2007; Goldberg et al., 2010; Keefe et al., 2006; Loewenstein et al., 2001; Sabbag et al., 2011). Such informant biases may include but are not limited to denial, minimization, or oversensitivity to perceived impairments. For example, informants who are very depressed or anxious may over-report functional deficits. Other informants such as friends or more distant relatives may not have sufficient opportunity to observe the patient to make reliable functional judgments. For example, we are finding that friends tend to overestimate the functional abilities of patients. This overestimation may reflect the fact that friends may themselves be prone to psychiatric illness and have a limited opportunity to observe specific functional behaviors.

Performance-based measures of functional outcomes

A widely used measure of functional capacity is the UPSA, which assesses an individual's performance on a variety of everyday tasks. There have been over 50 studies of the UPSA in schizophrenia. The UPSA includes tasks such as: communication (i.e., dialing the telephone to schedule a physician's appointment, obtaining and dialing a number from an information operator); finance (counting currency, paying a bill, and making change); transportation (using a bus schedule in planning a trip, understanding related charges, and obtaining needed travel information); comprehension/planning (reading and planning a recreational outing based on scenarios about a trip to the beach on a hot sunny day and the zoo on a cold rainy day); and household management skills (e.g., shopping for grocery items).

There is no doubt that performance-based measures such as the UPSA (Patterson et al., 2001) and shorter versions of the instrument, the UPSA-B (Mausbach et al., 2007), have provided invaluable information that are related to real-world outcomes such as vocational domains and the ability to live independently outside of psychiatric institutions. Indeed, the association between measures of functional capacity like the UPSA and neurocognitive performance in individuals with schizophrenia has been quite robust. There are at least ten published studies using various cognitive assessment methods that have resulted in correlation coefficients ranging from 0.6 to 0.7 between total scores on three versions of the UPSA and composite neuropsychological test scores (Loewenstein et al., 2012).

The UPSA has been endorsed as the best performance-based measure for use in clinical treatment studies (Green et al., 2011). The instrument has also been employed in studies of mild cognitive impairment and methamphetamine abuse (Goldberg et al., 2010; Henry et al., 2010). The psychometric properties of the UPSA are good, and it appears to be sensitive to a wide array of pathological conditions. One criticism that has been raised concerning the UPSA is whether it has potential ceiling effects that will make it difficult to measure changes in non-psychiatrically impaired healthy comparison groups that may be employed in studies of schizophrenia. In a recent report by Harvey et al. (in press), we observed considerable variability in the UPSA total and subscale scores of healthy non-psychiatric subjects. In addition, after regressing the UPSA total score on all of the neuropsychological test predictor variables in the study, it was found that the neuropsychological variables accounted for 40.6% of the total variability in functional performance after accounting for factors such as age and educational attainment. Thus, the UPSA appears to be sensitive to a range of performances among healthy normal subjects even though age and educational attainment did not appear to do so.

There have been other concerns that have been raised about performance-based functional measures such as the UPSA. First, functional capacity as assessed in the clinical and research setting is an essential element that underlies successful functional performance in the environment. However, successful real-world performance on a particular task includes person-, environmental-, and task-specific components. For example, an individual may have the functional capacity to manage one's finances based on the ability to pay bills and manage a checkbook. However, individual factors such as depression, apathy, or problems with prospective memory (remembering to remember an intended action) may still result in real-world difficulties in managing one's financial affairs.

Overall, existing measures do not reflect the situational complexity involved in everyday function (Czaja & Sharit, 2003). Current performance-based functional measures (similar to neuropsychological testing) require patients to perform functional tasks in a rather constrained manner that does not capture the complexities or potential barriers that exist in the everyday world that may alter task performance. For example, complex functional tasks that require multiple steps and place considerable demands on working memory, processing speed, and executive function may be more easily navigated on a simulated performance-based functional task format than in the real world. A patient might be individually able to manage each functional competency alone but have considerable difficulties in the real world when having to deal with multi-tasking and simultaneous functional demands. A further issue related to prospective memory is initiation. The cues to start a task are often quite subtle and self-generated, which is a major area of deficit in people with schizophrenia. Finally, cognitive and functional performance tests are administered in optimal testing conditions with few distractions, and are issues requiring further study.

As previously discussed, there are numerous issues associated with informant and patient reports. Although it is clear that patients greatly overestimate their functional performance (Harvey, 2011), knowledgeable informants may be in a position to observe what the patient can do in everyday life. On the other hand, informants are prone to reporter biases, inadequate opportunity to observe certain functional behaviors, and are likely not as accurate as experienced clinicians familiar with the patient (Sabbag et al., 2011). Finally, all types of informants are probably not equally as accurate in their assessments based on such parameters as time spent with the patient, opportunity to observe certain functional behaviors, and their relationship with the patient (friend versus relative). These are areas that are in need of further research. It may be that combining informant reports with objective functional measures would be the best approach to assess functional abilities in both patient and nonimpaired populations. However, ultimately, logical endpoints include prediction of successful vocational status and performance, independence in managing finances, medications, and other independent activities of daily living as well as residential status.

A final point is that high correlations between cognitive and functional performance outcomes in group analyses do not provide information about the predictive power for an individual case. It is well established that there is considerable performance variability in both patient and nonimpaired populations. For example, Mausbach et al. (2010) has shown that UPSA-B was related to residential and vocational outcomes; 76% of subjects residing independently scored 78 or above on the UPSA-B but 41% of subjects who were not residing independently also scored at or above this threshold. Similarly, 74% of those persons who were employed scored 82 or above on the UPSA-B but almost 43% scored at or above this threshold. While these numbers might be statistically significant, the sensitivity of the UPSA-B in detecting poor outcomes was exceedingly low. To raise the sensitivity to negative outcomes, one could adjust the cut-offs for impairment using Receiver Operator Curve (ROC) analyses, but this would invariably reduce specificity (those persons with positive real-world outcomes, which were correctly classified). Clearly, there is a need for multivariate models to provide the clinician with a better sense of predictors of real-world outcome at a given time-point or longitudinally. More importantly, true positive and negative predictive power of a test or series of tests (which will determine actual false positives and false negatives) is dependent on the base-rates of specific outcomes in certain patient populations. We believe that this is an area that is ripe for future research as we develop methods to better predict outcomes at an individual rather than merely a group level.

Conclusions

Coupled with population aging is the projected increase in the number of older adults with schizophrenia in the upcoming decades. Although the degree of symptom severity varies considerably across patients afflicted with this illness, most patients experience cognitive and functional decline and impairments in everyday living skills and social functioning. Thus, the illness is not only devastating to patients but also to families and society. It is also costly in terms of medical treatment and hospitalizations for these individuals and the impact on the dependency ratio – few patients with this illness are able to successfully engage in long-term employment.

Neurocognitive function is a defining feature of schizophrenia and the MATRICS cognitive battery has endpoints that are legitimate targets of emerging pharmacological and non-pharmacological interventions. Verbal and nonverbal memory deficits, impairments in attention and working memory, processing speed, and executive dysfunction are all important neurocognitive features that may impact real-world functioning. A knowledgeable informant or directly measurable vocational outcomes provide a rich source of information. However, patients are sometimes their own informants and the reports of friends and distant relatives may be biased and inaccurate. Performance-based measures such as the UPSA are highly related to neurocognitive performance, but like neuropsychological measures, are administered in optimal settings with minimal distractions. In real-world situations, successful performance of real-world tasks are a function of person variables (capacity, motivation), task-specific variables (complexity, familiarity), and environmental variables (competing cognitive demands). Thus, measures administered in clinical or research settings may not capture the complex determinants of a successful functional outcome. What is needed are multivariate models that not only show relationships at the group level but can allow a clinician to make accurate predictions at a more individual level.

Debilitating mental illnesses such as schizophrenia have been studied only to a limited degree among older adults. The data that are available are somewhat mixed but suggest that the impacts of the illness on cognitive and functional outcomes may be exacerbated in older adults, especially those with lower educational status, a history of hospitalization, persistent psychosis, or early onset of the disease. As there is accumulating evidence of progressive brain changes over the lifespan in patients with schizophrenia, understanding the course of cognitive deficits in later life will remain an important topic, both for understanding the lifetime course of schizophrenia and for developing interventions aimed at reduction of disability in the illness. What is particularly lacking are necessary longitudinal studies that will help to shed greater light on the determinants of specific cognitive and functional outcomes and their relationship with the underlying biology of brain function, and those interventions that will provide the greatest benefits for people suffering from schizophrenia and related disorders.

References

Administration on Aging. (2010). *A Profile of Older Americans*. Washington, DC: Department of Health and Human Services.

American Psychiatric Association. (1994). *Diagnostic and Statistical Manual of Mental Disorders* (4th edn.). Washington, DC: Author.

Bartels, S. J. & Pratt, S. I. (2009). Psychosocial rehabilitation and quality of life for older adults with serious mental illness: recent findings and future research directions. *Current Opinion in Psychiatry*, **22**, 381–385.

Bowie, C. R., Depp, C., McGrath, J. A., et al. (2010). Prediction of real-world functional disability in chronic mental disorders: a comparison of schizophrenia and bipolar disorder. *American Journal of Psychiatry*, **167**, 1116–1124.

Bowie, C. R., Leung, W. W., Reichenberg, A., et al. (2008a). Specificity of functional skills measures in schizophrenia: relationships to discrete neuropsychological and outcome measures. *Biological Psychiatry*, **63**, 505–511.

Bowie, C. R., Reichenberg, A., McClure, M. M., et al. (2008b). Age-associated differences in cognitive performance in older community dwelling schizophrenia patients: differential sensitivity of clinical neuropsychological and experimental information processing tests. *Schizophrenia Research*, **106**, 50–58.

Bowie, C. R., Reichenberg, A., Patterson, T. L., et al. (2006). Determinants of real-world functioning performance in schizophrenia: correlations with cognition, functional capacity, and symptoms. *American Journal of Psychiatry*, **163**, 418–425.

Bowie, C. R., Reichenberg A., Rieckmann, N., et al. (2004). Stability and functional correlates of memory-based classification in older schizophrenia patients. *American Journal of Geriatric Psychiatry*, **14**, 376–386.

Bowie, C. R., Twamley, E. W., Anderson, H., et al. (2007). Self-assessment of functional status in schizophrenia. *Journal of Psychiatric Research*, **41**, 1012–1018.

Brooks, L. G. & Loewenstein, D. A. (2010). Assessing the progression of mild cognitive impairment to Alzheimer's disease: current trends and future directions. *Alzheimer's Research and Therapy*, **2**, 28.

Czaja, S. J. & Sharit, J. (2003). Practically relevant research: capturing real world tasks, environments, and outcomes. *Gerontologist*, **43**, 9–18.

Czaja, S. J., Sharit, J., Hernandez, M. A., et al. (2010). Variability among older adults in internet health information–seeking performance. *Gerontechnology*, **9**, 46–55.

Czaja, S. J., Sharit, J., Ownby, D., et al. (2001). Examining age differences in performance of a complex information search and retrieval task. *Psychology and Aging*, **16**, 564–579.

Davis, K. L., Buchsbaum, M. S., Shihabuddin, L., et al. (1998). Ventricular enlargement in poor outcome schizophrenia. *Biological Psychiatry*, **43**, 783–793.

DeLisi, L. E. (1999). Defining the course of brain structural change and plasticity in schizophrenia. *Psychiatry Research*, **92**, 1–9.

De Vries, P. J., Honer, W. G., Kemp, P. M., et al. (2001). Dementia as a complication of schizophrenia. *Journal of Neurology, Neurosurgery & Psychiatry*, **70**, 588–596.

Diehl, M., Willis, S. L., & Schaie, K. W. (1995). Everyday problem solving in older adults: observational assessment and cognitive correlates. *Psychology and Aging*, **10**, 478–491.

Eyler-Zorrilla, L. T., Heaton, R. K., McAdams, L. A., et al. (2000). Cross-sectional study of older outpatients with schizophrenia and healthy comparison subjects: no differences in age-related cognitive decline. *American Journal of Psychiatry*, **157**, 1324–1326.

Friedman, J. I., Harvey, P. D., Coleman, T., et al. (2001). Six-year follow-up study of cognitive and functional status across the lifespan in schizophrenia: a comparison with Alzheimer's disease and normal aging. *American Journal of Psychiatry*, **158**, 1441–1448.

Fucetola, R., Seidman, L. J., Kremen, W. S., et al. (2000). Age and neuropsychologic function in schizophrenia: a decline in executive abilities beyond that observed in healthy volunteers. *Biology Psychiatry*, **48**, 137–146.

Granholm, E., Link, P., Fish, S., et al. (2010). Age-related practice effects across longitudinal neuropsychological assessments in older people with schizophrenia. *Neuropsychology*, **24**, 616–624.

Green, M. F., Nuechterlein, K. H., Gold, J. M., et al. (2004). Approaching a consensus cognitive battery for clinical trials in schizophrenia: the NIMH-MATRICS conference to select cognitive domains and test criteria. *Biology Psychiatry*, **56**, 301–307.

Green, M. F., Schooler, N. R., Kern, R. D., et al. (2011). Evaluation of functionally-meaningful measures for clinical trials of cognition enhancement in schizophrenia. *American Journal of Psychiatry*, **168**, 400–407.

Goldberg, T. E., Koppel, J., Keehlisen, L., et al. (2010). Performance-based measures of everyday function in mild cognitive impairment. *American Journal of Psychiatry*, **167**, 845–853.

Harvey, P. D. (2011). Assessment of everyday functioning in schizophrenia. *Innovations in Clinical Neuroscience*, **8**, 21–24.

Harvey, P. D., Bertisch, H., Friedman, J. I., et al. (2003). The course of functional decline in geriatric patients with schizophrenia: cognitive-functional and clinical symptoms as determinants of change. *American Journal of Geriatric Psychiatry*, **11**, 610–619.

Harvey, P. D., Howanitz, E., Parrella, M., et al. (1998). Symptoms, cognitive functioning, and adaptive skills in geriatric patients with lifelong schizophrenia: a comparison across treatment sites. *American Journal of Psychiatry*, **155**, 1080–1086.

Harvey, P. D., Loewenstein, D. A., & Czaja, S. (2012). Hospitalization and psychosis: influences on the course of cognition and everyday functioning in people with schizophrenia. *General Hospital Psychiatry*. [in press].

Harvey, P. D., Reichenberg, A., & Bowie, C. R. (2006). Cognition and aging in psychopathology: focus on schizophrenia and depression. *Annual Review of Clinical Psychology*, **2**, 389–409.

Harvey, P. D., Silverman, J. M., Mohs, R. C., et al. (1999). Cognitive decline in late-life schizophrenia: a longitudinal study of geriatric chronically hospitalized patients. *Biology Psychiatry*, **45**, 32–40.

Heaton, R. K., Gladsjo, J. A., Palmer, B. W., et al. (2001). Stability and course of neuropsychological deficits in schizophrenia. *Archives of General Psychiatry*, **58**, 24–32.

Henry, B. L., Minassian, A., & Perry, W. (2010). Effect of methamphetamine dependence on everyday functional ability. *Addictive Behaviors*, **35**, 593–598.

Hijman, R., Hulshoff Pol, H. E., Sitskoorn, M. M., et al. (2003). Global intellectual impairment does not accelerate with age in patients with schizophrenia: a cross-sectional analysis. *Schizophrenia Bulletin*, **29**, 509–517.

Hultsch, D. F., Hertzog, C., & Dixon, R. A. (1990). Ability correlates of memory performance in adulthood and aging. *Psychology and Aging*, **5**, 356–368.

Jellinger, K. (2001). Dementia as a complication of schizophrenia. *Journal of Neurology, Neurosurgery and Psychiatry*, **71**, 707–708.

Jeste, D. V., Alexopoulos, G. S., Bartels, S. J., et al. (1999). Consensus statement on the upcoming crisis in geriatric mental health. *Archives of General Psychiatry*, **56**, 848–853.

Kazui, H., Yoshida, T., Takaya, M., et al. (2011). Different characteristics of cognitive impairment in elderly schizophrenia and Alzheimer's disease in the mild cognitive impairment stage. *Dementia and Geriatric Cognitive Disorders*, **1**, 20–30.

Keefe, R. S. E., Poe, M., Walker, T. M., et al. (2006). The schizophrenia cognition rating scale: an interview-based assessment and its relationship to cognition, real-world functioning, and functional capacity. *American Journal of Psychiatry*, **163**, 426–432.

Kline, D. W. & Schieber, F. J. (1985). Vision and aging. In J. E. Birren and K. W. Schaie (eds.), *Handbook of the Psychology of Aging*. New York, NY: Van Nostrand Reinhold, pp. 296–331.

Leifker, F. R., Patterson, T. L., Heaton, R. K., et al. (2011). Validating measures of real-world outcome: the results of the VALERO Expert Survey and RAND Panel. *Schizophrenia Bulletin*, **37**, 334–343.

Loewenstein, D. A., Argüelles, S., Bravo, M., et al. (2001). Caregivers' judgments of the functional abilities of the Alzheimer's disease patient: a comparison of proxy reports and objective measures. *Journal of Gerontology Series B Psychological Sciences and Social Sciences*, **56**, P78–84.

Loewenstein, D. A., Czaja, S. J., Bowie, C. R., et al. (2012). Age-associated differences in cognitive performance in older patients with schizophrenia: a comparison with healthy older adults. *The American Journal of Geriatric Psychiatry*, **20**, 29–40.

Mausbach, B. T., Harvey, P. D., Goldman, S. R., et al. (2007). Development of a brief scale of everyday functioning in persons with serious mental illness. *Schizophrenia Bulletin*, **33**, 1364–1372.

Mausbach, B. T., Harvey, P. D., Pulver, A. E., et al. (2010). Relationship between the UCSD Performance-Based Skills Assessment (UPSA-B) and multiple indicators of functioning in people with schizophrenia and bipolar disorder. *Bipolar Disorder*, **12**, 45–55.

McClure, M. M., Bowie, C. R., Patterson, T. L., et al. (2007). Correlations of functional capacity and neuropsychological performance in schizophrenia: evidence for specificity of relationships? *Schizophrenia Research*, **89**, 330–338.

Mockler, D., Riordan, J., & Sharma, T. (1997). Memory and intellectual deficits do not decline with age in schizophrenia. *Schizophrenia Research*, **26**, 1–7.

National Institute on Aging. (2007). *Why Population Aging Matters: A Global Perspective*. Washington, DC: National Institute on Aging/National Institute of Health.

Nuechterlein, K. H., Green, M. F., Kern, R. S., et al. (2008). The MATRICS Consensus Cognitive Battery, part 1: test selection, reliability, and validity. *American Journal of Psychiatry*, **165**, 203–213.

Nuechterlein, K. H., Subotnik, K. L., Green, M. F., et al. (2011). Neurocognitive predictors of work outcome in recent-onset schizophrenia. *Schizophrenia Bulletin*, **37**, S33–40.

Ortiz-Gil, J., Pomarol-Clotet, E., Salvador, R., et al. (2011). Neural correlates of cognitive impairment in schizophrenia. *British Journal of Psychiatry*, **199**, 202–210.

Park, D. & Schwartz, N. (2000). *Cognitive Aging: A Primer*. Philadelphia, PA: Taylor and Francis (Psychology Press).

Patterson, T. L., Goldman, S., McKibbin, C. L., et al. (2001). UCSD performance-based skills assessment: development of a new measure of everyday functioning for severely mentally ill adults. *Schizophrenia Bulletin*, **27**, 235–245.

Petersen, R. C. (2003). Mild cognitive impairment: transition between aging and Alzheimer's disease. *Neurologia*, **15**, 93–101.

Prince, M., Patel, V., Saxena, S., et al. (2007). No health without mental health. *Lancet*, **370**, 859–877.

Sabbag, S., Twamley, E. M., Vella, L., et al. (2011). Assessing everyday functioning in schizophrenia: not all informants seem equally informative. *Schizophrenia Research*, **131**, 250–255.

Salgado-Pineda, P., Caclin, A., Baeza, I., et al. (2007). Schizophrenia and frontal cortex: where does it fail? *Schizophrenia Research*, 2007; **91**, 73–81.

Salva, G. N., Moore, D. J., Roesch, S. C., et al. (2006). An evaluation of longitudinal neurocognitive performance among middle-aged and older schizophrenic patients: use of mixed-model analyses. *Schizophrenia Research*, **83**, 215–233.

Schaie, K. W. (1996). *Intellectual Development in Adulthood: The Seattle Longitudinal Study*. Melbourne, VIC: Cambridge University Press.

Schieber, F., Fozard, J. L., Gordon-Salant, S., et al. (1991). Optimizing sensation and perception in older adults. *International Journal of Industrial Ergonomics*, 7, 133–162.

Schinka, J. A., Loewenstein, D. A., Raj, A., et al. (2010). Defining mild cognitive impairment: impact of varying decision criteria on neuropsychological diagnostic frequencies and correlates. *American Journal of Geriatric Psychiatry*, **18**, 684–691.

Sharit, J., Hernandez, M., Czaja, S. J., et al. (2009). Investigating the roles of knowledge and cognitive abilities in older adult information seeking on the web. *ACM Transactions of Computer-Human Interaction*, **15**, 1–25.

Valentijin, S. A. M., Boxtel, V., Van Hooren, S. A. H., et al. (2005). Change in sensory functioning predicts change in cognitive functioning: results from a 6-year follow-up in the Maastricht aging study. *Journal of the American Geriatrics Society*, **53**, 374–380.

World Health Organization. (2011). *Schizophrenia*. Available online at: http://www.who.int/mental_health/management/schizophrenia/en/

Social cognition and its relationship to neurocognition

Amy E. Pinkham

Introduction

Efforts to understand the role of cognition in schizophrenia have focused primarily on domains such as attention and memory that fall under the general category of neurocognition. Relatively recently however, social cognition has emerged as a major focus of study, with the number of publications devoted to this topic increasing substantially over the last 10 years (Green & Leitman, 2008). Factors supporting the importance of social cognition in schizophrenia are numerous, and primary among them is the fact that social cognitive abilities are directly related to functional outcomes including social competence, community functioning, and quality of life (Couture et al., 2006). Here, the available research on social cognition in schizophrenia will be broadly reviewed beginning with a definition of social cognition and a brief overview of identified social cognitive impairments in individuals with schizophrenia. The relationship between social cognition and neurocognition, or nonsocial cognition, will then be examined in detail by directly comparing the two and by examining the contribution of each to functional outcome.

Definition of social cognition

While definitions of social cognition are numerous, the concept refers broadly to the way in which individuals perceive, process, and utilize social information. Specific definitions include "the human ability and capacity to perceive the intentions and dispositions of others" (Brothers, 1990, p. 28) and "the processes that subserve behavior in response to conspecifics, and, in particular, to those higher cognitive processes subserving the extreme, diverse, and flexible social behaviors that are seen in primates" (Adolphs, 1999, p. 469). Combining several such definitions, an NIMH workshop on social cognition in schizophrenia characterized social cognition as "the mental operations that underlie social interactions, including perceiving, interpreting, and generating responses to the intentions, dispositions, and behaviors of others" (Green et al., 2008, p. 1211). Essential components of these definitions are the direct link to social behavior and the indication that social cognitive abilities affect social function. As applied to schizophrenia, these definitions suggest that impaired social cognition may be a primary mechanism through which individuals show poor social and community functioning.

While this chapter will focus primarily on the relationship between social cognition and neurocognition in schizophrenia, it should be noted that several lines of evidence,

Cognitive Impairment in Schizophrenia, ed. Philip D. Harvey. Published by Cambridge University Press. © Cambridge University Press 2013.

independent from the schizophrenia literature, suggest that social cognition is generally separable and distinct from neurocognition. First, at a basic level, the stimuli implicated in each type of cognition differ in their degree of emotionality and content. Neurocognitive tasks tend to utilize affect-neutral stimuli such as numbers or objects while social cognitive tasks use emotionally laden social stimuli such as images of individuals expressing different emotions or social scenarios.

Second, evidence for the relative independence of social cognition from traditional neurocognitive skills can be garnered from both lesion studies and examinations of clinical populations. Individuals with either frontal or prefrontal cortex damage show impaired social behavior and functioning despite the retention of intact cognitive skills such as memory and language (Anderson et al., 1999; Blair & Cipolotti, 2000; Fine et al., 2001). Similarly, individuals with lesions in the somatic marker circuitry show low emotional and social intelligence and disturbances in social functioning regardless of normative levels of cognitive intelligence (Bar-On et al., 2003). Some clinical disorders such as autism and Williams syndrome also demonstrate the independence of social cognition from neurocognition in that individuals with these disorders can show impairments in one domain but relatively intact functioning in the other. Many high-functioning individuals with autism demonstrate significant impairments in social cognition despite testing in the normal or above normal range on IQ (Heavey et al., 2000; Klin, 2000). Likewise, individuals with Williams syndrome tend to be outgoing and social, even though most show below normal intelligence (Jones et al., 2000), and these individuals also appear to have relatively preserved basic social cognitive skills (i.e., facial processing and simple theory of mind (ToM) abilities [Karmiloff-Smith et al., 1995]), despite having deficits in spatial cognition (Bellugi et al., 2000; Tager-Flusberg et al., 1998).

Third, neurobiological models have long posited that social cognition may be subserved by a specialized neural network composed of modules that are specifically devoted to processing social stimuli and distinct from those regions primarily responsible for processing nonsocial stimuli (Adolphs, 2001; Brothers, 1990; Phillips et al., 2003a). While these models had their foundations in lesion studies, recent work examining the neural basis of social cognitive impairments in disorders such as autism and schizophrenia have linked these impairments to abnormal functioning of the particular brain regions that appear to be critically involved in the processing of social stimuli (Pelphrey et al., 2004; Pinkham et al., 2003, 2008a). Such findings provide strong evidence for the independence of social and nonsocial cognitive systems.

Social cognition in schizophrenia

Within schizophrenia, investigations of social cognition can be roughly categorized into five domains including ToM (the ability to represent the mental states of others and to make inferences about another's intentions), social perception (the ability to identify social roles, societal rules, and social context), social knowledge (awareness of the rules and goals that govern and characterize social situations and interactions), attributional style (the way in which one explains the causes of life events), and emotional processing (the ability to perceive and use emotions) (Green et al., 2008). While these domains are good representations of the existing work, it should be noted that they are not empirically derived and considerable overlap is present between them. These domains also do not cover the entirety of social cognition. Topics such as counterfactual thinking, self-perception, and empathy all fall under the general heading of social cognition but have received only very limited attention in schizophrenia. Nevertheless, these listed categories do highlight the multidimensional nature of social cognition and provide a useful framework for organizing our current understanding of social cognitive abilities in individuals with the illness. The three domains that have been most heavily studied and that will be reviewed here are ToM, emotion perception, and attributional style.

Theory of mind

Individuals with schizophrenia display impairments in several skills that rely upon ToM such as understanding false beliefs (Ba et al., 2008; Brune et al., 2007; Corcoran & Frith, 2003; Langdon et al., 2006a; Pickup & Frith, 2001), deciphering hints (Bertrand et al., 2007; Marjoram et al., 2005; Pinkham & Penn, 2006), identifying the intentions of another individual (Brunet et al., 2003; Sarfati & Hardy-Bayle, 1999; Sarfati et al., 1997), identifying the mental state of another individual (Bora et al., 2008; Kelemen et al., 2005; Kington et al., 2000), and understanding faux pas (Martino et al., 2007; Zhu et al., 2007). Two recent meta-analyses by Sprong et al. (2007) and Bora et al. (2009) report large overall effect sizes of 1.25 and 1.10, respectively, when comparing the performance of patients and healthy individuals. These deficits are well established in chronic samples, and it appears that similar deficits are apparent in first-episode (Bertrand et al., 2007; Green et al., 2011; Kettle et al., 2008; Koelkebeck et al., 2010) and high-risk samples (Chung et al., 2008; Green et al., 2011; see Gibson et al., 2010 for an exception).

Two remaining areas of debate pertain to the characteristics of the reported deficits. First, evidence is mixed regarding whether these are state- or trait-related impairments. Several studies provide support for a state-dependent process in which individuals in remission show more normative levels of performance (Corcoran, 2003; Corcoran et al., 1995; Drury et al., 1998; Frith & Corcoran; 1996; Pousa et al., 2008); however, both previously mentioned meta-analyses noted that ToM deficits persist in remitted patients. This combination of evidence may suggest that impairments are primarily trait-related but are likely to become more pronounced during periods of acute symptom exacerbation. Second, is it unclear whether these deficits are related to particular symptoms. Some studies, including the meta-analysis by Sprong and colleagues (2007), indicate that individuals with symptoms of disorganization show the greatest impairments (Abdel-Hamid et al., 2009; Pilowsky et al., 2000; Sarfati & Hardy-Bayle, 1999; Sarfati et al., 1999). Yet, other studies suggest that the impairment may be most highly related to negative symptoms (Corcoran et al., 1995; Pickup & Frith, 2001), although these findings also remain controversial as more recent and larger studies have failed to find an association between ToM and negative symptoms (Couture et al., 2011). For now, it may be sufficient to conclude that both disorganization and negative symptoms show important relationships to ToM abilities (Ventura et al., 2011), but that one may not be more important than the other.

Emotion perception

While studies of emotion perception have examined multiple modalities of communicating emotion such as prosody (for reviews see Edwards et al., 2002; Hoekert et al., 2007) and bodily expressions (Bigelow et al., 2006), the majority of research attention has been devoted to the recognition of emotion in the faces of others. This work has been relatively consistent in demonstrating that individuals with schizophrenia are impaired in both facial affect identification and discrimination, and a recent meta-analysis reports a large effect size of 0.91 for the comparison of patients and healthy controls (Kohler et al., 2010).

Reviews of this literature are numerous and direct attention to the following general conclusions (Edwards et al., 2002; Kohler et al., 2010; Mandal et al., 1998; Pinkham et al., 2007a). First, the emotion recognition deficits seen in individuals with schizophrenia continue to be evident even when compared to individuals with other psychiatric disorders such as depression (Gaebel & Wolwer, 1992; Weniger et al., 2004). Performance deficits are less consistently shown, however, when disorders that can also include psychotic symptoms (i.e., bipolar disorder) are used as the comparison group (Addington & Addington, 1998; Bellack et al., 1996). Second, recognition impairments appear to be greater for negative emotions (e.g., fear, anger) than for positive emotions (e.g., happiness), and among the negative emotions, patients have the most difficulty accurately recognizing fear (Bigelow et al., 2006; Edwards et al., 2001; Kohler et al., 2003). Patients also tend to misattribute negative emotions to neutral faces (Kohler et al., 2003), and this pattern is related to the presence of active paranoid ideation (Pinkham et al., 2011a). Third, longitudinal studies examining abilities during times of symptom exacerbation and remission demonstrate stability suggesting a trait deficit (Addington & Addington, 1998; Kee et al., 2003; Kucharska-Pietura & Klimkowski, 2002; see Penn et al., 2000 for evidence that impairments may abate during remission). Fourth, in regard to course, it appears that emotion processing impairments are evident in the first episode (Edwards et al., 2001), extending into early psychosis (Kucharska-Pietura & Klimkowski, 2002; Pinkham et al., 2007b), and are likely present during the prodromal phase of illness as well (Addington et al., 2008; Amminger et al., 2011; Eack et al., 2010). Thus, these are long-standing impairments that do not appear to be the result of a degenerative process after illness onset. Fifth, emotion recognition abilities may be related to specific symptoms. Studies are mixed on the role of paranoia, with some suggesting that paranoid individuals may be more skilled than non-paranoid individuals and others showing an opposite pattern (reviewed in Pinkham et al., 2011a). Negative symptoms have also been implicated (Mandal et al., 1999; Sachs et al., 2004), with one recent study demonstrating that flat affect uniquely predicted emotion processing abilities (Gur et al., 2006). Finally, individuals with schizophrenia tend to show abnormal visual scanning of faces that includes reduced time looking at the most salient features of the face (e.g., eyes and mouth) (Loughland et al., 2002; Sasson et al., 2007; Streit et al., 1997), which may contribute to emotion recognition impairments.

Attributional style

The majority of work on attributional style in schizophrenia has focused on the two biases most commonly seen in individuals with paranoid or persecutory delusions. The first is a self-serving bias in which individuals take credit for successful outcomes and deny responsibility for negative outcomes. This bias was first identified by Kaney and Bentall (1989) and received early support from a few additional studies. Overall however, support for a self-serving bias has been somewhat limited with several subsequent studies reporting only the tendency to make external attributions for negative outcomes without the concomitant internal attribution for positive events (Fear et al., 1996; Garety & Freeman, 1999; Kinderman & Bentall, 1997; Krstev et al., 1999; Lyon et al., 1994; Sharp et al., 1997). More recent studies have therefore adopted the term "externalizing bias" when reporting similar results (Janssen et al., 2006; Langdon et al., 2006b, 2010). The second bias, the personalizing bias, can been seen largely as a clarification of the externalizing bias. Specifically, when making an external attribution, individuals can either attribute the event to a person (i.e., an external personal attribution) or to situational factors (i.e., an external situational attribution). A growing body of evidence suggests that individuals with persecutory delusions may be prone to committing a personalizing bias by most often attributing negative events to others (Aakre et al., 2009; Bentall et al., 2001; Garety & Freeman, 1999; Langdon et al., 2010).

One important question in this area is why paranoid individuals display a personalizing bias. As reviewed by Penn and colleagues (2008), blaming an individual for negative events may serve a protective function that allows the patient to maintain a positive self-image. The drawback, however, is that such a tendency fosters negative perceptions of others, consistent with paranoid ideation, that are not corrected even in light of contradictory evidence. Bentall and colleagues (2001) propose that impairments in ToM and a strong need for closure (i.e., an intolerance of ambiguity) may play important roles in preventing the correction of inaccurate perceptions and maintaining paranoid ideation. Of note, other biases such as the tendency to "jump to conclusions" and to show a confirmation bias have also been linked to paranoid ideation (reviewed in Freeman, 2007; Merrin et al., 2007) and suggest that, in addition, social cognitive biases other than those specific to attributional style may be critical to understanding schizophrenia.

Relationships between social cognition and neurocognition

The relationship between social cognition and neurocognition has been of interest to many in the research community with the primary debate focusing on the independence of the two constructs. As noted previously, ample evidence is available from disparate reports in the literature suggesting that social cognition and neurocognition are distinct; however, in light of the prominent neurocognitive impairments evident in schizophrenia, it is tempting to think that social cognitive abnormalities may simply be a result of deficits in more core cognitive processes. In an effort to address this possibility and to clarify the nature of the relationship between these constructs in schizophrenia, researchers have utilized four primary strategies: direct examination of the correlations between social cognition and neurocognition, factor analytical techniques, paradigms designed to test for generalized versus specific impairments, and examinations of the contributions of social cognition and neurocognition to functional outcome.

Correlations between social cognition and neurocognition

The studies that have examined zero-order correlations between performance on neuro-cognitive and social cognitive tasks are too numerous to detail here; however, a recent meta-analysis by Ventura et al. (2011) provides an excellent summary of this literature. In their work, Ventura and colleagues analyzed data from 35 studies and reported overall effect sizes for the relationships between three domains of social cognition (i.e., emotion perception and processing, social perception and knowledge, and ToM) and the six neurocognitive domains identified by the Measurement and Treatment Research to Improve Cognition in Schizophrenia (MATRICS) initiative (Green et al., 2004). The relationships between emotion perception and processing and the neurocognitive domains were all of moderate size and fairly similar, ranging from 0.22 to 0.30. More variability was seen in the correlations between social perception/knowledge and ToM and the neurocognitive domains (i.e., 0.17

to 0.37 and 0.18 to 0.34 for social perception/knowledge and ToM, respectively), but again, all were of medium size. Additionally, no relationship between any particular social cognitive and neurocognitive pair was markedly stronger than the remaining combinations. Based on these results, the authors conclude that social cognition and neurocognition are related but primarily separate constructs.

Factor analyses

While varied, studies using factor analytical techniques have been consistent in supporting the separability of social cognition and neurocognition. In an interesting approach, Allen and colleagues (2007) utilized confirmatory factor analysis to examine the structure of the Wechsler Adult Intelligence Scale (WAIS-R), a widely used IQ test that includes several subtests that incorporate social scenarios and stimuli. Data from 169 males with schizophrenia provided support for a four-factor model composed of verbal comprehension, perceptual organization, working memory, and social cognition, with picture arrangement and picture completion loading on this last factor. The authors speculate that because both subtests require the perception and analysis of social situations and people, they likely map best onto the social cognitive domains of social perception and social knowledge.

Similarly, studies using structural equation modeling have also supported the distinction between social cognition and neurocognition. Vauth and colleagues (2004) found that data from 133 individuals with schizophrenia fit their model well when social cognitive and basic cognitive abilities were separated, but not when the two domains were combined into a single factor. Utilizing different measures, and most notably a more comprehensive battery of social cognitive tasks, Sergi et al. (2007) provided complementary findings. They found that a two-factor model that separated social cognition and neurocognition yielded a significantly better model fit than a single factor model.

Finally, it does not appear that the distinction between social cognition and neurocognition is specific to individuals with schizophrenia. Rather, it seems to span a spectrum of vulnerability. From a large sample of 149 individuals that included 44 individuals with psychosis, 47 non-psychotic first-degree relatives, 41 healthy individuals who reported high levels of psychotic experiences, and 54 healthy controls, van Hooren and colleages (2008) reported that, with the exception of one ToM task, social cognitive and neurocognitive tasks loaded on different factors. Interestingly, multiple social cognitive factors emerged, also suggesting that social cognition may be best understood as a multidimensional construct.

Generalized versus specific impairments

Differential deficit designs involve the inclusion of a control task that is matched for difficulty with the experimental task. It is assumed that poor performance on both tasks is representative of a generalized deficit and that poor performance on the experimental task combined with intact performance on the control task is indicative of a specific impairment. As applied to the question of the independence of social cognition, the experimental task should assess a domain of social cognition, and the control task should assess a presumably related neurocognitive domain. Impairments on both tasks would therefore provide evidence for a singular cognitive construct whereas differential performance would suggest separable constructs.

Such designs have most commonly been implemented in investigations of facial affect recognition, and somewhat surprisingly, the findings have been mixed. As excellently reviewed by Penn and colleagues (1997), eight out of 10 early studies reported poorer performance for patients relative to controls on both emotion and general perception tasks, suggesting a generalized deficit. An important caveat, however, is that in the majority of these studies, the control task was either a task of facial identity recognition or an age recognition task. While not requiring the processing of emotion, both tasks still utilize social stimuli and require the processing of faces. Thus, this early work remains inconclusive as one could argue that the requirements of a true differential deficit design were not met and that both tasks assessed social cognition.

The findings of recent work have been more consistent despite the fact that the lack of an ideal control task continues to be a problem. For example, Schneider and colleagues (2006) compared individuals with schizophrenia to healthy controls and found that patients were impaired on emotion recognition but not on age discrimination or face memory. Similarly, Kosmidis et al. (2007) reported that patients performed worse than controls on an affect matching task, but that groups did not differ on an identity matching task. Finally, Silver et al. (2009) noted that patients showed greater impairment on a task of emotion recognition than a task of identity recognition. Each of these studies provides evidence for a specific impairment in social facial emotion perception, and therefore supports the view that social cognition is independent from neurocognition. However, each study also used social stimuli in the control task. It remains to be seen whether a specific deficit would continue to be evident in a more rigorous differential deficit design, and additional work is therefore warranted.

Contribution of neurocognition and social cognition to functional outcome

As a means of understanding the general importance of neurocognition and social cognition, as well as the relationship between them, investigators have focused a good deal of energy on examining how both relate to social and occupational functioning. An early review demonstrated that between 20% and 60% of the variance in functional outcome can be accounted for by neurocognitive abilities (Green et al., 2000), and while these numbers are compelling, it is important to note that a good portion of variance remains unexplained. Reports that social cognition shows clear associations with functional outcome (Couture et al., 2006) suggest that social cognitive abilities may fill this gap. Indeed, numerous studies have demonstrated that social cognitive performance contributes variance to models of functional outcome above and beyond that accounted for by general cognitive abilities. For example, ToM has been found to account for more variance in social behavioral problems (Brune, 2005), social functioning (Bora et al., 2006; Roncone et al., 2002), and social competence (Brune et al., 2007) than neurocognition.

This pattern also appears to be evident for emotion processing (Meyer & Kurtz, 2009), although the findings are less robust. A recent meta-analysis by Fett and colleagues (2011) examined data from 52 studies and reported that ToM showed significantly stronger correlations to community functioning than all assessed neurocognitive domains, but that emotion processing was only more strongly related to functioning than were attention and vigilance. For all other domains of neurocognition, emotion perception and neurocognitive abilities showed correlations of approximately equal strengths.

Perhaps more importantly, when multiple domains of social cognition and neurocognition are investigated, social cognition continues to uniquely predict social functioning. In the first study to concurrently assess emotion perception, ToM, and social knowledge, neurocognitive variables (i.e., overall intellectual functioning and executive function) predicted 15% of the variance in social skill, but the addition of the group of social cognitive variables to the model contributed an additional 26% of variance. This incremental gain was significant, indicating that social cognitive ability uniquely predicted social skill above and beyond neurocognitive abilities (Pinkham and Penn, 2006).

In addition to studies that have examined both neurocognition and social cognition as predictors of functional outcome, several recent studies have asked whether social cognition might mediate the relationship between neurocognition and functioning. Such investigations provide support for this hypothesis by first establishing that social cognition is significantly correlated with both neurocognition and functioning and then by demonstrating that the direct relationship between neurocognition and functioning is reduced or eliminated when social cognition is included in the model. As reviewed by Schmidt and colleagues (2011), of the 15 studies testing mediation models, only one failed to support the effect. These studies varied widely in sample characteristics and tasks used; however, a large degree of consistency was present across studies. Directly comparing domains within social cognition also revealed that social knowledge and social perception showed the largest effect sizes, 0.28 and 0.21, respectively, with emotion perception (0.19) and ToM (0.14) following. Unfortunately, no studies have examined attributional biases as a mediator. From these reports, we can conclude that neurocognition may therefore exert its effects on outcome through social cognition.

On the whole, the studies mentioned earlier highlight the importance of social cognition for understanding social behavior in schizophrenia. Additionally, given that social cognition contributes variance to functional outcome above and beyond neurocognition and that social cognitive performance mediates the relationship between neurocognition and outcome, these studies support the relative independence of social cognition from neurocognition.

Conclusions and future directions

From the information presented in this chapter, three primary conclusions come to the forefront. First, individuals with schizophrenia display deficits or biases in all investigated domains of social cognition. Second, social cognitive deficits in schizophrenia cannot be attributed solely to impaired neurocognitive abilities, and in fact, social cognition and neurocognition appear to be largely independent of one another. Third, social cognitive deficits are critically important for understanding impaired social and vocational functioning in individuals with schizophrenia. The combination of these factors leaves little question about the importance of social cognition for furthering our understanding of schizophrenia and highlights several promising avenues for future investigation.

Perhaps most importantly, the work reviewed here has provided a solid foundation for efforts aimed at improving social cognitive abilities in patients, and at present, both pharmacological and psychosocial treatment strategies have been implemented. Most current pharmacological treatments have utilized the typical and atypical antipsychotics, and unfortunately, have not yielded encouraging results. After reviewing eight studies including seven clinical trials and one case-control study, Hempel and colleagues (2010) concluded that antipsychotic medication had little effect on emotion recognition abilities and that the few improvements that were reported (Fakra et al., 2009; Gaebel & Wolwer, 1992) were likely due to the indirect effects of symptom reduction. While these findings are somewhat disheartening, recent work with the nonapeptide oxytocin offers a more optimistic view of pharmacological remediation strategies. Specifically, oxytocin administration has demonstrated significant improvements in ToM (Pedersen et al., 2011) and emotion recognition (Averbeck et al., 2011) in individuals with schizophrenia. It remains unclear if these improvements are secondary to symptom reduction, as oxytocin has also been associated with improvements in positive and negative symptoms (Feifel et al., 2010; Rubin et al., 2010); however, the latter study noted improved emotion recognition following acute administration suggesting that oxytocin does have independent effects.

Behavioral treatments also offer promise for ameliorative change and range from targeted treatments that focus on only one social cognitive skill such as affect recognition (Wolwer et al., 2005) to broad, integrative treatments that incorporate a variety of psychosocial strategies with social cognition among them (Bell et al., 2001; Hogarty et al., 2004). In general, both types of treatment programs have demonstrated significant improvements across multiple domains of social cognition; however, the targeted treatments result in fewer questions about the mechanisms driving these improvements and therefore seem more straightforward (reviewed in Horan et al., 2008). One targeted treatment that has recently gained attention is Social Cognition and Interaction Training (SCIT) developed by David Penn and colleagues at the University of North Carolina (Penn et al., 2005). Social cognition and interaction training is a 20-week, manualized intervention that targets dysfunctional social cognition including problems with emotion processing, ToM, and biased attributions. Through a systematized series of studies, SCIT has been shown to result in significant improvements in social cognitive abilities in inpatients (Penn et al., 2005), forensic inpatients (Combs et al., 2007), and outpatients (Roberts & Penn, 2009; Roberts et al., 2009). Moreover, in a few of these studies, improvements have also generalized to indices of social behavior such as reductions in aggressive incidents and increased social network size (Combs et al., 2007) and improved social skills (Roberts & Penn, 2009). Longitudinal studies are needed to determine the stability of these improvements, and more comprehensive assessment batteries will need to be included to determine the full generalizability of social cognitive improvements to functional outcome. Nevertheless, these findings offer considerable promise for remediating social cognitive impairments, and together with the findings from pharmacological studies, suggest that augmenting a behavioral intervention like SCIT with oxytocin may be particularly fruitful.

The work reviewed in this chapter also emphasizes the need for a comprehensive model of social cognitive impairment in schizophrenia that links brain and behavior. As noted previously, ample evidence indicates that a specialized neural network is implicated in social cognition (Adolphs, 2001) and that individuals with schizophrenia show abnormal functioning in these brain regions (Phillips et al., 2003b; Pinkham et al., 2003, 2008a). A full review of this work is well outside the scope of this chapter; however, two findings from our recent work are worthy of note. In separate studies, we found that activation of social cognitive brain regions in individuals with schizophrenia was significantly correlated with social functioning (Pinkham et al., 2008b) and occupational functioning (Pinkham et al., 2011b). These findings suggest a potential neurobiological mechanism for social and functional impairments in schizophrenia and that remediation of abnormal neural responding may result in improved social cognition and functional outcome. Thus, in moving forward, a greater understanding of the mechanisms underlying social cognitive impairments will likely be necessary to optimally develop pharmacological and behavioral remediation strategies.

Finally, brief mention of measurement is also warranted. The relative youth of the field of social cognition in schizophrenia and the complex, multi-faceted nature of social cognition itself have resulted in a lack of consensus on key domains comprising social cognition and the appropriate means of assessing social cognitive performance. First, despite providing the field with a definition of social cognition, the NIMH workshop on social cognition in schizophrenia still concluded that there is no field-wide agreement on which abilities define the construct (Green et al., 2008). This is in part due to the fact that the currently defined domains have considerable conceptual and measurement-related overlap. Contributing, in addition, is the relative lack of studies implementing multiple measures of social cognition with sample sizes large enough to allow for either exploratory or confirmatory factor analyses. Second, multiple measures are often used to assess the same domain of social cognition (Bora et al., 2009), and there is little agreement about which measure provides the most accurate assessment. More importantly, there is little psychometric data upon which to base such a decision. Many of the existing tasks have only limited psychometric data, and those that do highlight several problems such as ceiling effects (e.g., hinting task, Bertrand et al., 2007; Marjoram et al., 2005; Versmissen et al., 2008) and poor internal consistency (e.g., FEIT and FEDT, Kee et al., 2004; Penn et al., 2000). These problems, both in consensus and in measure quality, currently restrict the utility of social cognition as a treatment target and outcome in treatment trials (Penn et al., 2009) and may also preclude a complete appreciation of the relationships between neurocognition, social cognition, and functional outcome. Large-scale psychometric studies and refined measures will therefore be necessary before the full importance of social cognition can be gleaned. This limitation notwithstanding, social cognition is recognized as a high priority in the study of schizophrenia and offers a critical addition to our understanding of cognitive impairment in this illness.

References

Aakre, J. M., Seghers, J. P., St-Hilaire, A., et al. (2009). Attributional style in delusional patients: a comparison of remitted paranoid, remitted nonparanoid, and current paranoid patients with nonpsychiatric controls. *Schizophrenia Bulletin*, 35, 994–1002.

Abdel-Hamid, M., Lehmkamper, C., Sonntag, C., et al. (2009). Theory of mind in schizophrenia: the role of clinical symptomatology and neurocognition in understanding other people's thoughts and intentions. *Psychiatry Research*, 165, 19–26.

Addington, J. & Addington, D. (1998). Facial affect recognition and information processing in schizophrenia and bipolar disorder. *Schizophrenia Research*, 32, 171–181.

Addington, J., Penn, D., Woods, S. W., et al. (2008). Facial affect recognition in individuals at clinical high risk for psychosis. *British Journal of Psychiatry*, 192, 67–68.

Adolphs, R. (1999). Social cognition and the human brain. *Trends in Cognitive Sciences*, 3, 469–479.

Adolphs, R. (2001). The neurobiology of social cognition. *Current Opinion in Neurobiology*, 11, 231–239.

Allen, D. N., Strauss, G. P., Donohue, B., et al. (2007). Factor analytic support for social cognition as a separable cognitive domain in schizophrenia. *Schizophrenia Research*, 93, 325–333.

Amminger, G. P., Schafer, M. R., Papageorgiou, K., et al. (2011). Emotion recognition in individuals at clinical high-risk for schizophrenia. *Schizophrenia Bulletin*. [Epub ahead of print].

Anderson, S. W., Bechara, A., Damasio, H., et al. (1999). Impairment of social and moral behavior related to early damage in human prefrontal cortex. *Nature Neuroscience*, 2, 1032–1037.

Averbeck, B. B., Bobin, T., Evans, S., et al. (2011). Emotion recognition and oxytocin in patients with schizophrenia. *Psychological Medicine*. [Epub ahead of print].

Ba, M. B., Zanello, A., Varnier, M., et al. (2008). Deficits in neurocognition, theory of mind, and social functioning in patients with schizophrenic disorders: are they related? *Journal of Nervous and Mental Disease*, **196**, 153–156.

Bar-On, R., Tranel, D., Denburg, N. L., et al. (2003). Exploring the neurological substrate of emotional and social intelligence. *Brain*, **126**, 1790–1800.

Bell, M., Bryson, G., Greig, T., et al. (2001). Neurocognitive enhancement therapy with work therapy: effects on neuropsychological test performance. *Archives of General Psychiatry*, **58**, 763–768.

Bellack, A. S., Blanchard, J. J., & Mueser, K. T. (1996). Cue availability and affect perception in schizophrenia. *Schizophrenia Bulletin*, **22**, 535–544.

Bellugi, U., Lichtenberger, L., Jones, W., et al. (2000). I. The neurocognitive profile of Williams syndrome: a complex pattern of strengths and weaknesses. *Journal of Cognitive Neuroscience*, **12**, S7–29.

Bentall, R. P., Corcoran, R., Howard, R., et al. (2001). Persecutory delusions: a review and theoretical integration. *Clinical Psychology Review*, **21**, 1143–1192.

Bertrand, M. C., Sutton, H., Achim, A. M., et al. (2007). Social cognitive impairments in first episode psychosis. *Schizophrenia Research*, **95**, 124–133.

Bigelow, N. O., Paradiso, S., Adolphs, R., et al. (2006). Perception of socially relevant stimuli in schizophrenia. *Schizophrenia Research*, **83**, 257–267.

Blair, R. J. & Cipolotti, L. (2000). Impaired social response reversal. A case of 'acquired sociopathy'. *Brain*, **123**, 1122–1141.

Bora, E., Eryavuz, A., Kayahan, B., et al. (2006). Social functioning, theory of mind and neurocognition in outpatients with schizophrenia; mental state decoding may be a better predictor of social functioning than mental state reasoning. *Psychiatry Research*, **145**, 95–103.

Bora, E., Gokcen, S., & Veznedaroglu, B. (2008). Empathic abilities in people with schizophrenia. *Psychiatry Research*, **160**, 23–29.

Bora, E., Yucel, M., & Pantelis, C. (2009). Theory of mind impairment in

schizophrenia: meta-analysis. *Schizophrenia Research*, **109**, 1–9.

Brothers, L. (1990). The social brain: a project for integrating primate behaviour and neuropsychology in a new domain. *Concepts in Neuroscience*, **1**, 27–51.

Brune, M. (2005). Emotion recognition, 'theory of mind,' and social behavior in schizophrenia. *Psychiatry Research*, **133**, 135–147.

Brune, M., Abdel-Hamid, M., Lehmkamper, C., et al. (2007). Mental state attribution, neurocognitive functioning, and psychopathology: what predicts poor social competence in schizophrenia best? *Schizophrenia Research*, **92**, 151–159.

Brunet, E., Sarfati, Y., & Hardy-Bayle, M. C. (2003). Reasoning about physical causality and other's intentions in schizophrenia. *Cognitive Neuropsychiatry*, **8**, 129–139.

Chung, Y. S., Kang, D. H., Shin, N. Y., et al. (2008). Deficit of theory of mind in individuals at ultra-high-risk for schizophrenia. *Schizophrenia Research*, **99**, 111–118.

Combs, D. R., Adams, S. D., Penn, D. L., et al. (2007). Social Cognition and Interaction Training (SCIT) for inpatients with schizophrenia spectrum disorders: preliminary findings. *Schizophrenia Research*, **91**, 112–116.

Corcoran, R. (2003). Inductive reasoning and the understanding of intention in schizophrenia. *Cognitive Neuropsychiatry*, **8**, 223–235.

Corcoran, R. & Frith, C. D. (2003). Autobiographical memory and theory of mind: evidence of a relationship in schizophrenia. *Psychological Medicine*, **33**, 897–905.

Corcoran, R., Mercer, G., & Frith, C. D. (1995). Schizophrenia, symptomatology and social inference: investigating "theory of mind" in people with schizophrenia. *Schizophrenia Research*, **17**, 5–13.

Couture, S. M., Granholm, E. L., & Fish, S. C. (2011). A path model investigation of neurocognition, theory of mind, social competence, negative symptoms and real-world functioning in schizophrenia. *Schizophrenia Research*, **125**, 152–160.

Couture, S. M., Penn, D. L., & Roberts, D. L. (2006). The functional significance of social cognition in schizophrenia: a review. *Schizophrenia Bulletin*, **32**, S44–63.

Drury, V. M., Robinson, E. J., & Birchwood, M. (1998). 'Theory of mind' skills during an acute episode of psychosis and following recovery. *Psychological Medicine*, **28**, 1101–1112.

Eack, S. M., Mermon, D. E., Montrose, D. M., et al. (2010). Social cognition deficits among individuals at familial high risk for schizophrenia. *Schizophrenia Bulletin*, **36**, 1081–1088.

Edwards, J., Jackson, H. J., & Pattison, P. E. (2002). Emotion recognition via facial expression and affective prosody in schizophrenia: a methodological review. *Clinical Psychology Review*, **22**, 789–832.

Edwards, J., Pattison, P. E., Jackson, H. J., et al. (2001). Facial affect and affective prosody recognition in first-episode schizophrenia. *Schizophrenia Research*, **48**, 235–253.

Fakra, E., Salgado-Pineda, P., Besnier, N., et al. (2009). Risperidone versus haloperidol for facial affect recognition in schizophrenia: findings from a randomised study. *World Journal of Biological Psychiatry*, **10**, 719–728.

Fear, C., Sharp, H., & Healy, D. (1996). Cognitive processes in delusional disorders. *British Journal of Psychiatry*, **168**, 61–67.

Feifel, D., Macdonald, K., Nguyen, A., et al. (2010). Adjunctive intranasal oxytocin reduces symptoms in schizophrenia patients. *Biological Psychiatry*, **68**, 678–680.

Fett, A. K., Viechtbauer, W., Dominguez, M. D., et al. (2011). The relationship between neurocognition and social cognition with functional outcomes in schizophrenia: a meta-analysis. *Neuroscience and Biobehavioral Reviews*, **35**, 573–588.

Fine, C., Lumsden, J., & Blair, R. J. (2001). Dissociation between 'theory of mind' and executive functions in a patient with early left amygdala damage. *Brain*, **124**, 287–298.

Freeman, D. (2007). Suspicious minds: the psychology of persecutory delusions. *Clinical Psychological Review*, **27**, 425–457.

Frith, C. D. & Corcoran, R. (1996). Exploring 'theory of mind' in people with schizophrenia. *Psychological Medicine*, **26**, 521–530.

Gaebel, W. & Wolwer, W. (1992). Facial expression and emotional face recognition in schizophrenia and depression. *European Archives of Psychiatry and Clinical Neuroscience*, **242**, 46–52.

Garety, P. A. & Freeman, D. (1999). Cognitive approaches to delusions: a critical review of theories and evidence. *Britich Journal of Clinical Psychology*, **38**, 113–154.

Gibson, C. M., Penn, D. L., Prinstein, M. J., et al. (2010). Social skill and social cognition in adolescents at genetic risk for psychosis. *Schizophrenia Research*, **122**, 179–184.

Green, M. F., Bearden, C. E., Cannon, T. D., et al. (2011). Social cognition in schizophrenia, Part 1: performance across phase of illness. *Schizophrenia Bulletin*. [Epub ahead of print].

Green, M. F., Kern, R. S., Braff, D. L., et al. (2000). Neurocognitive deficits and functional outcome in schizophrenia: are we measuring the "right stuff"? *Schizophrenia Bulletin*, **26**, 119–136.

Green, M. F. & Leitman, D. I. (2008). Social cognition in schizophrenia. *Schizophrenia Bulletin*, **34**, 670–672.

Green, M. F., Nuechterlein, K. H., Gold, J. M., et al. (2004). Approaching a consensus cognitive battery for clinical trials in schizophrenia: the NIMH-MATRICS conference to select cognitive domains and test criteria. *Biological Psychiatry*, **56**, 301–307.

Green, M. F., Penn, D. L., Bentall, R., et al. (2008). Social cognition in schizophrenia: an NIMH workshop on definitions, assessment, and research opportunities. *Schizophrenia Bulletin*, **34**, 1211–1220.

Gur, R. E., Kohler, C. G., Ragland, J. D., et al. (2006). Flat affect in schizophrenia: relation to emotion processing and neurocognitive measures. *Schizophrenia Bulletin*, **32**, 279–287.

Heavey, L., Phillips, W., Baron-Cohen, S., et al. (2000). The Awkward Moments Test: a naturalistic measure of social understanding in autism. *Journal of Autism and Developmental Disorders*, **30**, 225–236.

Hempel, R. J., Dekker, J. A., van Beveren, N. J., et al. (2010). The effect of antipsychotic medication on facial affect recognition in schizophrenia: a review. *Psychiatry Research*, **178**, 1–9.

Hoekert, M., Kahn, R. S., Pijnenborg, M., et al. (2007). Impaired recognition and expression of emotional prosody in schizophrenia: review and meta-analysis. *Schizophrenia Research*, **96**, 135–145.

Hogarty, G. E., Flesher, S., Ulrich, R., et al. (2004). Cognitive enhancement therapy for schizophrenia: effects of a 2-year randomized trial on cognition and behavior. *Archives of General Psychiatry*, **61**, 866–876.

Horan, W. P., Kern, R. S., Green, M. F., et al. (2008). Social cognition training for individuals with schizophrenia: emerging evidence. *American Journal of Psychiatric Rehabilitation*, **11**, 205–252.

Janssen, I., Versmissen, D., Campo, J. A., et al. (2006). Attribution style and psychosis: evidence for an externalizing bias in patients but not individuals at high risk. *Psychological Medicine*, **36**, 771–778.

Jones, W., Bellugi, U., Lai, Z., et al. (2000). II. Hypersociability in Williams syndrome. *Journal of Cognitive Neuroscience*, **12**, S30–46.

Kaney, S. & Bentall, R. P. (1989). Persecutory delusions and attributional style. *British Journal of Medical Psychology*, **62**, 191–198.

Karmiloff-Smith, A., Klima, E., Bellugi, U., et al. (1995). Is there a social module? Language, face processing, and theory of mind in individuals with Williams syndrome. *Journal of Cognitive Neuroscience*, **7**, 196–208.

Kee, K. S., Green, M. F., Mintz, J., et al. (2003). Is emotion processing a predictor of functional outcome in schizophrenia? *Schizophrenia Bulletin*, **29**, 487–497.

Kee, K. S., Horan, W. P., Mintz, J., et al. (2004). Do the siblings of schizophrenia patients demonstrate affect perception deficits? *Schizophrenia Research*, **67**, 87–94.

Kelemen, O., Erdelyi, R., Pataki, I., et al. (2005). Theory of mind and motion perception in schizophrenia. *Neuropsychology*, **19**, 494–500.

Kettle, J. W., O'Brien-Simpson, L., & Allen, N. B. (2008). Impaired theory of mind in first-episode schizophrenia: comparison with community, university and depressed controls. *Schizophrenia Research*, **99**, 96–102.

Kinderman, P. & Bentall, R. P. (1997). Causal attributions in paranoia and depression: internal, personal, and situational attributions for negative events. *Journal of Abnormal Psychology*, **106**, 341–345.

Kington, J. M., Jones, L. A., Watt, A. A., et al. (2000). Impaired eye expression recognition in schizophrenia. *Journal Psychiatry Research*, **34**, 341–347.

Klin, A. (2000). Attributing social meaning to ambiguous visual stimuli in higher-functioning autism and Asperger syndrome: the Social Attribution Task. *Journal of Child Psychological Psychiatry*, **41**, 831–846.

Koelkebeck, K., Pedersen, A., Suslow, T., et al. (2010). Theory of mind in first-episode schizophrenia patients: correlations with cognition and personality traits. *Schizophrenia Research*, **119**, 115–123.

Kohler, C. G., Turner, T. H., Bilker, W. B., et al. (2003). Facial emotion recognition in schizophrenia: intensity effects and error pattern. *American Journal of Psychiatry*, **160**, 1768–1774.

Kohler, C. G., Walker, J. B., Martin, E. A., et al. (2010). Facial emotion perception in schizophrenia: a meta-analytic review. *Schizophrenia Bulletin*, **36**, 1009–1019.

Kosmidis, M. H., Bozikas, V. P., Giannakou, M., et al. (2007). Impaired emotion perception in schizophrenia: a differential deficit. *Psychiatry Research*, **149**, 279–284.

Krstev, H., Jackson, H., & Maude, D. (1999). An investigation of attributional style in first-episode psychosis. *British Journal of Clinical Psychology*, **38**, 181–194.

Kucharska-Pietura, K. & Klimkowski, M. (2002). Perception of facial affect in chronic schizophrenia and right brain damage. *Acta Neurobiologiae Experimentalis (Warsaw)*, **62**, 33–43.

Langdon, R., Coltheart, M., & Ward, P. B. (2006a). Empathetic perspective-taking is impaired in schizophrenia: evidence from a study of emotion attribution and theory of mind. *Cognitive Neuropsychiatry*, **11**, 133–155.

Langdon, R., Corner, T., McLaren, J., et al. (2006b). Externalizing and personalizing biases in persecutory delusions: the relationship with poor insight and theory-of-mind. *Behavior Research Therapy*, **44**, 699–713.

Langdon, R., Ward, P. B., & Coltheart, M. (2010). Reasoning anomalies associated with delusions in schizophrenia. *Schizophrenia Bulletin*, **36**, 321–330.

Loughland, C. M., Williams, L. M., & Gordon, E. (2002). Visual scanpaths to positive and negative facial emotions in an outpatient schizophrenia sample. *Schizophrenia Research*, **55**, 159–170.

Lyon, H. M., Kaney, S., & Bentall, R. P. (1994). The defensive function of persecutory delusions. Evidence from attribution tasks. *British Journal of Psychiatry*, **164**, 637–646.

Mandal, M. K., Jain, A., Haque-Nizamie, S., et al. (1999). Generality and specificity of emotion-recognition deficit in schizophrenic patients with positive and negative symptoms. *Psychiatry Research*, **87**, 39–46.

Mandal, M. K., Pandey, R., & Prasad, A. B. (1998). Facial expressions of emotions and schizophrenia: a review. *Schizophrenia Bulletin*, **24**, 399–412.

Marjoram, D., Gardner, C., Burns, J., et al. (2005). Symptomatology and social inference: a theory of mind study of schizophrenia and psychotic affective disorder. *Cognitive Neuropsychiatry*, **10**, 347–359.

Martino, D. J., Bucay, D., Butman, J. T., et al. (2007). Neuropsychological frontal impairments and negative symptoms in schizophrenia. *Psychiatry Research*, **152**, 121–128.

Merrin, J., Kinderman, P., & Bentall, R. P. (2007). 'Jumping to conclusions' and attributional sytle in persecutory delusions. *Cognitive Therapy and Research*, **31**, 741–758.

Meyer, M. B. & Kurtz, M. M. (2009). Elementary neurocognitive function, facial affect recognition and social-skills in schizophrenia. *Schizophrenia Research*, **110**, 173–179.

Pedersen, C. A., Gibson, C. M., Rau, S. W., et al. (2011). Intranasal oxytocin reduces psychotic symptoms and improves Theory of Mind and social perception in schizophrenia. *Schizophrenia Research*, **132**, 50–53.

Pelphrey, K., Adolphs, R., & Morris, J. P. (2004). Neuroanatomical substrates of social cognition dysfunction in autism. *Mental Retardation and Developmental Disability Research Review*, **10**, 259–271.

Penn, D., Roberts, D. L., Munt, E. D., et al. (2005). A pilot study of social cognition and interaction training (SCIT) for schizophrenia. *Schizophrenia Research*, **80**, 357–359.

Penn, D. L., Combs, D. R., Ritchie, M., et al. (2000). Emotion recognition in schizophrenia: further investigation of generalized versus specific deficit models. *Journal of Abnormal Psychology*, **109**, 512–516.

Penn, D. L., Corrigan, P. W., Bentall, R. P., et al. (1997). Social cognition in schizophrenia. *Psychological Bulletin*, **121**, 114–132.

Penn, D. L., Keefe, R. S. E., Davis, S. M., et al. (2009). The effects of antipsychotic medications on emotion perception in patients with chronic schizophrenia in the CATIE trial. *Schizophrenia Research*, **115**, 17–23.

Penn, D. L., Sanna, L. J., & Roberts, D. L. (2008). Social cognition in schizophrenia: an overview. *Schizophrenia Bulletin*, **34**, 408–411.

Phillips, M. L., Drevets, W. C., Rauch, S. L., et al. (2003a). Neurobiology of emotion perception I: the neural basis of normal emotion perception. *Biological Psychiatry*, **54**, 504–514.

Phillips, M. L., Drevets, W. C., Rauch, S. L., et al. (2003b). Neurobiology of emotion perception II: implications for major psychiatric disorders. *Biological Psychiatry*, **54**, 515–528.

Pickup, G. J. & Frith, C. D. (2001). Theory of mind impairments in schizophrenia:

symptomatology, severity and specificity. *Psychological Medicine*, **31**, 207–220.

Pilowsky, T., Yirmiya, N., Arbelle, S., et al. (2000). Theory of mind abilities of children with schizophrenia, children with autism, and normally developing children. *Schizophrenia Research*, **42**, 145–155.

Pinkham, A. E., Brensinger, C., Kohler, C., et al. (2011a). Actively paranoid patients with schizophrenia over attribute anger to neutral faces. *Schizophrenia Research*, **125**, 174–178.

Pinkham, A. E., Gur, R. E., & Gur, R. C. (2007a). Affect recognition deficits in schizophrenia: neural substrates and psychopharmacological implications. *Expert Review of Neurotherapeutics*, **7**, 807–816.

Pinkham, A. E., Hopfinger, J. B., Pelphrey, K. A., et al. (2008a). Neural bases for impaired social cognition in schizophrenia and autism spectrum disorders. *Schizophrenia Research*, **99**, 164–175.

Pinkham, A. E., Hopfinger, J. B., Ruparel, K., et al. (2008b). An investigation of the relationship between activation of a social cognitive neural network and social functioning. *Schizophrenia Bulletin*, **34**, 688–697.

Pinkham, A. E., Loughead, J., Ruparel, K., et al. (2011b). Abnormal modulation of amygdala activity in schizophrenia in response to direct- and averted-gaze threat-related facial expressions. *American Journal of Psychiatry*, **168**, 293–301.

Pinkham, A. E. & Penn, D. L. (2006). Neurocognitive and social cognitive predictors of interpersonal skill in schizophrenia. *Psychiatry Research*, **143**, 167–178.

Pinkham, A. E., Penn, D. L., Perkins, D. O., et al. (2003). Implications for the neural basis of social cognition for the study of schizophrenia. *American Journal of Psychiatry*, **160**, 815–824.

Pinkham, A. E., Penn, D. L., Perkins, D. O., et al. (2007b). Emotion perception and social skill over the course of psychosis: a comparison of individuals 'at-risk' for psychosis and individuals with early and chronic schizophrenia spectrum illness. *Cognitive Neuropsychiatry*, **12**, 198–212.

Pousa, E., Duno, R., Brebion, G., et al. (2008). Theory of mind deficits in chronic schizophrenia: evidence for state dependence. *Psychiatry Research*, **158**, 1–10.

Roberts, D. L. & Penn, D. L. (2009). Social cognition and interaction training (SCIT) for outpatients with schizophrenia: a preliminary study. *Psychiatry Research*, **166**, 141–147.

Roberts, D. L., Penn, D. L., Labate, D., et al. (2009). Transportability and feasibility of Social Cognition and Interaction Training (SCIT) in community settings. *Behavioural and Cognitive Psychotherapy*, **38**, 35–47.

Roncone, R., Falloon, I. R., Mazza, M., et al. (2002). Is theory of mind in schizophrenia more strongly associated with clinical and social functioning than with neurocognitive deficits? *Psychopathology*, **35**, 280–288.

Rubin, L. H., Carter, C.S., Drogos, L., et al. (2010). Peripheral oxytocin is associated with reduced symptom severity in schizophrenia. *Schizophrenia Research*, **124**, 13–21.

Sachs, G., Steger-Wuchse, D., Kryspin-Exner, I., et al. (2004). Facial recognition deficits and cognition in schizophrenia. *Schizophrenia Research*, **68**, 27–35.

Sarfati, Y. & Hardy-Bayle, M. C. (1999). How do people with schizophrenia explain the behaviour of others? A study of theory of mind and its relationship to thought and speech disorganization in schizophrenia. *Psychological Medicine*, **29**, 613–620.

Sarfati, Y., Hardy-Bayle, M. C., Besche, C., et al. (1997). Attribution of intentions to others in people with schizophrenia: a non-verbal exploration with comic strips. *Schizophrenia Research*, **25**, 199–209.

Sarfati, Y., Hardy-Bayle, M. C., Brunet, E., et al. (1999). Investigating theory of mind in schizophrenia: influence of verbalization in disorganized and non-disorganized patients. *Schizophrenia Research*, **37**, 183–190.

Sasson, N., Tsuchiya, N., Hurley, R., et al. (2007). Orienting to social stimuli differentiates social cognitive impairment in autism and schizophrenia. *Neuropsychologia*, **45**, 2580–2588.

Schmidt, S. J., Mueller, D. R., & Roder, V. (2011). Social cognition as a mediator variable between neurocognition and functional outcome in schizophrenia: empirical review and new results by structural equation modeling. *Schizophrenia Bulletin*, **37**, S41–54.

Schneider, F., Gur, R. C., Koch, K., et al. (2006). Impairment in the specificity of emotion processing in schizophrenia. *American Journal Psychiatry*, **163**, 442–447.

Sergi, M. J., Rassovsky, Y., Widmark, C., et al. (2007). Social cognition in schizophrenia: relationships with neurocognition and negative symptoms. *Schizophrenia Research*, **90**, 316–324.

Sharp, H., Fear, C., & Healy, D. (1997). Attributional style and delusions: an investigation based on delusional content. *European Psychiatry*, **12**, 1–7.

Silver, H., Bilker, W., & Goodman, C. (2009). Impaired recognition of happy, sad and neutral expressions in schizophrenia is emotion, but not valence, specific and context dependent. *Psychiatry Research*, **169**, 101–106.

Sprong, M., Schothorst, P., Vos, E., et al. (2007). Theory of mind in schizophrenia: meta-analysis. *British Journal of Psychiatry*, **191**, 5–13.

Streit, M., Wolwer, W., & Gaebel, W. (1997). Facial-affect recognition and visual scanning behaviour in the course of schizophrenia. *Schizophrenia Research*, **24**, 311–317.

Tager-Flusberg, H., Boshart, J., & Baron-Cohen, S. (1998). Reading the windows to the soul: evidence of domain-specific sparing in Williams syndrome. *Journal of Cognitive Neuroscience*, **10**, 631–639.

van Hooren, S., Versmissen, D., Janssen, I., et al. (2008). Social cognition and neurocognition as independent domains in psychosis. *Schizophrenia Research*, **103**, 257–265.

Vauth, R., Rusch, N., Wirtz, M., et al. (2004). Does social cognition influence the relation between neurocognitive deficits and vocational functioning in schizophrenia? *Psychiatry Research*, **128**, 155–165.

Ventura, J., Wood, R. C., and Hellemann, G. S. (2011). Symptom domains and neurocognitive functioning can help differentiate social cognitive processes in schizophrenia: a meta-analysis. *Schizophrenia Bulletin*. [Epub ahead of print].

Versmissen, D., Janssen, I., Myin-Germeys, I., et al. (2008). Evidence for a relationship between mentalising deficits and paranoia over the psychosis continuum. *Schizophrenia Research*, **99**, 103–110.

Weniger, G., Lange, C., Ruther, E., et al. (2004). Differential impairments of facial affect recognition in schizophrenia subtypes and major depression. *Psychiatry Research*, **128**, 135–146.

Wolwer, W., Frommann, N., Halfmann, S., et al. (2005). Remediation of impairments in facial affect recognition in schizophrenia: efficacy and specificity of a new training program. *Schizophrenia Research*, **80**, 295–303.

Zhu, C. Y., Lee, T. M., Li, X. S., et al. (2007). Impairments of social cues recognition and social functioning in Chinese people with schizophrenia. *Psychiatry Clinical Neuroscience*, **61**, 149–158.

Chapter

9

Cognitive functioning and awareness of illness in schizophrenia: a review and meta-analysis

Akshay Nair, André Aleman, and Anthony S. David

Introduction

Insight or awareness of illness has been a major topic of research for at least 20 years. Lack of insight was once considered to be the *sine qua non* of schizophrenia. While it is commonly observed in both acute and chronic patients, in the developed as well as the less developed world, lack of insight is seen more as a matter of degree than an absolute and in fact can be viewed as a rather complex set of intersecting beliefs and attitudes (Amador & David, 2004).

It is possible to caricature insight as mere "agreeing with the doctor." However, most serious clinicians and researchers formulate the core of insight as an awareness that one is ill, but using the person's own frame of reference. This in turn is shaped and influenced by family background, culture, education, personality, and many other factors. It is not possible to quantify the influence of each of these, but a representation is given in Figure 9.1, with "unknown" being the largest factor followed by psychotic psychopathology, which tends to correlate (inversely) with insight measures but not to a degree that suggests that measuring insight is redundant (Amador & David, 2004).

Our own model (David, 1990) separates this overarching view of illness from a more specific awareness of particular experiences or potentially psychopathological symptoms. Here, insight implies an awareness that the experience in question is peculiar, exceptional, or worthy of note at the very least, which then prompts an attribution that it is abnormal, disordered, or explained by some other factor. Finally, insight implies an appreciation of the wider effects of one's state or experiences on functioning in the world, relationships, well being, etc.

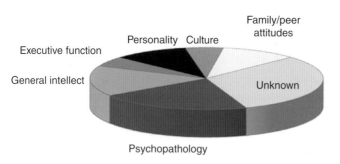

Figure 9.1. Pictorial representation of the multiple contributors to the insight construct.

Cognitive Impairment in Schizophrenia, ed. Philip D. Harvey. Published by Cambridge University Press. © Cambridge University Press 2013.

The interest in the present context is the extent to which insight as a process is cognitive, that it can be broken down into a series of information processing steps, that it is (or is not) capacity limited, and that it may be subject to dysfunction. Formulating insight as based upon self-appraisal or self-evaluation would seem to be a useful point of departure. Self-processing has attracted attention recently among cognitive neuroscientists and some preliminary models have been put forward, which can, intuitively at least, be adapted to our purposes. Self-processing can also be viewed as normative – that is, it does not have to stand or fall on a definition of pathology or "what the doctor says" but exists *sui generis*.

Referring to an outline model (Figure 9.2), people in the world experience events, memories, perceptions, actions, and interactions with others (social cognition) all the time. Self-appraisal may be defined as the self-directed or prompted offline re-experiencing of such events. The aim of this re-experiencing includes reality monitoring – did this really happen?; was it my imagination? – or some other meta-cognitive task, such as: was my judgment accurate or fair? In the case of illness awareness of the general kind, self-reflection may amount to the comparison of and adjudication between clinical views (you are ill, you are experiencing hallucinations, etc.) and personal views (there is nothing wrong with me; my voices are talking to me). The output from this comparator mechanism then leads to an action, which might be to seek further information, to seek help, to avoid clinicians, to mitigate the experiences, etc.

Clearly there are many points at which the process may fail or go awry. Initiation of the self-appraisal process may not occur. Presumably this is governed by executive functions as with any other intentional, goal-driven processes. Next, the self-appraisal process may be hard to sustain especially, as conceived, if it entails the weighing of two or more sets of information and hence would rely on working memory. If one such source of information is stored memories or knowledge (semantic memory) then the "quality" of any conclusion drawn will depend on this store of knowledge being accurate and uncorrupted. Finally, action based on the process may be hampered by problems with planning and by processing speed. The whole system is attentionally demanding and presumably capacity limited such that it would be vulnerable to any general diminution in processing efficiency. Put this way, we might postulate that executive function, semantic memory, working memory, processing speed, and overall IQ might all be expected to impair self-processing and clinical insight.

This formulation is rather general and is not refined enough to be confirmed or refuted experimentally. At this stage, it simply serves as a way to organize and consider published data examining the relationship between cognitive performance and insight in schizophrenia. When one begins such an examination, it soon becomes evident that there is an overwhelming pool of material to draw upon. We have previously subjected this to a meta-analysis (Aleman et al., 2006). This showed that there was a reliable although small association between general intellectual functioning and insight measures, with a slightly greater effect when studies of executive function, particularly the Wisconsin Card Sorting Test, were used. Since that publication, there have been almost as many new studies to consider. Hence, we undertook a second comprehensive meta-analysis on all studies. The main purpose was to examine whether particular cognitive functions were more or less related to insight. We also sought to explore whether diagnostic precision had any effect (i.e., where schizophrenia as opposed to psychosis

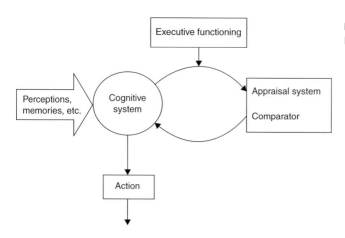

Figure 9.2. An information processing model for self-appraisal.

was specified) and whether the different insight scales or measures lead to differing estimates of the association with cognition.

Methods

Methods used in this chapter reflect those used in our previous meta-analysis on this subject (Aleman et al., 2006) in order to produce comparable results and hopefully a significant update on the topic.

Study selection

Our study identification strategy had three phases. First, we searched databases PubMed and Web of Science for relevant papers using the key words: insight OR unawareness, combined with psychosis OR schizophrenia, combined with cogniti*OR neuropsycholog* OR neurocogniti* OR intelligence, memory OR WCST (Wisconsin Card Sorting Test). The previous meta-analysis had used the same search strategy to locate papers prior to April 2004; therefore, in this study we searched papers published from 2004 up until September 2011. This generated 376 results from PubMed and 591 results from Web of Science. A review of these results was then conducted to determine which papers met our inclusion criteria. In total 34 new papers were identified and added to the collection of 35 identified by Aleman et al. (2006) to bring the total in this analysis to 69 studies. The inclusion criteria for the papers were as follows:

1. Correlations between insight scales and cognitive performance were reported in the study or sufficient information was reported to enable us to compute effect sizes.
2. The sample comprised patient groups with a psychotic disorder, whether affective or nonaffective.
3. The article had been published in a peer-reviewed English-language journal.
4. A valid measure of insight was used such as, but not exclusively, the insight item from the Positive and Negative Syndrome Scale (PANSS-G12), the Schedule for the Assessment Of Insight (SAI), the Scale to Assess Unawareness of Mental Disorder (SUMD) and the Insight and Treatment Attitudes Questionnaire (ITAQ).

5. A valid measure of cognitive function that represented one of five cognitive domains, described later: (1) total cognition, (2) IQ, (3) memory, (4) executive function, and (5) WCST–categories achieved or preservative errors.

The five cognitive domains were defined in the same manner as in Aleman et al. (2006). "Total cognition" represented the pooled mean correlation of all cognitive tests examined in a paper; this category also included correlations with "composite" cognitive scores. The second domain was measures of IQ, including the Wechsler Adult Intelligence Scale (WAIS) and National Adult Reading Test (NART). In cases where only a number of WAIS subtests were included, these subtests were pooled. The third domain, memory, included measures of verbal, visual, and working memory performance. Fourth was frontal executive function, which included the Trail Making Test, Part B (TMT-B), Verbal Fluency Test, and Wisconsin Card Sorting Test (WCST). Finally, a separate analysis limited to the WCST was included. In the WCST analysis we included categories achieved as well as perseverative errors, which were pooled when both were reported. For further details, please refer to Aleman et al. (2006).

Wherever necessary, the direction of correlation between insight and cognitive measures was reversed such that all included effect sizes represented the correlation between better cognitive function and better insight. For example, this was often required where SUMD and PANSS scales were used as higher scores represented poorer insight or WCST-PE where higher scores represented poorer executive function.

Data analysis

This study used the mean correlation coefficients (r) weighted for sample size as the effect size. Where precise correlation coefficients were not given, they were calculated using techniques detailed in Lipsey & Wilson (2001). One problem faced by those conducting the meta-analysis is that of studies not reporting nonsignificant data. There are numerous strategies designed to deal with this problem when the original data are not available: (1) exclude these studies from the analysis; however, this is not desirable as it introduces bias; (2) replace the missing results with a correlation coefficient of 0. This is an extremely conservative approach and runs the risk of masking small overall effect sizes; (3) one may replace the missing effect sizes with the mean effect of those studies that do report nonsignificant data. This may, however, be seen as overly generous and may exaggerate small effect sizes. A compromise struck in the previous meta-analysis was to replace the missing effect sizes with the lowest value of the 95% confidence interval of the mean effect size of those studies that report nonsignificant data. This conservative approach aims at striking a balance between over- and underestimating the underlying relationship and to allow us to include as many papers as possible. A separate non-published analysis replacing missing values with 0 (zero) was also conducted to assess whether this affected the significance of any of the relationships found, but it did not. After inputting the effect size for each study, meta-analytical techniques were applied to obtain a combined effect weighted for sample size. The Z and P values provide an indication as to the statistical significance of the association. In order to account for the heterogeneity of measures, samples, and concepts that these studies examined, a random-effects model was used. Publication bias was examined by using a funnel plot of standard error and Fisher Z score. Using the Duval and Tweedie's Trim and Fit (Rothstein et al., 2005) analysis, missing studies were imputed and added to the funnel plot. Rosenthal's fail safe n was also calculated. All analyses were completed using the Comprehensive Meta-analysis package, version 2 (http://www.meta-analysis.com).

Results

Appendix 9.1 details the studies included in this analysis. Table 9.1 shows the first analyses of insight versus cognitive measures for the whole sample, all psychoses, and for those studies that reported results for only patients with schizophrenia. Overall the mean weighted correlation coefficient between insight and all cognitive measures pooled was r=0.16 (95% CI=0.13–0.18, P<0.001). This analysis included 69 studies and combined data from 5127 participants. For IQ, the mean weighted r=0.16 (n=2745, 95% CI=0.12–0.19, P<0.001); for memory, r=0.13 (n=2078, 95% CI=0.09–0.18, P<0.001); for all executive function tests, pooled r=0.14 (n=3730, 95% CI=0.11–0.18, P<0.001); and for WCST results (categories completed and perseverative errors), r=0.13 (n=2263, 95% CI=0.08–0.172). Further statistics are available in Table 9.1. Of note, all results were statistically significant and effect sizes were not heterogeneous between studies. Figure 9.3 shows the forest plot for total cognition analyses by effect size.

For studies that used samples consisting of only patients with schizophrenia, we conducted this analysis again. Overall, the mean weighted correlation coefficient for insight and all cognitive measures pooled together was r=0.17 (95% CI=0.12–0.22, P<0.001). This analysis included 33 studies and combined data from 1708 participants. For IQ, the mean weighted r=0.19 (n=951, 95% CI=0.13–0.26, P<0.001); for memory, r=0.14 (n=594, 95%

Table 9.1. Results of meta-analyses of the insight–cognition relationship in patients with psychosis (mixed diagnoses) and those with the diagnosis of schizophrenia

	Participants (n)	Studies (n)	R^1	95% CI		Z	P	Q	P	I^2
Psychosis										
Total cognition	5127	69	0.16	0.13	0.18	10.97	<0.001	52.42	0.92	<0.001
IQ	2745	43	0.16	0.12	0.19	8.01	<0.001	36.92	0.69	<0.001
Memory	2078	29	0.13	0.09	0.18	5.93	<0.001	27.91	0.47	<0.001
Executive function	3730	53	0.14	0.11	0.18	8.61	<0.001	37.33	0.94	<0.001
WCST	2263	31	0.13	0.08	0.17	5.18	<0.001	35.89	0.21	16.41
Schizophrenia										
Total cognition	1708	33	0.17	0.12	0.22	6.87	<0.001	31.03	0.52	<0.001
IQ	951	19	0.19	0.13	0.26	5.88	<0.001	13.36	0.77	<0.001
Memory	594	13	0.14	0.03	0.25	2.52	0.01	19.98	0.07	39.95
Executive function	1220	24	0.16	0.11	0.22	5.52	<0.001	20.19	0.63	<0.001
WCST	792	13	0.15	0.05	0.24	2.90	<0.005	21.34	0.05	43.76

R^1, mean weighted correlation coefficient; WCST, Wisconsin Card Sorting Test.

Table 9.2. Correlation between insight and total cognition by insight scale

	Participants (n)	Studies (n)	R[1]	95% CI		Z	P	Q	P	I[2]
Insight scales										
SUMD	1523	25	0.14	0.09	0.19	5.18	<0.001	17.30	0.84	<0.001
SAI	1031	15	0.18	0.12	0.24	5.82	<0.001	13.77	0.47	<0.001
PANSS	1261	11	0.14	0.08	0.19	4.84	<0.001	6.44	0.78	<0.001
ITAQ	510	7	0.18	0.08	0.27	3.73	<0.001	6.33	0.39	5.14
Other	802	11	0.17	0.10	0.24	4.79	<0.001	6.33	0.79	<0.001

R[1], mean weighted correlation coefficient; SUMD, Scale to Assess Unawareness of Mental Disorder; SAI, Schedule for Assessment of Insight; PANSS, Positive and Negative Syndrome Scale; ITAQ, Insight and Treatment Attitudes Questionnaire.

CI=0.03–0.25, P=0.01); for all executive function tests, pooled r=0.16 (n=1220, 95% CI=0.11–0.22, P<0.001); and for WCST results (categories achieved and perseverative errors), r=0.15 (n=792, 95% CI=0.05–0.24, P<0.01). For the WCST analysis, the heterogeneity between studies was of borderline statistical significance (Q=21.3, P=0.05, I^2=43.8) and for the memory analysis, heterogeneity was close to statistical significance (Q=20.0, P=0.07, I^2=40.0). In comparison to the "all psychoses" analysis described earlier, all relationships were found to be slightly stronger in this group. In both analyses the effect sizes show a small overall effect and, in contrast to our previous analysis, the IQ–insight relationships appear marginally stronger than insight–executive function relationships in both "all psychoses" and schizophrenia analyses.

We also compared the relationship between total cognition and insight as measured by the different insight scales used. The four most commonly used scales – SUMD, SAI, ITAQ, and PANSS – were analyzed individually with all other scales being analyzed together as "other". The results can be found in Table 9.2. All scales were significantly correlated with general cognition with effect sizes ranging from r=0.14 for SUMD to r=0.18 for SAI. There was no significant within-group heterogeneity or between-group heterogeneity (Q=2.3, P=0.69) indicating that there was no significant difference between the scales used in this respect.

Publication bias in the literature can undermine the validity of a meta-analysis. This bias can be investigated in a number of ways. First, the construction of a funnel plot, as seen in Figure 9.4, where a measure of effect size, here Fisher's Z, and study size, here as standard error, are plotted. Ideally the funnel plot should be symmetrical across the mean weighted effect size. In an effort to objectively assess this symmetry, a number of statistical techniques have been developed. One such technique is the Duval and Tweedie's Trim and Fit analysis. Using this technique (described in detail in Rothstein et al., 2005), studies that are presumed missing from the forest plot are imputed. In our analysis, three studies were imputed as missing, represented as black circles, all lying close to the null effect. Including these studies results in a marginal shift of the overall mean weighted effect size. Another commonly used statistic is the "fail safe n," which was devised as a way of assessing how many studies of effect size 0 would be required to render the overall effect size of the study nonsignificant.

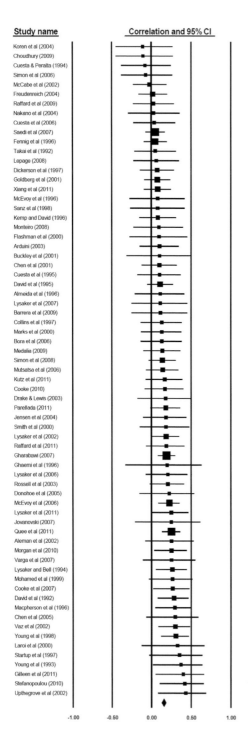

Figure 9.3. Forest plot showing all the effect sizes and 95% confidence intervals for total cognition using the random effects model. Chart is ordered by effect size and squares are proportional to the study size.

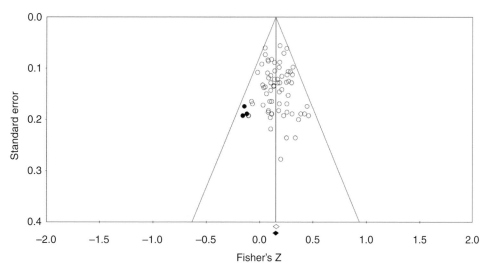

Figure 9.4. Funnel plot of standard error by Fisher's Z for total cognition, based on Duval and Tweedie's Trim and Fit Analysis, showing imputed missing studies (filled circles). Filled diamond represents the change in overall effect size if imputed studies are used for comparison.

In this meta-analysis, Rosenthal's fail safe n was calculated as 1889 studies. It is almost impossible that this number of studies are unpublished, therefore it is highly likely that the effect size we have found is not due to chance or publication bias alone.

Discussion

This meta-analysis sought to provide a comprehensive overview and summary of research into the relationship between insight and neurocognition in psychosis. Overall we found a small but statistically significant correlation between measures of insight and neurocognition across a variety of cognitive domains. We will first consider possible methodological reasons for our results, and second, the implications these findings have for a "neurocognitive theory of insight."

Limitations of meta-analysis

Meta-analysis is a powerful tool in quantitative research; however, there are a number of limitations, which should be considered when interpreting our results. First, results of a meta-analysis depend entirely on the included studies. While every effort to include all relevant studies was taken, we acknowledge that some relevant studies may, unfortunately, have been missed. There is also the concern that smaller studies, especially those that do not find significant results, may not get published and hence it is not possible to include their findings. Based on the analyses conducted in the previous section, we do not feel that this publication bias is significant but acknowledge that it cannot be excluded entirely.

By bringing together results from smaller studies, meta-analysis helps provide an overview of a complex field. As a result, however, our sample is a fairly heterogeneous population both demographically and based on clinical parameters such as diagnosis, illness duration, phase of illness, and the use of antipsychotic medication. This is a significant limitation as it may dilute stronger correlations between insight and neurocognition that may exist in certain better-defined sub-populations. We also acknowledge that our categorization of cognitive tests may appear somewhat crude given the wide variety of tests used in the included papers, and it is possible that in doing so, we introduced bias in favor of the null hypothesis by aggregating potentially stronger correlations with weaker ones. This categorization was performed in an effort to summarize a large body of literature for the reader.

Limitations of studies included in this analysis

Aside from limitations specific to the technique of meta-analysis, any meta-analysis to some extent inherits the limitations of its included papers. While we sought to include high quality papers, there were a few common limitations across a number of the included studies that are worth highlighting. A number of studies included fairly heterogeneous samples themselves, and much like the implications for our meta-analysis discussed earlier, this may result in a weakening of the overall results from the individual study. Many studies also conducted a large array of neurocognitive tests on their samples. This may have been in an effort to be thorough; however, as a previous review (Cooke et al., 2005) points out, it may also be because a number of studies do not formulate a clear and testable hypothesis between insight and a specific cognitive domain. Aside from the statistical implications of repeated testing on the same sample, it is clear from the documentation of the results that very rarely did all subjects complete the entire battery. This introduces bias into studies, as it is not always clear which participants could not complete which tasks, and it also adversely affects the power of the studies, weakening the overall result. Finally, it is worth mentioning that the consideration of confounding factors varied significantly between studies and this may have implications for overall results.

Measurement of insight

Interest in insight has been growing exponentially over the last two decades. In our review alone we found nearly as many papers were published on neurocognition and insight after 2004 as were published in all the preceding years. The concept of insight has also evolved over time. Initially it was considered a binary concept that patients were deemed to have or not have. Now it is clear that insight is a multifactorial complex concept. This complexity is reflected in the construction of scales designed to measure it, such as the SUMD that includes over 70 items. This begs the question, however – how does this complex concept relate to neurocognition? As an example, it has been hypothesized (Morgan et al., 2010) that poor neurocognitive functioning would be related primarily to the misattribution of symptoms. If this hypothesis is true then this correlation will be hidden or diminished when neurocognition is tested against scales that include other components of insight. The wide variety in the reporting of insight results, from breakdown of components to the creation of composite scores, means that it is not possible to undertake domain-specific analysis in this paper; however, this would be an interesting next step.

Measurement of neurocognition

The studies included in this paper have mostly used standardized and accepted measures of neurocognition. Aside from the limitations associated with over-testing, as described earlier, it may be worth asking what these tests are actually measuring and what implications this has for our results. A review and meta-analysis by Alvarez & Emory (2006) demonstrates that common tests such as the WCST or Stroop do not simply localize as frontal lobe tests. They conclude that these tests are sensitive rather than specific measures of frontal lobe activity. While they may test a neuropsychological concept such as "set-shifting," if they do not definitively localize neuroanatomically then one should be cautious when using them to frame hypotheses that may be neuroanatomically based. Ideally, experiments on the subject in the future should try and connect disease-specific functional imaging with relevant neurocognitive tasks and then seek to test their relationship with insight.

All of these points are possible methodological reasons why our meta-analysis does not demonstrate a strong correlation between insight and neurocognition. Putting all of these methodological limitations to one side, it is important to ask the following: if our findings do truly represent the relationship between neurocognition and insight, what implications does this have for the theory of insight? It is clear from the data that this small effect is highly significant and is unlikely to be a result of chance. In the introduction to this chapter, we presented some of the theories as to why poor neurocognition may be related to poor insight. If we take these results at face value, it is clear that these theories do not tell the whole story. There is not enough space within the confines of this chapter to review all the current theories related to insight (this has been done previously by Cooke et al. [2005], for example), but it is worth noting that in this field there are several competing theories of insight, such as the psychological denial theory, the symptom theory, and the neurocognitive theory. It is unlikely that any one theory alone will explain the complex concept of insight as it now stands and our results may indicate that the neurocognitive hypothesis stands alongside other models in explaining poor insight. In fact, a number of studies (Cooke et al., 2007; Aleman et al., 2006) have shown a curvilinear relationship between insight and neurocognition and have posited that more than one mechanism is responsible for this relationship.

It may also be that neurocognitive theory is more applicable to certain populations as opposed to 'psychosis' in general. Our results indicate a slightly stronger relationship in the schizophrenia subgroup than the "all psychoses" sample, for example. Equally, within the nosological entity of schizophrenia, there may be a subgroup for which cognitive deficits are more related to the loss of insight than are others.

When compared to the previous meta-analysis on neurocognitive functioning and insight in psychosis, published six years ago (Aleman et al., 2006), the effect sizes in the current meta-analysis are in the same range. The most notable difference was the somewhat smaller effect size observed for WCST perseverative errors compared to the previous meta-analysis ($r=0.13$ vs. $r=0.23$). However, the current analysis was based on 31 studies (2263 patients) whereas the previous analysis was based on 13 studies (712 patients). The specificity of a stronger correlation between poor insight and mental flexibility as measured by set shifting ability compared to other cognitive functions is therefore less secure. However, it remains possible that a stronger and more specific relationship exists between poor insight and meta-cognitive processes such as awareness of making errors and incorporating feedback in changing strategy (David et al., 2012; Koren et al., 2004, Lysaker et al., 2011). Another specific cognitive process that may be linked more strongly to poor insight is closely related to such meta-cognitive monitoring and concerns self-evaluation; for example, in relationship to theory of mind (van der Meer et al., 2010).

After all, insight may depend more on the ability "to see ourselves as others see us" (Aleman et al., 2002; David, 1999) than on general cognitive ability.

In summary, this chapter has presented data from a comprehensive, up-to-date meta-analysis of the literature on the relationship between insight and neurocognition in psychosis. Overall, our results indicate that there is a small but significant relationship between insight and neurocognition as measured by classical neuropsychological tests. It is difficult to be clear what this correlation represents due to a variety of limitations, both in this meta-analysis and the study of which it comprises. Perhaps a more robust hypothesis-led approach, using the sort of cognitive neuropsychological model proffered in the introduction, and bringing in findings from functional neuro-imaging, may help elucidate this complex relationship. That model is compatible with our results, which show small but robust effects across the board with respect to component cognitive functions but require a more precise experimental or case-study approach to pin down which components are affected and how. Future studies should also investigate the clinical implications of these findings, such as whether cognitive rehabilitation improves insight.

Appendix 9.1. List of all studies included in analysis (n = 69)

Study name	Sample size	Insight scale	Neurocognitive measure
Aleman et al. (2002)	38	PANSS	Digit span, visual elevator task, source memory
Almeida et al. (1996)	40	SAI	Digit span, NART, recognition memory test, spatial span, verbal fluency
Arduini et al. (2003)	64	SUMD	WCST
Barrera et al. (2009)	31	Other	Brixton Test (similar to WCST), cognitive estimates, Hayling Sentence Completion, MSE
Bora et al. (2007)	58	SUMD	Digit span, Letter Number Working Memory Test, verbal fluency, WAIS, WCST
Buckley et al. (2001)	24	SUMD	TMT
Chen et al. (2001)	80	SAI	WCST
Chen et al. (2005)	31	SAI	WMS-R
Choudhury et al. (2009)	30	SUMD	WCST
Collins et al. (1997)	58	PANSS	WCST
Cooke et al. (2010)	64	PANSS	CPT, BADS score, Brixton Test, verbal fluency, Hayling Sentence Completion, HVLT, Stroop TMT, WAIS-IQ, WCST

Appendix 9.1. *(cont.)*

Study name	Sample size	Insight scale	Neurocognitive measure
Cooke et al. (2007)	67	Other	Quick IQ test
Cuesta & Peralta (1994)	40	Other	Bender visual motor tests, immediate & delayed verbal and visual memory, Luria's test of premotor praxia, MMSE, Rey's complex figure, TMT, verbal fluency, WAIS
Cuesta et al. (1995)	52	Other	WCST
Cuesta et al. (2006)	56	SUMD, ITAQ, other	Immediate and delayed verbal memory, verbal fluency, Stroop, TMT, WAIS, WCST
David et al. (1992)	91	SAI, other	NART
David et al. (1995)	150	SAI	NART, TMT
Dickerson et al. (1997)	87	PANSS	Chicago word fluency, Halstead-Wepman aphasia screening, logical memory of WMS-R, Rey-Osterrieth complex figure, TMT, WAIS-R, WCST
Donohoe et al. (2005)	30	Other	NART-IQ, Stroop, letter-number, sustained attention task, visual elevator task, WAIS, WMS logical memory
Drake & Lewis (2003)	33	PANSS, SAI, ITAQ, SUMD	Sentences test, triads, NART-IQ, quick test for IQ, TMT, Hayling, frontal lobe score, Brixton Test, Theory of Mind Test
Fennig et al. (1996)	189	Other	Quick test for IQ
Flashman et al. (2000)	29	SUMD	Full-scale IQ test
Freudenreich et al. (2004)	122	SUMD	CVLT, digit span, full-scale IQ, Stroop, WCST
Ghaemi et al. (1996)	16	ITAQ	Full-scale IQ test, WMS memory passages immediate & delayed recall, WMS visual reproduction immediate and delayed recall, similarities (WAIS-R)
Gharabawi et al. (2007)	323	PANSS	CogTest battery evaluating: attention, reasoning/problem solving, declarative memory, visual memory, working memory
Gilleen et al. (2011)	31	SAI	Key search, letter number span, modified six elements, RMBT, TMT, WAIS-IQ
Goldberg et al. (2001)	146	PANSS	RBANS, WCST, WAIS-III, WRAT-R

Appendix 9.1. (*cont.*)

Study name	Sample size	Insight scale	Neurocognitive measure
Jensen et al. (2004)	50	PANSS	Tests for long-term memory and selective attention from "Automated Psychological Test System"
Jovanovski et al. (2007)	21	SUMD	BADS, WASI
Kemp & David (1996)	74	SAI, PSE	Cognitive estimates, NART, TMT, verbal fluency
Koren et al. (2004)	30	SUMD	WAIS-R block design and similarities, WCST
Kutz & Tolman (2011)	71	PANSS	CVLT, digit span, Penn conditional exclusion test, verbal fluency, WAIS-R vocabulary
Laroi et al. (2000)	21	SUMD	Kimura Figure Test, TMT-B, WAIS-R (block design and vocabulary), WCST
Lepage et al. (2008)	47	PANSS	WMS-III (logical memory, visual reproduction, spatial span), WAIS-III (digit span, digit symbol, block design), TMT-B, Tower of London
Lysaker & Bell (1994)	92	PANSS	WCST
Lysaker et al. (2002)	132	SUMD	WAIS-III, WCST
Lysaker et al. (2006)	53	SUMD	Verbal fluency, sorting task, Stroop, TMT, Tower task, word context
Lysaker et al. (2007)	31	SUMD	WCST
Lysaker et al. (2011)	65	SUMD	WCST, WAIS-III (vocabulary and digit symbol), HVLT recalled, CPT omissions
Macpherson et al. (1996)	64	SAI	MMSE, NART
Marks et al. (2000)	59	SUMD, PANSS, SAI	HTLV, letter number sequencing, logical memory from WMS-R, NART, similarities Stroop, WCST
McCabe et al. (2002)	89	SAI	Luria-Nebraska neuropsychological battery
McEvoy et al. (1996)	32	ITAQ	Figural fluency, WCST, WAIS-R vocabulary, Rey-Osterrieth complex figure
McEvoy et al. (2006)	203	ITAQ	Composite score derived from wide ranging neurocognitive battery
Medalia & Thysen (2008)	71	SUMD	BACS (Tower of London, verbal fluency, verbal memory, digit sequencing)

Appendix 9.1. *(cont.)*

Study name	Sample size	Insight scale	Neurocognitive measure
Mohamed et al. (1999)	46	SUMD	Verbal fluency, design fluency, TMT, modified WCST
Monteiro et al. (2008)	40	SUMD	CPT, Stroop, TMT, WAIS-R, WCST
Morgan et al. (2010)	82	SAI	NART, WAIS-R, Raven's colored progressive matrices, AVLT (immediate, verbal learning), visual reproduction, LNS, verbal fluency, TMT-B
Mutsatsa et al. (2006)	94	SAI	WAIS-R, NART, planning task, set shifting task, spatial span working memory test
Nakano et al. (2004)	37	SAI	WAIS-R, WCST
Parellada et al. (2011)	57	SUMD	WCST, Stroop, controlled verbal fluency test, TMT-B, digit span, letter-number sequencing, WAIS
Quee et al. (2011)	270	Other	Composite neurocognitive variable
Raffard et al. (2009)	60	SUMD	NART-IQ
Raffard et al. (2011)	64	PANSS	NART-IQ
Rossell et al. (2003)	78	SAI	NART, controlled oral word association test, WAIS-R, WCST
Saeedi et al. (2007)	278	PANSS	Category fluency, delayed verbal memory, immediate verbal memory, TMT, WCST
Sanz et al. (1998)	33	ITAQ, SAI, PANSS	MMSE, NART, Star Cancellation Test, TMT WCST
Simon et al. (2006)	38	SUMD	BADS, Stroop, TMT verbal fluency – letters and semantic, WCST
Simon et al. (2009)	131	Other	Letter number sequencing, TMT, WCST
Smith et al. (2000)	38	SUMD	CVLT, Digit Span Distractibility Test, verbal fluency, WAIS-R, WCST
Startup (1996)	28	ITAQ	Spot the word (estimate of verbal intelligence)
Stefanopoulou et al. (2009)	36	ITAQ	WAIS-III (full scale, performance, verbal)
Takai et al. (1992)	57	Other	WAIS
Upthegrove et al. (2002)	30	SAI	Digit span
Varga et al. (2007)	32	SUMD	AVLT verbal learning and delayed recall, digit span, WAIS-III, Stroop, TMT-B, WCST

Appendix 9.1. (cont.)

Study name	Sample size	Insight scale	Neurocognitive measure
Vaz et al. (2002)	82	SAI	Cognitive factor of PANSS
Xiang et al. (2012)	139	ITAQ	WCST
Young et al. (1993)	31	SUMD	TMT, verbal fluency, WAIS-R, WCST
Young et al. (1998)	108	SUMD	WAIS-R, WCST

PANSS, Positive and Negative Syndrome Scale – insight item G12; SAI, Schedule for Assessment of Insight; SUMD, Scale to Assess Unawareness of Mental Disorder; ITAQ, Insight and Treatment Attitudes Questionnaire; PSE, Present State Examination; NART, National Adult Reading Test; WCST, Wisconsin Card Sorting Test; MSE, Modified Six Elements Test; WAIS, Wechsler Adult Intelligence Test; TMT, Trail Making Test (Part B only); WMS, Wechsler Memory Test; CPT, Continuous Performance Test; BADS, Behavioural Assessment of the Dysexecutive Syndrome; HVLT, Hopkins Verbal Learning Test; MMSE, Mini-Mental State Examination; CVLT, California Verbal Learning Test; RMBT, Rivermead Behavioural Test; RBANS, Repeatable Battery for the Assessment of Neuropsychological Status; WRAT, Wide Range Achievement Test; WASI, Wechsler Abbreviated Scale of Intelligence; BACS, Brief Assessment into Cognition in Schizophrenia; AVLT, Auditory Verbal Learning Test; LNS, letter number sequencing.

References

Aleman, A., Agrawal, N., Morgan, K. D., et al. (2006). Insight in psychosis and neuropsychological function: meta-analysis. *British Journal of Psychiatry*, **189**, 204–212.

Aleman, A., de Haan, E. H. F., & Kahn, R. S. (2002). Insight and neurocognitive function in schizophrenia. *Journal of Neuropsychiatry and Clinical Neuroscience*, **14**, 241–242.

Almeida, O. P., Levy, R., Howard, R. J., et al. (1996). Insight and paranoid disorders in late life (late paraphenia). *International Journal of Geriatric Psychiatry*, **11**, 653–658.

Alvarez, J. A. & Emory, E. (2006). Executive function and the frontal lobes: a meta-analytic review. *Neuropsychology Review*, **16**, 17–42.

Amador, X. F. & David, A. S. (eds.). (2004). *Insight and Psychosis: Awareness of Illness in Schizophrenia and Related Disorders* (2nd edn.). Oxford: Oxford University Press.

Arduini, L., Kalyvoka, A., Stratta, P., et al. (2003). Insight and neuropsychological function in patients with schizophrenia and bipolar disorder with psychotic features. *Canadian Journal of Psychiatry*, **48**, 338–341.

Barrera, A., McKenna, P. J., & Berrios, G. E. (2009). Formal thought disorder, neuropsychology and insight in schizophrenia. *Psychopathology*, **42**, 264–269.

Bora, E., Sehitoglu, G., Aslier, M., et al. (2007). Theory of mind and unawareness of illness in schizophrenia: is poor insight a mentalizing deficit? *European Archives of Psychiatry and Clinical Neuroscience*, **257**, 104–111.

Buckley, P. F., Hasan, S., Friedman, L., et al. (2001). Insight and schizophrenia. *Comprehensive Psychiatry*, **42**, 39–41.

Chen, E. Y., Kwok, C. L., Chen, R. Y., et al. (2001). Insight changes in acute psychotic episodes: a prospective study of Hong Kong Chinese patients. *Journal of Nervous and Mental Disease*, **189**, 24–30.

Chen, K. C., Chu, C. L., Yang, Y. K., et al. (2005). The relationship among insight, cognitive function of patients with schizophrenia and their relatives' perception. *Psychiatry and Clinical Neuroscience*, **59**, 657–660.

Choudhury, S., Khess, C. R., Bhattacharyya, R., et al. (2009). Insight in schizophrenia and its association with executive functions. *Indian Journal of Psychological Medicine*, **31**, 71–76.

Collins, A. A., Remington, G. J., Coulter, K., et al. (1997). Insight, neurocognitive function and symptom clusters in chronic schizophrenia. *Schizophrenia Research*, **27**, 37–44.

Cooke, M. A., Peters, E. R., Fannon, D., et al. (2010). Cognitive insight in psychosis: the relationship between self-certainty and self-reflection dimensions and neuropsychological measures. *Psychiatry Research*, **178**, 284–289.

Cooke, M. A., Peters, E. R., Greenwood, K. E., et al. (2007). Insight in psychosis: influence of cognitive ability and self-esteem. *British Journal of Psychiatry*, **191**, 234–237.

Cooke, M. A., Peters, E. R., Kuipers, E., et al. (2005). Disease, deficit or denial? Models of poor insight in psychosis. *Acta Psychiatrica Scandinavica*, **112**, 4–17.

Cuesta, M. J. & Peralta, V. (1994). Lack of insight in schizophrenia. *Schizophrenia Bulletin*, **20**, 359–366.

Cuesta, M. J., Peralta, V., Caro, F., et al. (1995). Is poor insight in psychotic disorders associated with poor performance on the Wisconsin Card Sorting Test? *American Journal of Psychiatry*, **152**, 1380–1382.

Cuesta, M. J., Peralta, V., Zarzuela, A., et al. (2006). Insight dimensions and cognitive function in psychosis: a longitudinal study. *BMC Psychiatry*, **6**, 26.

David, A., Buchanan, A., Reed, A., et al. (1992). The assessment of insight in psychosis. *British Journal of Psychiatry*, **161**, 599–602.

David, A., van Os, J., Jones, P., et al. (1995). Insight and psychotic illness. Cross-sectional and longitudinal associations. *British Journal of Psychiatry*, **167**, 621–628.

David, A. S. (1990). Insight and psychosis. *British Journal of Psychiatry*, **156**, 798–808.

David, A. S. (1999). "To see ourselves as others see us". Aubrey Lewis's insight. *British Journal of Psychiatry*, **175**, 210–216.

David, A. S., Bedford, N., Wiffen, B., et al. (2012). Failures of metacognition and lack of insight in neuropsychiatric disorders. *Philosophical Transactions of the Royal Society of London. Series B: Biological Sciences*, **367**, 1379–1390.

Dickerson, F. B., Boronow, J. J., & Ringel, N. (1997). Lack of insight among outpatients with schizophrenia. *Psychiatric Services*, **48**, 195–199.

Donohoe, G., Corvin, A., & Robertson, I. H. (2005). Are the cognitive deficits associated with impaired insight in schizophrenia specific to executive task performance? *Journal of Nervous and Mental Disorders*, **193**, 803–808.

Drake, R. J. & Lewis, S. W. (2003). Insight and neurocognition in schizophrenia. *Schizophrenia Research*, **62**, 165–173.

Fennig, S., Everett, E., Bromet, E. J., et al. (1996). Insight in first-admission psychotic patients. *Schizophrenia Research*, **22**, 257–263.

Flashman, L. A., McAllister, T. W., Andreasen, N. C., et al. (2000). Smaller brain size associated with unawareness of illness in patients with schizophrenia. *American Journal of Psychiatry*, **157**, 1167–1169.

Freudenreich, O., Deckersbach, T., & Goff, D. C. (2004). Insight into current symptoms of schizophrenia. Association with frontal cortical function and affect. *Acta Psychiatrica Scandinavica*, **110**, 14–20.

Ghaemi, S. N., Hebben, N., Stoll, A. L., et al. (1996). Neuropsychological aspects of lack of insight in bipolar disorder: a preliminary report. *Psychiatry Research*, **65**, 113–120.

Gharabawi, G., Bossie, C., Turkoz, I., et al. (2007) The impact of insight on functioning in patients with schizophrenia or schizoaffective disorder receiving risperidone long-acting injectable. *Journal of Nervous and Mental Disorders*, **195**, 976–982.

Gilleen, J., Greenwood, K., & David, A. S. (2011). Domains of awareness in schizophrenia. *Schizophrenia Bulletin*, **37**, 61–72.

Goldberg, R. W., Green-Paden, L. D., Lehman, A. F., et al. (2001). Correlates of insight in serious mental illness. *Journal of Nervous and Mental Disorders*, **189**, 137–145.

Jensen, J., Nilsson, L. L., & Levander, S. (2004). Neurocognitive and psychopathological correlates of self-monitoring ability in schizophrenia. *European Achives of Psychiatry and Clinical Neuroscience*, **254**, 312–317.

Jovanovski, D., Zakzanis, K. K., Young, D. A., et al. (2007). Assessing the relationship between insight and everyday executive deficits in schizophrenia: a pilot study. *Psychiatry Research*, **151**, 47–54.

Kemp, R. & David, A. (1996). Psychological predictors of insight and compliance in psychotic patients. *British Journal of Psychiatry*, **169**, 444–450.

Koren, D., Seidman, L. J., Poyurovsky, M., et al. (2004). The neuropsychological basis of insight in first-episode schizophrenia: a pilot metacognitive study. *Schizophrenia Research*, **70**, 195–202.

Kurtz, M. M. & Tolman, A. (2011). Neurocognition, insight into illness and subjective quality-of-life in schizophrenia: what is their relationship? *Schizophrenia Research*, **127**, 157–162.

Laroi, F., Fannemel, M., Ronneberg, U., et al. (2000). Unawareness of illness in chronic schizophrenia and its relationship to structural brain measures and neuropsychological tests. *Psychiatry Research*, **100**, 49–58.

Lepage, M., Buchy, L., Bodnar, M., et al. (2008). Cognitive insight and verbal memory in first episode of psychosis. *European Psychiatry*, **23**, 368–374.

Lipsey, M. W. & Wilson, D. B. (2001). *Practical Meta-Analysis*. Thousand Oaks, CA: Sage.

Lysaker, P. & Bell, M. (1994). Insight and cognitive impairment in schizophrenia. Performance on repeated administrations of the Wisconsin Card Sorting Test. *Journal of Nervous and Mental Disorders*, **182**, 656–660.

Lysaker, P. H., Bryson, G. J., & Bell, M. D. (2002). Insight and work performance in schizophrenia. *Journal of Nervous and Mental Disorders*, **190**, 142–146.

Lysaker, P. H., Daroyanni, P., Ringer, J. M., et al. (2007). Associations of awareness of illness in schizophrenia spectrum disorder with social cognition and cognitive perceptual organization. *Journal of Nervous and Mental Disorders*, **195**, 618–621.

Lysaker, P. H., Dimaggio, G., Buck, K. D., et al. (2011). Poor insight in schizophrenia: links between different forms of metacognition with awareness of symptoms, treatment need, and consequences of illness. *Comprehensive Psychiatry*, **52**, 253–260.

Lysaker, P. H., Whitney, K. A., & Davis L. W. (2006). Awareness of illness in schizophrenia: associations with multiple assessments of executive function. *Journal of Neuropsychiatry and Clinical Neuroscience*, **18**, 516–520.

Macpherson, R., Jerrom, B., & Hughes, A. (1996). Relationship between insight, educational background and cognition in schizophrenia. *British Journal of Psychiatry*, **168**, 718–722.

Marks, K. A., Fastenau, P. S., Lysaker, P. H., et al. (2000). Self-Appraisal of Illness Questionnaire (SAIQ): relationship to researcher-rated insight and neuropsychological function in schizophrenia. *Schizophrenia Research*, **45**, 203–211.

McCabe, R., Quayle, E., Beirne, A. D., et al. (2002). Insight, global neuropsychological functioning, and symptomatology in chronic schizophrenia. *Journal of Nervous and Mental Disorders*, **190**, 519–525.

McEvoy, J. P., Hartman, M., Gottlieb, D., et al. (1996). Common sense, insight, and neuropsychological test performance in schizophrenia patients. *Schizophrenia Bulletin*, **22**, 635–640.

McEvoy, J. P., Johnson, J., Perkins, D., et al. (2006). Insight in first-episode psychosis. *Psychological Medicine*, **36**, 1385–1393.

Medalia, A. & Thysen, J. (2008). Insight into neurocognitive dysfunction in schizophrenia. *Schizophrenia Bulletin*, **34**, 1221–1230.

Mohamed, S., Fleming, S., Penn, D. L., et al. (1999). Insight in schizophrenia: its relationship to measures of executive functions. *Journal of Nervous and Mental Disorders*, **187**, 525–531.

Monteiro, L. C., Silva, V. A., & Louza, M. R. (2008). Insight, cognitive dysfunction and symptomatology in schizophrenia. *European Archives of Psychiatry and Clinical Neuroscience*, **258**, 402–405.

Morgan, K. D., Dazzan, P., Morgan, C., et al. (2010). Insight, grey matter and cognitive function in first-onset psychosis. *British Journal of Psychiatry*, **197**, 141–148.

Mutsatsa, S. H., Joyce, E. M., Hutton, S. B., et al. (2006). Relationship between insight, cognitive function, social function and symptomatology in schizophrenia: the West London first episode study. *European Archives of Psychiatry and Clinical Neuroscience*, **256**, 356–363.

Nakano, H., Terao, T., Iwata, N., et al. (2004). Symptomatological and cognitive predictors of insight in chronic schizophrenia. *Psychiatry Research*, **127**, 65–72.

Parellada, M., Boada, L., Fraguas, D., et al. (2011). Trait and state attributes of insight in first episodes of early-onset schizophrenia and other psychoses: a 2-year longitudinal study. *Schizophrenia Bulletin*, **37**, 38–51.

Quee, P. J., van der Meer, L., Bruggeman, R., et al. (2011). Insight in psychosis: relationship with neurocognition, social cognition and clinical symptoms depends on phase of illness. *Schizophrenia Bulletin*, **37**, 29–37.

Raffard, S., Bayard, S., Gely-Nargeot, M. C., et al. (2009). Insight and executive functioning in schizophrenia: a multidimensional approach. *Psychiatry Research*, **167**, 239–250.

Raffard, S., Capdevielle, D., Gely-Nargeot, M. C., et al. (2011). Insight is not associated with insensitivity to future consequences in schizophrenia. *Psychiatry Research*, **187**, 307–309.

Rossell, S. L., Coakes, J., Shapleske, J., et al. (2003). Insight: its relationship with cognitive function, brain volume and symptoms in schizophrenia. *Psychological Medicine*, **33**, 111–119.

Rothstein, H., Sutton, A., & Borenstein, M. (eds.). (2005). *Publication Bias in Meta-Analysis: Prevention, Assessment and Adjustments*. Chichester: Wiley-Blackwell.

Saeedi, H., Addington, J., & Addington, D. (2007). The association of insight with psychotic symptoms, depression, and cognition in early psychosis: a 3-year follow-up. *Schizophrenia Research*, **89**, 123–128.

Sanz, M., Constable, G., Lopez-Ibor, I., et al. (1998). A comparative study of insight scales and their relationship to psychopathological and clinical variables. *Psychological Medicine*, **28**, 437–446.

Simon, A. E., Berger, G. E., Giacomini, V., et al. (2006). Insight, symptoms and executive functions in schizophrenia. *Cognitive Neuropsychiatry*, **11**, 437–451.

Simon, V., De Hert, M., Wampers, M., et al. (2009). The relation between neurocognitive dysfunction and impaired insight in patients with schizophrenia. *European Psychiatry*, **24**, 239–243.

Smith, T. E., Hull, J. W., Israel, L. M., et al. (2000). Insight, symptoms, and neurocognition in schizophrenia and schizoaffective disorder. *Schizophrenia Bulletin*, **26**, 193–200.

Startup, M. (1996). Insight and cognitive deficits in schizophrenia: evidence for a curvilinear relationship. *Psychological Medicine*, **26**, 1277–1281.

Stefanopoulou, E., Lafuente, A. R., Saez Fonseca, J. A., et al. (2009). Insight, global functioning and psychopathology amongst in-patient clients with schizophrenia. *Psychiatry Quarterly*, **80**, 155–165.

Takai, A., Uermatsu, M., & Ueki, H. (1992). Insight and its related factors in chronic schizophrenic patients: a preliminary study. *European Journal of Psychiatry*, **6**, 159–170.

Upthegrove, R., Oyebode, F., George, M., et al. (2002). Insight, social knowledge and working memory in schizophrenia. *Psychopathology*, **35**, 341–346.

van der Meer, L., Costafreda, S., Aleman, A., et al. (2010). Self-reflection and the brain: a theoretical review and meta-analysis of neuroimaging studies with implications for schizophrenia. *Neuroscience and Biobehavioral Review*, **34**, 935–946.

Varga, M., Magnusson, A., Flekkoy, K., et al. (2007). Clinical and neuropsychological correlates of insight in schizophrenia and bipolar I disorder: does diagnosis matter? *Comprehensive Psychiatry*, **48**, 583–591.

Vaz, F. J., Béjar, A., & Casado, M. (2002). Insight, psychopathology, and interpersonal relationships in schizophrenia. *Schizophrenia Bulletin*, **28**, 311–317.

Xiang, Y. T., Wang, Y., Wang, C. Y., et al. (2012). Association of insight with sociodemographic and clinical factors, quality of life, and cognition in Chinese patients with schizophrenia. *Comprehensive Psychiatry*, **53**, 140–144.

Young, D. A., Davila, R., & Scher, H. (1993). Unawareness of illness and neuropsychological performance in chronic schizophrenia. *Schizophrenia Research*, **10**, 117–124.

Young, D. A., Zakzanis, K. K., Bailey, C., et al. (1998). Further parameters of insight and neuropsychological deficit in schizophrenia and other chronic mental disease. *Journal of Nervous and Mental Disorders*, **186**, 44–50.

Chapter

10

Genetic influences on cognition in schizophrenia

Katherine E. Burdick, Benjamin Glicksberg, and
Gary Donohoe

Heritability of schizophrenia

Family and twin studies have consistently reported a high heritability for schizophrenia (Sullivan et al., 2003). In the largest family-based study to date, Lichtenstein et al. (2009) assessed recurrence risk for schizophrenia within more than two million nuclear families, including approximately nine million unique individuals from Sweden's multi-generation database and hospital discharge registries. Heritability was high (64%) and the relative risk (RR) was consistent with prior reports (schizophrenic sibling RR=9.0) indicating a strong genetic component to schizophrenia.

More than two decades of research into the molecular underpinnings of schizophrenia have begun to reveal the level of its genetic complexity. Early studies indicated that the disorder could not be attributed to a single genetic locus (O'Rourke et al., 1982) or accounted for by additive effects of noninteracting multiple single loci (Risch, 1990). Progress has been made with recent large-scale genome-wide association studies (GWAS) contributing important initial evidence of replicable schizophrenia risk alleles, in the form of single nucleotide polymorphisms (SNPs) (Ripke et al., 2011). Association data from SNP-based analyses have confirmed at least eight convincing risk variants for schizophrenia (Ripke et al., 2011), many of which are nonspecific to schizophrenia, influencing risk more broadly for major psychiatric illnesses including bipolar disorder (Williams et al., 2011). In addition to single-locus effects, convergent data suggest that there is a polygenic component underlying risk for schizophrenia, involving thousands of common alleles, in aggregate, each with very small effect (Purcell et al., 2009; Ripke et al., 2011; Ruderfer et al., 2011).

The combined effect of common variation assayed by GWAS allelic variants and polygenic aggregate scores, although substantial, does not account for all of the heritability for schizophrenia, implicating an important role for *rare* variation. Several reports now confirm a strong relationship between risk for schizophrenia and structural variations in the genome, in the form of rare copy number variants (CNVs) (Kirov et al., 2009; Stefansson et al., 2008; Walsh et al., 2008; Xu et al., 2008). Copy number variant associations in schizophrenia include both recurrent individual CNV loci (e.g., 22q11.2 deletions) as well as an overall increased frequency, or burden, of rare CNVs (Doherty et al., 2012).

Despite the recent advances in psychiatric genetics, the search for disease susceptibility genes has had limited success, due in part to the notable complexity of both the phenotype

Cognitive Impairment in Schizophrenia, ed. Philip D. Harvey. Published by Cambridge University Press. © Cambridge University Press 2013.

and underlying genetic architecture (Gottesman & Gould, 2003). Hence, the need to deconstruct the illness into its most basic elements has become fundamental to elucidating its neurobiological substrates (Lenox et al., 2002). Molecular genetic efforts have sought to identify and validate intermediate phenotypes of complex psychiatric disorders; that is, those phenomena falling between the grossly manifest signs of psychopathology and their likely genetic correlates. The use of such biomarkers in molecular genetic studies may enhance power to detect susceptibility loci first by reducing the complexity of the phenotype through dissecting it into its component parts, and second by assaying a trait that is believed to be more proximal to gene action (Braff et al., 2007). In schizophrenia, impaired cognitive function has been shown to have a familial or genetic component, suggesting that this trait may serve as a powerful assay to elucidate basic mechanisms that underlie core illness features (Bates & Malhotra, 2002; Egan, 2001).

Cognition in schizophrenia

Cognitive impairment has long been recognized as a core feature of schizophrenia (Bleuler, 1950; Elvevåg & Goldberg, 2000), with significant, diffuse dysfunction that includes intellectual deterioration as well as more specific deficits in individual cognitive domains, such as working memory and executive functioning (Keefe & Fenton, 2007). Although the underlying etiology of cognitive impairment in schizophrenia has not yet been elucidated, data support a neurodevelopmental model in which genetic factors play a significant role (Fatemi & Folsom, 2009; Glahn et al., 2006).

The use of the intermediate phenotype or endophenotype approach has become an important aspect of schizophrenia genetics research. Gottesman and colleagues (Gottesman & Gould, 2003; Gottesman & Shields, 1972, 1973) first articulated the concept of utilizing an "endophenotype" in psychiatry as a biological marker to obtain "simpler clues to genetic underpinnings than the disease syndrome itself." The four primary criteria that make a disease-related trait a good candidate as an endophenotype include: (1) it is consistently present in probands with the disorder; (2) it is not state-related, but is measurable very early in the course of the disease and/or during periods of remission; (3) it is heritable; and (4) it is found, albeit to a lesser extent, in healthy (unaffected) relatives of probands when compared with unrelated healthy individuals (Gottesman & Shields, 1973).

Neurocognitive dysfunction has received substantial attention as a candidate endophenotype in schizophrenia and may be particularly useful in the context of large-scale molecular genetic studies, as it is relatively easy to implement and is noninvasive. Moreover, cognitive deficits appear to be closely linked with genetic susceptibility for several major mental illnesses and fulfill the basic "endophenotype" criteria previously set out. As such, a growing body of evidence suggests that both global (i.e., intelligence quotient [IQ]) and specific (e.g., working memory) measures of neurocognitive function may have utility in genetic studies by enhancing power and/or elucidating gene function at the endophenotype level. Selecting cognitive endophenotypes for schizophrenia is complicated by the number of deficits involved, different theories about their neurocognitive basis (including the separability of these deficits), and differences in assessment. Deficits in lower stages of information processing have been assessed using neurophysiological indices (e.g., mismatch negativity) (Javitt et al., 1997). Higher stages of information processing have been variously targeted in terms of general cognitive functioning, prefrontal function (characterized as deficits in attention or working memory), and memory function.

Cognitive deficits as stable traits in schizophrenia

The prevalence and course of cognitive deficits in schizophrenia is described in detail in Chapter 7. In summary, cognitive deficits are present from an early stage of the disorder and often predate the emergence of clinical symptoms (Erlenmeyer-Kimling et al., 2000; Niendam et al., 2003). They are relatively stable over time and are closely related to functional outcome (Green et al., 2004). While cognitive deficits are somewhat correlated with clinical symptoms (e.g., negative symptoms in schizophrenia), the amount of variance shared by these variables appears to be small, and cognitive function often emerges as a separate factor from clinical symptoms in factor analysis (Donohoe & Robertson, 2003; Donohoe et al., 2006; Good et al., 2004). The early emergence and relative independence from state-related illness fluctuations support a strong genetic contribution to the cognitive impairment in patients with schizophrenia.

Heritability of cognitive deficits in schizophrenia

A large body of literature has investigated the heritability of cognitive deficits in schizophrenia using family and twin study designs. The proportion of individual variation in a given phenotype in a population due to genetic differences (termed heritability, [h^2]) can be estimated based on the fact that different classes of relatives share more or less genetic material. For example, monozygotic (MZ) twins share, on average, 100% of their DNA, dizygotic (DZ) twins/siblings share 50%, and half-siblings 25%. In classical twin study designs, heritability is investigated in terms of phenotypic similarity/differences between MZ twins and DZ twins. The effects of environmental factors can also be investigated by comparing MZ twins reared together versus apart and DZ twins reared together/apart (see Sternberg & Grigorenko, 1997, for the application of this approach to the phenotype of intelligence). In the case of cognitive deficits in schizophrenia, because of practical sampling constraints, demonstration of cognitive deficit in relatives of schizophrenic probands at a higher rate than in controls is usually taken as evidence of heritability, and a number of family studies of this type have been performed. These studies generally support the concept that the cognitive deficits associated with these disorders are inherited, including general cognitive ability, working memory, and episodic memory (Cannon et al., 2000; Goldberg et al., 1990, 1995; Kremen et al., 2006; Touloupoulou et al., 2007, 2010). The heritability of deficits in general cognitive ability and working memory in particular appear to overlap strongly with the heritability of illness risk in schizophrenia (Touloupoulou et al., 2007), although not to the point of suggesting a complete overlap between the genetic architecture of schizophrenia and cognition.

Attention

Attention involves the controlled or voluntary focusing of awareness. As such it requires both active maintenance of focus on relevant stimuli and the equally active suppression or ignoring of nonrelevant stimuli. In contemporary neuropsychology, attention is often fractionated into more specific components (e.g., sustained, selective, and divided [controlled]), each crucial for maintaining coherent behavior in the face of multiple action or response alternatives. Inheritance of attentional deficits in schizophrenia has typically been measured by various Continuous Performance Tasks (CPT)(Cornblatt et al., 1994). Family studies have tended to use the more demanding versions of the CPT, which include either increased perceptual load or selective attention elements. Four studies found that relatives of patients were impaired using the degraded stimulus (DS) version (Chen et al., 1998, 2004; Laurent et al., 2000; Saoud et al., 2000), and three using the identical pairs (IP) version (Appels et al., 2003; Franke et al., 1994; Laurent et al., 1999). Among studies failing to find evidence of a genetic contribution to CPT task deficits, one found that performance was not predictive of genetic loading for schizophrenia (Keefe et al., 1997), and one smaller study by Jones et al. (2001) using the CPT-DS found that neither schizophrenia relatives nor patients differed significantly from controls in CPT performance. The single reported twin study of CPT did not support a genetic contribution to CPT performance (Cannon, 2000).

Donohoe et al. (2009) reported that effect sizes for family studies of CPT performance were heterogeneous, probably relating to different versions of the task (e.g., the 1–9 and 3–7 versions showing smaller effect sizes), but possibly also to differences in sample characteristics and sample size. While effect sizes were in the small to medium range, the confidence intervals contained 0.00 for eight of the 12 studies for which effect sizes were calculated. This suggests that the actual size of the difference between unaffected relatives of patients with schizophrenia and controls may be quite small, consistent with previous evidence suggesting that the CPT may be of limited utility for molecular studies (Heinrichs, 2004; Keri & Janka, 2004).

Working memory

Working memory (WM) is involved in a wide range of cognitive operations that require simultaneous storage and processing of information (Baddeley, 1990). Conceptualized in terms of storage subsystems coordinated by a central executive, this function represents an active system of maintaining and manipulating information that provides the basis for many complex cognitive abilities. Of nine family studies measuring WM in relatives using a well-established task (e.g., the spatial delayed response task or one of the Wechsler WM tasks), almost all found evidence for impaired working memory performance across the range of tests used (Conklin et al., 2000, 2005; Glahn et al., 2003; Goldberg et al., 2003; Keri et al., 2001; Krabbendam et al., 2001; Myles-Worsley & Park, 2002; Park et al., 1995; Tuulio-Henriksson et al., 2003). The single twin study, based on the Finnish twin register, included 48 discordant twin pairs (18 MZ and 30 DZ twins) and eight pairs concordant for schizophrenia. This study reported significant statistical evidence for a linear decrease in performance on a spatial working memory task as genetic risk of schizophrenia increased (Cannon et al., 2000).

These studies suggest significant heritability of working memory deficits, with unaffected first-degree relatives holding an intermediate position between patients and controls in severity of WM deficits (Krabbendam et al., 2001; Myles-Worsley & Park, 2002; Tuulio-Henriksson et al., 2003). Even when the performance of unaffected relatives is matched against that of controls, there is evidence from a functional imaging study by Callicott et al. (2003) that relatives are "working harder" than controls (at the level of cortical activation) to achieve similar accuracy scores on the task. We estimated effect for deficits in working memory in a previous review (Donohoe et al., 2009). In general, there were moderate effect sizes observed, despite the range of tasks used involving both verbal and spatial modalities. The largest effects were seen for the spatial delayed response paradigm, with Park et al.'s (1995) study showing large effect sizes for both versions of the task used. The study by Tuulio-Henriksson et al. (2003) is interesting in its comparison of singleton relatives versus relatives from multiplex families (families with more than one affected member), where multiplex families showed greater spatial WM deficits than simplex family members but less significant verbal WM differences. Together the family and twin data strongly support a genetic contribution to measures of spatial WM, but do not allow an estimation of heritability (h^2), not least because of the diversity of tasks employed. Such diversity in the behavioral and cognitive demands of various working memory tasks, and hence in the brain regions implicated, is a significant problem for interpreting the resulting genetic associations.

Memory

Memory functioning has been one of the most widely reported cognitive deficits in schizophrenia (Aleman et al., 1999; Cirillo & Seidman, 2003). Deficits in episodic memory, mnemonic processes that record, retain, and retrieve autobiographical knowledge about experiences that occurred at a specific time and place (Tulving, 1985), have received particular attention in genetic studies of schizophrenia. Krabbendam et al. (2001) reported that this aspect of memory, rather than semantic memory (memory for facts), distinguished patients with schizophrenia and their first-degree relatives from controls. Since the earliest investigations of memory impairments (Scoville & Milner, 1957), lesion studies have consistently associated impaired episodic memory with bilateral medial temporal lobe (including the hippocampus, parahippocampus, and entorhinal and perirhinal cortices) function (Fernandez et al., 1999; Squire & Zola, 1996). The distinct roles of these brain structures have been parsed on the basis of the information modality being encoded (verbal, visual, and spatial), encoding versus retrieval processes (Squire et al., 2004), and how memory retrieval is elicited (item retrieval versus associative processing, recollection versus familiarity). A number of tasks have been used to study verbal episodic memory in studies investigating the genetic basis of memory deficits in families with schizophrenia. Most have used verbal list learning tasks (especially the California Verbal Learning Task, CVLT), and story recall (using the Logical Memory subtest from the Wechsler Memory Scale [WMS]; Wechsler, 1997). Visual tasks that have also been included in genetics studies have included mainly visual reproduction (using the WMS Visual Reproduction subtest) and facial recognition (using either the WMS or Warrington Facial Recognition subtest).

Epidemiological studies have consistently found evidence for impaired episodic memory performance in samples of MZ twins (Goldberg, 1990, 1993, 1995; Gourovitch et al., 1999) and first-degree relatives of patients with schizophrenia (Cannon et al., 1994, 2000; Conklin 2002; Egan et al., 2001; Staal et al., 2000; Toulopoulou et al., 2003a,b). Largest effect sizes are seen in twin studies (Goldberg et al., 1995) and in a study comparing unaffected relatives from multiplex versus simplex families (Faraone et al., 2000). Evidence of significant differences between relatives and controls is found across the variety of memory tasks used, despite differences in memory modality (verbal versus visual) and type of retrieval (recall versus recognition). Verbal memory deficits show a medium effect size for differences between unaffected relatives and matched control samples (Donohoe et al., 2009). Effect sizes for visual memory deficits tend to be smaller, and a number of studies that reported statistical difference between relatives and controls on verbal memory tasks failed to find a similar association on visual memory tasks (Egan et al., 2001; Faraone et al., 1996; Toulopoulou et al., 2003a). Additionally, verbal list learning but not visual reproduction contributed to discrimination of degree of genetic loading for unaffected MZ and DZ twins of patients with schizophrenia (Cannon et al., 2000). There is also evidence of a larger effect size for free immediate recall than for delayed recall deficits or recognition deficits, consistent with the evidence that this is the more impaired modality in schizophrenia (Heinrichs & Zakzanis, 1998). However, simple distinctions between recall and recognition for the purposes of phenotypic utility are probably not warranted (Cannon et al., 1994; Conklin et al., 2002; Gourovitch et al., 1999).

General cognitive ability or intelligence

General cognitive ability and intelligence has received the most attention of any human trait in terms of its underlying genetic basis. While this history has not been without controversy (cf. the eugenics movement), the genetic contributions to intelligence have been widely studied both in the general population and across psychiatric disorders. Given the heritability of both schizophrenia and IQ, it is perhaps not surprising that family studies have also found evidence of significantly greater IQ impairments in unaffected relatives of schizophrenia probands than in healthy controls (Cannon et al., 2000; Hughes et al., 2005; Kremen et al., 1998; McIntosh et al., 2005). This is consistent with evidence, discussed later, that genetic variants identified as mediating schizophrenia risk have been associated with variation in both general cognitive ability and more specific aspects of neurocognitive functioning (Donohoe et al., 2009; Zhang et al., 2010).

Genetic association studies

In addition to heritability and family-based studies, a growing literature supports the hypothesis that genetic markers that influence risk for schizophrenia may be acting through their effects on brain functions, measurable via neuropsychological tasks. Early data from candidate gene studies implicated several genes/alleles as influencing both risk for illness and cognitive performance (e.g., dystrobrevin binding protein-1 [DTNBP1, Burdick et al., 2006, 2007; Zhang et al., 2010] and disrupted in schizophrenia-1 [DISC1, Callicott et al., 2004; Burdick et al., 2005]). Variation within DTNBP1 has been shown to influence cognitive performance in patients with schizophrenia and in healthy subjects. Previous work by our group indicated that the six-locus DTNBP1 haplotype (CTCTAC) that was associated with an increased risk for schizophrenia and schizoaffective disorder (Funke et al., 2004) also resulted in a substantial decrement in general cognitive ability (g) in both patients with schizophrenia and healthy controls (Burdick et al., 2006). Carriers of the risk haplotype performed worse than non-carriers in every cognitive domain, including attention, memory, and executive function, indicative of a generalized effect on cognition. Additionally, in a second study (Burdick et al., 2007) we found that when compared with non-carriers, schizophrenia patients who carried the DTNBP1 risk haplotype were more likely to evidence a cognitive decline from premorbid estimated IQ to current level of functioning.

Our DTNBP1 data are consistent with linkage results suggesting that the chromosomal region that encompasses DTNBP1 is associated with IQ in healthy subjects (Posthuma et al., 2005) and cognitive deficits in schizophrenia (Hallmayer et al., 2005), as well as a candidate gene study demonstrating that a protective DTNBP1 haplotype was associated with higher educational attainment (Williams et al., 2004). Several subsequent candidate gene studies of DTNBP1 have reported similar results (Donohoe et al., 2007; Hashimoto et al., 2010;

Luciano et al., 2009; Stefanis et al., 2007; Wolf et al., 2011; Zinkstok et al., 2007), with a recent meta-analysis supporting these findings (Zhang et al., 2011).

More recently, GWAS have reached beyond the candidate gene level in very large samples made possible through consortium-based efforts (Ripke et al., 2011) and have identified several novel risk variants. Nine loci harboring SNPs associated with increased schizophrenia risk have been identified by GWAS with substantial validity (O'Donovan et al., 2008; Ripke et al., 2011; Stefansson et al., 2009). These include the zinc finger protein 804A (*ZNF804A*) gene on chromosome 2q32; multiple variants within the major histo-compatibility complex (MHC) region on chromosome 6p21–6p22; a variant in the pro-moter region of the neurogranin (*NRGN*) gene on chromosome 11q24; a variant within the transcription factor 4 (*TCF4*) gene on chromosome 18q21; a variant downstream from microRNA miRNA137 on chromosome 1p21.3; a 0.5 Mb gene-rich region on chromosome 10q24.32; an intronic SNP in the *CUB* and sushi multiple domains 1 (*CSMD1*) gene; and common variants in gene deserts on chromosomes 2q32.3 and 8p21.3.

Additionally, there is substantial evidence for trans-disorder effects, particularly between schizophrenia and mood disorders, as the schizophrenia risk variant at *ZNF804A* has also been implicated in bipolar disorder (Williams et al., 2011). The strongest risk locus identified to date in bipolar disorder is the gene coding for the alpha subunit 1C of the L-type voltage-gated calcium channel (*CACNA1C*) (Sklar et al., 2011), a variant which also influences risk for schizophrenia and recurrent major depression (Green et al., 2009). Indeed, a recent cross-phenotype study reported that six of the eight SNPs most robustly associated with either schizophrenia or bipolar disorder show trans-disorder effects (Williams et al., 2011). It is therefore likely that these genetic variants that influence risk for multiple neuropsychiatric disorders do so via their effects on overlapping intermediate brain phenotypes such as neurocognitive dysfunction. Several studies have now evaluated the effects of GWAS-identified risk loci on neurocognitive functions that may underlie this broad susceptibility; we will review two of the genes that have been most widely studied to date (*ZNF804A* and *CACNA1C*).

ZNF804A

Esslinger and colleagues investigated the influence of the *ZNF804A* risk variant (rs1344706) on cortical activity within and connectivity between regions during working memory (N-back task) and on emotional recognition in a sample of 115 healthy controls. Differences in functional connectivity but not regional activation were observed. They reported reduced connectivity in the dorsolateral prefrontal cortex (DLPFC) between and within hemi-spheres, but also increased connectivity between the hippocampal formation (HF) and the DLPFC, and between the amygdala and the HF, orbitofrontal cortex, and prefrontal cortex. This evidence of *ZNF804A*'s effects on brain function during cognitive task per-formance has since been partially replicated (Paulus et al., 2011; Rasetti et al., 2011). At the level of neuropsychological performance; however, the interpretation of *ZNF804A* as deleteriously affecting cognitive performance has been questioned. In a study from our group (Walters et al., 2010), we found and then replicated evidence that the *ZNF804A* risk allele was associated with better cognitive performance on working memory and episodic memory tasks – which involve the DLPFC and HF. This effect was present in patients but not controls, suggesting that the *ZNF804A* risk variant may identify a patient subgroup with relatively spared cognitive performance. In a subsequent study of a different patient group, we found relatively larger hippocampal volumes in risk allele carriers, consistent with our earlier behavioral findings (Donohoe et al., 2011). While several smaller equivocal studies have also been reported (Balog et al., 2011; Lencz et al., 2010), a recent study in Han Chinese supports the view that *ZNF804A* may be particularly associated with a schizophrenia subgroup characterized by relatively spared performance (Chen et al., 2012).

Following their original connectivity paper, Esslinger and colleagues have proposed that *ZNF804A* may be particularly important for processing socially relevant information. This proposal is based on data suggesting the involvement of the *ZNF804A* risk variant in aberrant brain activation during social information processing using a theory of mind (TOM) task (Walter et al., 2009) and in state-independent interhemispheric processing (Esslinger et al., 2011). Partially supporting these data, we recently reported that, on a measure of causal attributions in social situations (attribution positive and negative events to self, others, or situational factors), healthy control risk allele carriers were more biased than non-carriers (Hargreaves et al., 2012). Further sufficiently powered studies of cognitive studies would be useful to confirm this characterization of *ZNF804A* as associated with relatively spared cognitive function on the one hand and with problems with social cognition on the other. This is of particular interest in schizophrenia, where social cognitive deficits have become increasingly noted as strong predictors of functional outcome (Horan et al., 2011).

CACNA1C

An SNP (rs1006737) in the calcium channel gene, *CACNA1C*, initially associated with bipolar illness (Ferreira et al., 2008; Sklar et al., 2008, 2011), has also been linked with schizophrenia (Green et al., 2009; Nyegaard et al., 2010) and recurrent major depression (Green et al., 2009). Several subsequent studies have evaluated the effects of *CACNA1C* variation on neurocognitive capacity.

CACNA1C rs1006737 has been shown to affect neural networks underlying reward and emotional processing (Bigos et al., 2010; Wessa et al., 2010), verbal fluency (Krug et al., 2010), alerting and orienting aspects of attention (Thimm et al., 2011), and executive functions (Bigos et al., 2010). *CACNA1C* is responsible for coding the L-type voltage-gated calcium channel Cav1.2, which has been shown to be involved in synaptic plasticity, learning, and memory in an NMDA-independent manner (Moosmang et al., 2005; White et al., 2008; Woodside et al., 2004), and *CACNA1C* knock-out mice show notable deficits in long-term potentiation (Striessnig et al., 2006). These convergent data suggest that variation within *CACNA1C* may play a critical role in the development of neurocognitive deficits associated with schizophrenia, and may point toward a novel treatment strategy targeting calcium channel dysfunction for these disabling symptoms.

As noted in the introduction to this chapter, common variation in the form of SNPs is not the only form of genomic variation that influences schizophrenia susceptibility. Rare variation is also known to play a role; however, because of the very low frequency of many structural variants, there are fewer studies that directly implicate this type of genomic variation in cognitive dysfunction associated with schizophrenia. Substantial data exist in other clinical samples that suggest that many of the identified CNVs are associated with cognitive developmental disorders (Morrow, 2010). Moreover, a recent prospective study characterized the broader spectrum of phenotypes related to recurrent schizophrenia-associated CNVs in a clinically referred sample of 38 779 individuals (Sahoo et al., 2011).

Microarrays confirmed the presence of a CNV from one of the six recurrent schizophrenia loci (1q21.1; 15q11.2; 15q13.3; 16p11.2; 16p13.11; and 22q11.2) in 1150 individuals. Among CNV carriers, referrals for genetic testing had been made for a wide variety of indications including developmental delay, intellectual disability, autism, and several congenital abnormalities related to neurocognitive impairment (Morrow, 2010).

Summary

Recent data have highlighted the complexity of the genetic architecture underlying several of the major mental illnesses, including schizophrenia. There are rare genetic abnormalities, in the form of copy number variations, that are likely to explain a large percentage of the variance in susceptibility to these illnesses in a small subgroup of individuals, but it is also true that multiple risk alleles across a large number of candidate genes will be implicated, each with a very small effect. As a result, the search for susceptibility loci has proven difficult.

Neurocognitive dysfunction has been utilized as an important intermediate phenotype in efforts to understand the molecular underpinnings of schizophrenia. Family data alongside genetic association studies converge to suggest that cognitive impairment in schizophrenia is strongly genetic and directly related to the predisposition for the disease (Touloupolou et al., 2007, 2010). Efforts to treat the cognitive deficits in patients with schizophrenia will be vastly aided by elucidating the biological etiologies of the impairment, and genetics approaches will continue to be a critical component toward this understanding.

References

Aleman, A., Hijman R., de Haan E. H., et al. (1999). Memory impairment in schizophrenia: a meta-analysis. *American Journal of Psychiatry*, **156**, 1358–1366.

Appels, M. C., Sitskoorn, M. M., Westers, P., et al. (2003). Cognitive dysfunctions in parents of schizophrenic patients parallel the deficits found in patients. *Schizophrenia Research*, **63**, 285–293.

Baddeley, A. D. (1990). The development of the concept of working memory: implications and contributions of neuropsychology. In G. Vallar & T. Shallice (eds.), *Neuropsychological Impairments of Short-term Memory*. New York, NY: Cambridge University Press, pp. 54–73. Balog, Z., Kiss, I., & Kéri, S. (2011). ZNF804A may be associated with executive control of attention. *Genes, Brain and Behavior*, **10**, 223–227.

Bates, J. A. & Malhotra, A. K. (2002). Genetic factors and neurocognitive traits. *CNS Spectrums*, 7, 274–280, 283–284.

Bigos, K. L., Mattay, V. S., Callicott, J. J., et al. (2010). Genetic variation in CACNA1C affects brain circuitries related to mental illness. *Archives of General Psychiatry*, **67**, 939–945.

Bleuler, E. (1950). *Dementia Praecox or the Group of Schizophrenias*. Oxford: International Universities Press.

Braff, D. L., Freedman, R., Schork, N. J., et al. (2007). Deconstructing schizophrenia: an overview of the use of endophenotypes in order to understand a complex disorder. *Schizophrenia Bulletin*, **33**, 21–32.

Burdick, K. E., Goldberg, T. E., Funke, B., et al. (2007). DTNBP1 genotype influences cognitive decline in schizophrenia. *Schizophrenia Research*, **89**, 169–172.

Burdick, K. E., Lencz, T., Funke, B., et al. (2006). Genetic variation in DTNBP1 influences general cognitive ability. *Human Molecular Genetics*, **15**, 1563–1568.

Callicott, J. H., Mattay, V. S., Verchinski, B. A., et al. (2003). Complexity of prefrontal cortical dysfunction in schizophrenia: more than up or down. *American Journal of Psychiatry*, **160**, 2209–2215.

Cannon, T. D., Huttunen, M. O., Lonnqvist, J., et al. (2000). The inheritance of neuropsychological dysfunction in twins discordant for schizophrenia. *American Journal of Human Genetics*, **67**, 369–382.

Cannon, T. D., Zorilla, L. E., Shtasel, D., et al. (1994). Neuropsychological functioning in siblings discordant for schizophrenia and healthy volunteers. *Archives of General Psychiatry*, **51**, 651–661.

Chen, W. J., Chang, C-H., Liu, S. K., et al. (2004). Sustained attention deficits in nonpsychotic relatives of schizophrenia patients: a recurrence risk ratio analysis. *Biological Psychiatry*, **55**, 995–1000.

Chen, W. J., Liu, S. K., Chang, C. J., et al. (1998). Sustained attention deficit and schizotypal personality features in nonpsychotic relatives of schizophrenic patients. *American Journal of Psychiatry*, **155**, 1214–1220.

Chen, M., Xu, Z., Zhai, J., et al. (2012). Evidence of IQ-modulated association between ZNF804A gene polymorphism and cognitive function in schizophrenia patients. *Neuropsychopharmacology*, **37**, 1572–1578.

Cirillo, M. A. & Seidman, L. J. (2003). Verbal declarative memory dysfunction in schizophrenia: from clinical assessment to genetics and brain mechanisms. *Neuropsychology Review*, **13**, 43–77.

Conklin, H. M., Calkins, M. E., & Anderson, C. W. (2002). Recognition memory for faces in schizophrenia patients and their first-degree relatives. *Neuropsychologia*, **40**, 2314–2324.

Conklin, H. M., Curtis, C. E., Calkins, M. E., et al. (2005). Working memory functioning in schizophrenia patients and their first-degree relatives: cognitive functioning shedding light on etiology. *Neuropsychologia*, **43**, 930–942.

Conklin, H. M., Curtis, C. E., Katsanis, J., et al. (2000). Verbal working memory impairment in schizophrenia patients and their first-degree relatives: evidence from the digit span task. *American Journal of Psychiatry*, **157**, 275–277.

Cornblatt, B. A. & Keilp, J. G. (1994). Impaired attention, genetics, and the pathophysiology of schizophrenia. *Schizophrenia Bulletin*, **20**, 31–46.

Doherty, J., O'Donovan, M., & Owen, M. (2012) Recent genomic advances in schizophrenia. *Clinical Genetics*, **81**, 103–109.

Donohoe, G., Clarke, S., Morris, D., et al. (2006). Are deficits in executive sub-processes simply reflecting more general cognitive decline in schizophrenia? *Schizophrenia Research*, **85**, 168–173.

Donohoe, G., Morris, D. W., Clarke, S. et al. (2007). Variance in neurocognitive performance is associated with dysbindin-1 in schizophrenia: a preliminary study. *Neuropsychologia*, **45**, 454–458.

Donohoe, G. & Robertson, I. H. (2003). Can specific deficits in executive functioning explain the negative symptoms of schizophrenia? A review. *Neurocase*, **9**, 97–108.

Donohoe, E., Rose, D., Morris, A., et al. (2011). S20–02 – Follow up of schizophrenia GWAS based on cognitive performance, high density EEG, and structural brain imaging. *European Psychiatry*, **26**, 2083.

Donohoe, G., Walters, J., Morris, D. W., et al. (2009). Influence of NOS1 on verbal intelligence and working memory in both patients with schizophrenia and healthy control subjects. *Archives of General Psychiatry*, **66**, 1045–1054.

Egan, M. F., Goldberg, T. E., Gscheidle, T., et al. (2001). Relative risk for cognitive impairments in siblings of patients with schizophrenia. *Biological Psychiatry*, **50**, 98–107.

Elevåg, B. & Goldberg, T. E. (2000). Cognitive impairment in schizophrenia is the core of the disorder. *Critical Review in Neurobiology*, **14**, 1–21.

Erlenmeyer-Kimling, L., Rock, D., Roberts, S. A., et al. (2000). Attention, memory, and motor skills as childhood predictors of schizophrenia-related psychoses: the New York high-risk project. *American Journal of Psychiatry*, **157**, 1416–1422.

Esslinger, C., Kirsch, P., Haddad, L., et al. (2011). Cognitive state and connectivity effects of the genome-wide significant psychosis variant in ZNF804A. *NeuroImage*, **54**, 2514–2523.

Faraone, S. V., Seidman, L. J., Kremen, W. S., et al. (1996). Neuropsychological functioning among the elderly nonpsychotic relatives of schizophrenic patients. *Schizophrenia Research*, **21**, 27–31.

Faraone, S. V., Seidman, L. J., Kremen, W. S., et al. (2000). Neuropsychologic functioning among the nonpsychotic relatives of schizophrenic patients: the effect of genetic loading. *Biological Psychiatry*, **48**, 120–126.

Fatemi, S. H. & Folsom, T. D. (2009). The neurodevelopmental hypothesis of schizophrenia, revisited. *Schizophrenia Bulletin*, **35**, 528–548.

Fernandez, T., Yan, W. L., Hamburger, S., et al. (1999). Apolipoprotein E alleles in childhood-onset schizophrenia. *American Journal of Medical Genetics*, **88**, 211–213.

Ferreira, M. A., O'Donovan, M. C., Meng, Y. A., et al. (2008). Collaborative genome-wide association analysis supports a role for *ANK3* and *CACNA1C* in bipolar disorder. *Nature Genetics*, **40**, 1056–1058.

Franke, P., Maier, W., Hardt, J., et al. (1994). Attentional abilities and measures of schizotypy: their variation and covariation in schizophrenic patients, their siblings, and normal control subjects. *Psychiatry Research*, **54**, 259–272.

Funke, B., Finn, C. T., Plocik, A. M., et al. (2004). Association of the DTNBP1 locus with schizophrenia in a U.S. population. *American Journal of Human Genetics*, **75**, 891–898.

Glahn, D. C., Bearden, C. E., Cakir, S., et al. (2006). Differential working memory impairment in bipolar disorder and schizophrenia: effects of lifetime history of psychosis. *Bipolar Disorder*, **8**, 117–123.

Glahn, D. C., Therman, S., Manninen, M., et al. (2003). Spatial working memory as an endophenotype for schizophrenia. *Biological Psychiatry*, **53**, 624–626.

Goldberg, T. E., Egan, M. F., Gscheidle, T., et al. (2003). Executive subprocesses in working memory: relationship to catechol-O-methyltransferase Val158Met genotype and schizophrenia. *Archives of General Psychiatry*, **60**, 889–896.

Goldberg, T. E., Ragland, J. D., Torrey, E. F., et al. (1990). Neuropsychological assessment of monozygotic twins discordant for schizophrenia. *Archives of General Psychiatry*, **47**, 1066–1072.

Goldberg, T. E., Torret, E. F., Gold, J. M., et al. (1993). Learning and memory in monozygotic twins discordant for schizophrenia. *Psychological Medicine*, **23**, 71–85.

Goldberg, T. E., Torrey, E. F., Gold, J. M., et al. (1995). Genetic risk of neuropsychological impairment in schizophrenia: a study of monozygotic twins discordant and concordant for the disorder. *Schizophrenia Research*, **17**, 77–84.

Good, K. P., Rabinowitz, J., Whitehorn, D., et al. (2004). The relationship of neuropsychological test performance with the PANSS in antipsychotic naïve, first-episode psychosis patients. *Schizophrenia Research*, **68**, 11–19.

Gottesman, I. I. & Gould, T. D. (2003). The endophenotype concept in psychiatry: etymology and strategic intentions. *American Journal of Psychiatry*, **160**, 636–645.

Gottesman, I. I. & Shields, J. (1972). *Schizophrenia and Genetics: A Twin Study Vantage Point*. Oxford: Academic Press.

Gottesman, I. I. & Shields, J. (1973). Genetic theorizing and schizophrenia. *British Journal of Psychiatry*, **122**, 15–30.

Gourovitch, M. L., Torrey, E. F., Gold, J. M., et al. (1999). Neuropsychological performance of monozygotic twins discordant for bipolar disorder. *Biological Psychiatry*, **45**, 639–646.

Green, E. K., Grozeva, D., Jones I., et al. (2009). The bipolar disorder risk allele at CACNA1C also confers risk of recurrent major depression and of schizophrenia. *Molecular Psychiatry*, **15**, 1016–1022.

Green, M. F., Kern, R. S., & Heaton, R. K. (2004). Longitudinal studies of cognition and functional outcome in schizophrenia: implications for MATRICS. *Schizophrenia Research*, **72**, 41–51.

Hallmayer, J. F., Kalaydjieva, L., Badcock, J., et al. (2005). Genetic evidence for a distinct subtype of schizophrenia characterized by pervasive cognitive deficit. *American Journal of Human Genetics*, 77, 468–476.

Hargreaves, A., Morris, D. W., Rose, E., et al. (2012). ZNF804A and social cognition in patients with schizophrenia and healthy controls. *Molecular Psychiatry*, 17, 118–119.

Hashimoto, R., Noguchi, H., Hori, H., et al. (2010). A genetic variation in the dysbindin gene (DTNBP1) is associated with memory performance in healthy controls. *World Journal of Biological Psychiatry*, 11, 431–438.

Heinrichs, R. W. (2004). Meta-analysis and the science of schizophrenia: variant evidence or evidence of variants? *Neuroscience and Biobehavioral Reviews*, 28, 379–394.

Heinrichs, R. W. & Zakzanis, K. K. (1998). Neurocognitive deficit in schizophrenia: a quantitative review of the evidence. *Neuropsychology*, 12, 426–445.

Horan, W. P., Green, M. F., Degroot, M., et al. (2011). Social cognition in schizophrenia, Part 2: 12-month stability and prediction of functional outcome in first-episode patients. *Schizophrenia Bulletin* [Epub ahead of print].

Hughes, C., Kumari, V., Das, M., et al (2005). Cognitive functioning in siblings discordant for schizophrenia. *Acta Psychiatrica Scandinavica*, 111, 185–192.

Javitt, D. C., Strous, R. D., Grochowski, S., et al. (1997). Impaired precision, but normal retention, of auditory sensory ("echoic") memory information in schizophrenia. *Journal of Abnormal Psychology*, 106, 315–324.

Jones, L. A., Cardno, A. G., Sanders, R. D., et al. (2001). Sustained and selective attention as measures of genetic liability to schizophrenia. *Schizophrenia Research*, 48, 263–272.

Keefe, R. S. & Fenton, W. S. (2007). How should DSM-V criteria for schizophrenia include cognitive impairment? *Schizophrenia Bulletin*, 33, 912–920.

Keefe, R. S., Silverman, J. M., Mohs, R. C., et al. (1997). Eye tracking, attention, and schizotypal symptoms in nonpsychotic relatives of patients with schizophrenia. *Archives of General Psychiatry*, 54, 169–176.

Kéri, S., Kelemen, O., Benedek, G., et al. (2001). Different trait markers for schizophrenia and bipolar disorder: a neurocognitive approach. *Psychological Medicine*, 31, 915–922.

Kéri, S. & Janka, Z. (2004). Critical evaluation of cognitive dysfunctions as endophenotypes of schizophrenia. *Acta Psychiatrica Scandinavica*, 110, 83–91.

Kirov, G., Grozeva, D., Norton, N., et al. (2009). Support for the involvement of large copy number variants in the pathogenesis of schizophrenia. *Human Molecular Genetics*, 18, 1497–1503.

Krabbendam, L., Marcelis, M., Delespaul, P., et al. (2001). Single or multiple familial cognitive risk factors in schizophrenia? *American Journal of Medical Genetics*, 105, 183–188.

Kremen, W.S., Faraone, S.V., Seidman, L.J., et al. (1998). Neuropsychological risk indicators for schizophrenia: A preliminary study of female relatives of schizophrenic and bipolar probands. *Psychiatry Research*, 3, 227–240.

Kremen, W. S., Lyons, M. J., Boake, C., et al. (2006). A discordant twin study of premorbid cognitive ability in schizophrenia. *Journal of Clinical and Experimental Neuropsychology*, 28, 208–224.

Krug, A., Nieratschker, V., Markov, V., et al. (2010). Effect of CACNA1C rs1006737 on neural correlates of verbal fluency in healthy individuals. *NeuroImage*, 49, 1831–1836.

Laurent, A., Biloa-Tang, M., Bougerol, T., et al. (2000). Executive/attentional performance and measures of schizotypy in patients with schizophrenia and in their nonpsychotic first-degree relatives. *Schizophrenia Research*, 46, 269–283.

Laurent, A., Saoud, M., Bougerol, T., et al. (1999). Attentional deficits in patients with schizophrenia and in their non-psychotic first-degree relatives. *Psychiatry Research*, 89, 147–159.

Lencz, T., Szeszko, P. R., DeRosse, P., et al. (2010). A schizophrenia risk gene, ZNF804A, influences neuroanatomical and neurocognitive phenotypes. *Neuropsychopharmacology*, 35, 2284–2291.

Lenox, R. H., Gould, T. D., Manji, H. K. (2002). Endophenotypes in bipolar disorder.

American Journal of Medical Genetics, **114**, 391–406.

Lichtenstein, P., Yip, B. H., Bjork, C., et al. (2009). Common genetic determinants of schizophrenia and bipolar disorder in Swedish families: a population-based study. *Lancet,* **373**, 234–239.

Luciano, M., Miyajima, F., Lind, P. A., et al. (2009). Variation in the dysbindin gene and normal cognitive function in three independent population samples. *Genes, Brain and Behavior,* **8**, 218–227.

McIntosh, A. M., Harrison, L. K., Forrester, K., et al. (2005). Neuropsychological impairments in people with schizophrenia or bipolar disorder and their unaffected relatives. *British Journal of Psychiatry,* **186**, 378–385.

Moosmang, S., Haider, N., Klugbauer, N., et al. (2005). Role of hippocampal Cav1.2 Ca^{2+} channels in NMDA receptor-independent synaptic plasticity and spatial memory. *Journal of Neuroscience,* **25**, 9883–9892.

Morrow, E. M. (2010). Genomic copy number variation in disorders of cognitive development. *Journal of the American Academy of Child and Adolescent Psychiatry,* **49**, 1091–1104.

Myles-Worsley, M. & Park, S. (2002). Spatial working memory deficits in schizophrenia patients and their first-degree relatives from Palau, Micronesia. *American Journal of Medical Genetics,* **114**, 609–615.

Niendam, T. A., Bearden, C. E., Rosso, I. M., et al. (2003). A prospective study of childhood neurocognitive functioning in schizophrenic patients and their siblings. *American Journal of Psychiatry,* **160**, 2060–2062.

Nyegaard, M., Demontis, D., Foldager, L., et al. (2010). CACNA1C (rs1006737) is associated with schizophrenia. *Molecular Psychiatry,* **15**, 119–121.

O'Donovan, M. C., Craddock, N., Norton, N., et al. (2008). Identification of loci associated with schizophrenia by genome-wide association and follow-up. *Nature,* **40**, 1053–1058.

O'Rourke, D. H., Gottesman, I. I., Suarez, B. K., et al. (1982). Refutation of the general single-locus model for the etiology of schizophrenia. *American Journal of Human Genetics,* **34**, 630–649.

Park, S., Holzman, P. S., Goldman-Rakic, P. S. (1995). Spatial working memory deficits in the relatives of schizophrenic patients. *Archives of General Psychiatry,* **52**, 821–828.

Paulus, F. M., Krach, S., Bedenbender, J., et al. (2011). Partial support for ZNF804A genotype-dependent alterations in prefrontal connectivity. *Human Brain Mapping* [Epub ahead of print].

Posthuma, D., Luciano, M., Geus, E. J., et al. (2005). A genomewide scan for intelligence identifies quantitative trait loci on 2q and 6p. *American Journal of Human Genetics,* **77**, 318–326.

Purcell, S. M., Wray, N. R., Stone, J. L., et al. (2009). Common polygenic variation contributes to risk of schizophrenia and bipolar disorder. *Nature,* **460**, 748–752.

Rasetti, R., Sambataro, F., Chen, Q., et al. (2011). Altered cortical network dynamics: a potential intermediate phenotype for schizophrenia and association with ZNF804A. *Archives of General Psychiatry,* **68**, 1207–1217.

Ripke, S., Sanders, A. R., Kendler, K. S., et al. (2011). The Schizophrenia Psychiatric Genome-Wide Association Study (GWAS) Consortium. Genome-wide association study identifies five new schizophrenia loci. *Nature Genetics,* **43**, 969–976.

Risch, N. (1990). Genetic linkage and complex diseases, with special reference to psychiatric disorders. *Genetic Epidemiology,* **7**, 3–16.

Ruderfer, D. M., Kirov, G., Chambert, K., et al. (2011). A family-based study of common polygenic variation and risk of schizophrenia. *Molecular Psychiatry,* **16**, 887–888.

Sahoo, T., Theisen, A., Rosenfeld, J. A., et al. (2011). Copy number variants of schizophrenia susceptibility loci are associated with a spectrum of speech and developmental delays and behavior problems. *Genetics in Medicine,* **13**, 868–880.

Saoud, M., d'Amato, T., & Gutknecht, C. (2000). Neuropsychological deficit in siblings discordant for schizophrenia. *Schizophrenia Bulletin,* **26**, 893–902.

Scoville, W. B. & Milner, B. (1957). Loss of recent memory after bilateral hippocampal lesions. *Journal of Neurology, Neurosurgery and Psychiatry*, **20**, 11–21.

Sklar, P., Ripke, S., Scott, L., et al. (2011). Large-scale genome-wide association analysis of bipolar disorder identifies a new susceptibility locus near ODZ4. *Nat Genet*, **43**, 877–983.

Sklar, P., Smoller, J. W., Fan, J., et al. (2008). Whole-genome association study of bipolar disorder. *Molecular Psychiatry*, **13**, 558–569.

Sullivan, P. F., Kendler, K. S., Neale, M. C. (2003). Schizophrenia as a complex trait: evidence from a meta-analysis of twin studies. *Archives of General Psychiatry*, **60**, 1187–1192.

Squire, L. R., Stark, C. E., Clark, R. E. (2004). The medial temporal lobe. *Annual Review of Neuroscience*, **27**, 279–306.

Squire, L. R. & Zola, S. M. (1996). Structure and function of declarative and nondeclarative memory systems. *Proceedings of the National Academy of Sciences of the United States of America*, **93**, 13515–13522.

Staal, W. G., Hijman, R., Hulshoff Pol, H. E., et al. (2000). Neuropsychological dysfunctions in siblings discordant for schizophrenia. *Psychiatry Research*, **95**, 227–235.

Stefanis, N. C., Trikalinos, T. A., Avramopoulos, D., et al. (2007). Impact of schizophrenia candidate genes on schizotypy and cognitive endophenotypes at the population level. *Biological Psychiatry*, **62**, 784–792.

Stefansson, H., Ophoff, R. A., Steinberg, S., et al. (2009). Common variants conferring risk of schizophrenia. *Nature*, **460**, 744–747.

Stefansson, H., Rujescu, D., Cichon, S., et al. (2008). Large recurrent microdeletions associated with schizophrenia. *Nature*, **455**, 232–236.

Sternberg, R. J. & Grigoreniko, E. L. (1997). The cognitive costs of physical and mental ill health: applying the psychology of the developed world to the problems of the developing world. *Eye on Psi Chi*, **2**, 20–27.

Striessnig, J., Koschak, A., Sinnegger-Brauns, M. J., et al. (2006). Role of voltage-gated L-type Ca^{2+} channel isoforms for brain function. *Biochemical Society Transactions*, **34**, 903–909.

Thimm, M., Kircher, T., Kellermann, T., et al. (2011). Effects of a CACNA1C genotype on attention networks in healthy individuals. *Psychological Medicine*, **41**, 1551–1561.

Toulopoulou, T., Goldberg, T. E., Mesa, I. R., et al. (2010). Impaired intellect and memory: a missing link between genetic risk and schizophrenia? *Archives of General Psychiatry*, **67**, 905–913.

Toulopoulou, T., Morris, R. G., Rabe-Hesketh, S., et al. (2003a). Selectivity of verbal memory deficit in schizophrenic patients and their relatives. *American Journal of Medical Genetics Part B: Neuropsychiatric Genetics*, **116**B, 1–7.

Toulopoulou, T., Picchioni, M., Rijsdijk, F., et al. (2007). Substantial genetic overlap between neurocognition and schizophrenia: genetic modeling twin samples. *Archives of General Psychiatry*, **64**, 1348–1355.

Toulopoulou, T., Rabe-Hesketh, S., King, H., et al. (2003b). Episodic memory in schizophrenic patients and their relatives. *Schizophrenia Research*, **63**, 261–271.

Tulving, E. (1985). How many memory systems are there? *American Psychologist*, **40**, 385–398.

Tuulio-Henriksson, A., Arajärvi, R., Partonen, T., et al. (2003). Familial loading associates with impairment in visual span among healthy siblings of schizophrenia patients. *Biological Psychiatry*, **54**, 623–628.

Walsh, T., McClellan, J. M., McCarthy, S. E., et al. (2008). Rare structural variants disrupt multiple genes in neurodevelopmental pathways in schizophrenia. *Science*, **320**, 539–543.

Walter, H., Ciaramidaro, A., Adenzato, M., et al. (2009). Dysfunction of the social brain in schizophrenia is modulated by intention type: an fMRI study. *Social Cognitive and Affective Neuroscience*, **4**, 166–176.

Walters, J. T., Corvin, A., Owen, M. J., et al. (2010). Psychosis susceptibility gene ZNF804A and cognitive performance in schizophrenia. *Archives of General Psychiatry*, **67**, 692–700.

Wechsler, D. (1997). *Wechsler Memory Scale-III.* San Antonio, TX: The Psychological Corporation.

Wessa, M., Linke, J., Witt, S. H., et al. (2010). The CACNA1C risk variant for bipolar disorder influences limbic activity. *Molecular Psychiatry*, **15**, 1126–1127.

White, J. A., McKinney, B. C., John, M. C., et al. (2008). Conditional forebrain deletion of the L-type calcium channel CaV1.2 disrupts remote spatial memories in mice. *Learning and Memory*, **15**, 1–5.

Williams, H. J., Norton, N., Dwyer, S., et al. (2011). Fine mapping of ZNF804A and genome-wide significant evidence for its involvement in schizophrenia and bipolar disorder. *Molecular Psychiatry*, **16**, 429–441.

Williams, N. M., Preece, A., Morris, D. W., et al. (2004). Identification in 2 independent samples of a novel schizophrenia risk haplotype of the dystrobrevin binding protein gene (DTNBP1). *Archives of General Psychiatry*, **61**, 336–344.

Wolf, C., Jackson, M. C., Kissling, C., et al. (2011). Dysbindin-1 genotype effects on emotional working memory. *Molecular Psychiatry*, **16**, 145–155.

Woodside, B. L., Borroni, A. M., Hammonds, M. D., et al. (2004). NMDA receptors and voltage-dependent calcium channels mediate different aspects of acquisition and retention of a spatial memory task. *Neurobiology of Learning and Memory*, **81**, 105–114.

Xu, B., Roos, J. L., Levy, S., et al. (2008). Strong association of de novo copy number mutations with sporadic schizophrenia. *Nature Genetics*, **40**, 880–885.

Zhang, J. P., Burdick, K. E., Lencz, T., et al. (2010). Meta-analysis of genetic variation in DTNBP1 and general cognitive ability. *Biological Psychiatry*, **68**, 1126–1133.

Zhang, F., Chen, Q., Ye, T., et al. (2011). Evidence of sex-modulated association of ZNF804A with schizophrenia. *Biological Psychiatry*, **69**, 914–917.

Zinkstok, J. R., de Wilde, O., van Amelsvoort, T. A., et al. (2007). Association between the DTNBP1 gene and intelligence: a case-control study in young patients with schizophrenia and related disorders and unaffected siblings. *Behavioral and Brain Functions*, **3**, 19.

Chapter

11

Neurobiological determinants of cognition

Daniel C. Javitt

Acknowledgments

Funding was provided in part by NIH grants R37MH49334 and P50MH086385.

Introduction

Dopaminergic models of schizophrenia were first proposed about 50 years ago, based upon both the fortuitous discovery of antipsychotic effects of the chlorpromazine and other D2 receptor antagonists in the late 1950s. Although it was originally hoped that dopaminergic models would account for all aspects of schizophrenia including cognitive dysfunction, limitations of the model have become increasingly clear over recent years, forcing an increased focus on alternative mechanisms (Howes & Kapur, 2009).

Recent neurochemical models of schizophrenia focus on disturbances of glutamatergic neurotransmission, particularly at N-methyl-D-aspartate (NMDA)-type glutamate receptors, based in large part upon actions of the NMDA receptor antagonists such as phencyclidine (PCP) and ketamine, both in animal models and normal volunteers. Glutamatergic models provide specific predictions regarding the nature and extent of cognitive dysfunction in schizophrenia that differ from those provided by other types of models. Such predictions have been significantly supported by recent behavioral, neurophysiological, and neuroimaging-type studies, implicating NMDA receptor dysfunction as a key neurobiological determinant of impaired cognition in schizophrenia.

Phencyclidine/N-methyl-D-aspartate model of schizophrenia

In early clinical studies, both PCP and ketamine were shown to induce positive and negative symptoms, as well as cognitive deficits that closely resembled those of schizophrenia. These deficits were subsequently shown to reflect their ability to block neurotransmission at NMDA receptors, suggesting that both symptoms and neurocognitive dysfunction may be accounted for parsimoniously by dysfunction of a single transmitter/receptor pathway. Since the original promulgation of the glutamate/NMDA hypothesis of schizophrenia in the late 1980s (Coyle, 1996; Javitt, 1987; Javitt and Zukin, 1991), significant progress has been made in delineating the potential role of NMDA-R dysfunction in the etiology of schizophrenia.

The NMDA receptors are one of several receptor types for the neurotransmitter glutamate. As opposed to other glutamate receptors, NMDA-R play a unique, functional

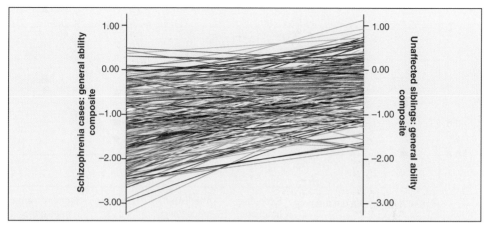

Figure 2.3. General cognitive performance in people with schizophrenia and their unaffected siblings (n=269 families). z-scores are calculated using control means and standard deviations. Each differently colored line shows the relative performance on the general cognitive ability composite of one schizophrenia case (on the left axis) and his/her unaffected sibling (on the right axis). The downward slope from right to left gives a sense of the consistency with which ill siblings underperform their unaffected siblings cognitively.

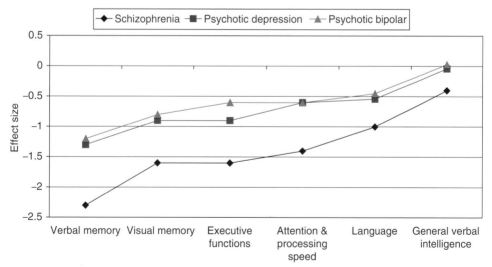

Figure 4.1. Neuropsychological performance profiles of schizophrenia, psychotic major depressive disorder, and psychotic bipolar disorder patients 24 months after first admission.

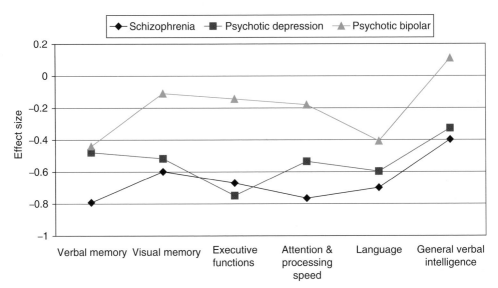

Figure 4.2. Neuropsychological performance profiles of schizophrenia, psychotic major depressive disorder, and psychotic bipolar disorder patients six months after first admission.

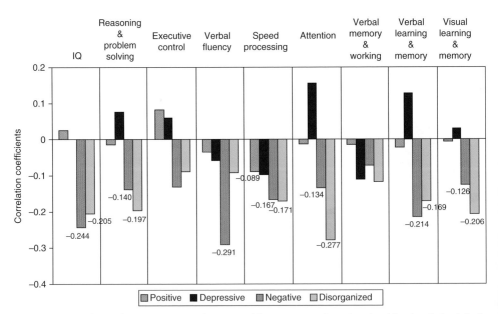

Figure 4.3. Correlations between cognitive domains and four symptom dimensions in schizophrenia (statistically significant relationships are those with reported values).

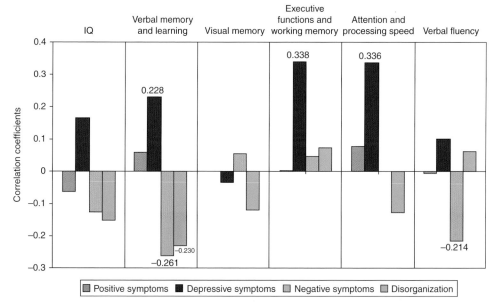

Figure 4.5. Pearson's correlations between symptom dimensions of psychoses and cognitive domains.

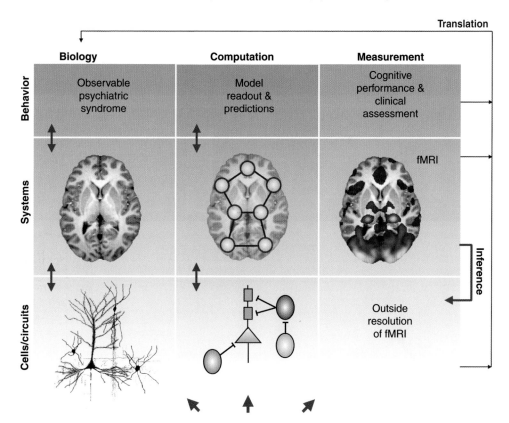

Figure 12.2. Framework for translational cognitive neuroscience of schizophrenia. The proposed framework combines pharmacological manipulation and cellular-level computational modeling with behavioral measurement and neural system read-out with state-of-the-art fMRI. This allows direct mechanism examination through manipulation of the underlying circuitry and comparing results with deficits observed in schizophrenia patients. This computational neuropsychiatry approach allows us to traverse levels of scientific explanation by establishing mechanistic links between cells, neural systems, and psychiatric symptoms.

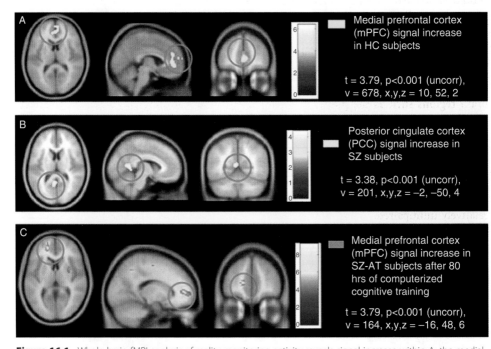

Figure 16.1. Whole brain fMRI analysis of reality-monitoring activity reveals signal increase within A: the medial prefrontal cortex (mPFC) in 15 healthy comparison subjects (HC); B: the posterior cingulate cortex, rather than the mPFC, in patients with schizophrenia (SZ) prior to computerized cognitive training; C: the mPFC in only the group of schizophrenia patients who completed 80 hours of active computerized cognitive training (SZ-AT), similar to the neural activation patterns observed in the HC sample. (Reproduced with permission from Subramaniam et al., 2012.)

role, in that they are blocked by Mg^{2+} in a voltage-dependent fashion, and are thus sensitive to both presynaptic glutamate release and postsynaptic membrane potential. This allows them to function in a "Hebbian" fashion to integrate information across multiple input paths. As opposed to neurons governed by other neurotransmitters such as dopamine, glutamatergic neurons are widely distributed in the brain and account for about 60% of all cortical neurons, including all cortical pyramidal neurons and all thalamic projection neurons to the cortex. Thus, PCP/NMDA models predict that cognitive deficits in schizophrenia should be distributed throughout the cortex, including both sensory and higher associative cortices. Within each region, however, only a subset of glutamatergic processes should be affected. Thus, specificity of cognitive dysfunction in schizophrenia may be based upon engagement of specific receptor types rather than in the region engaged.

Glutamatergic determinants of higher cognitive dysfunction

Deficits in complex cognitive functions such as executive processing have been abundantly demonstrated in schizophrenia and have been associated with impaired function of specific brain regions such as the prefrontal cortex. Deficits in learning and declarative memory, which localize to the hippocampus, have also been extensively documented (Barch, 2005; Reichenberg & Harvey, 2007). However, while it is clear that these processes are impaired, it is less clear why some processes – even within a single brain region – are impaired while others are preserved. A key prediction of glutamatergic models of schizophrenia is that NMDA receptor antagonists such as PCP or ketamine should be able to reproduce patterns of deficit observed in schizophrenia, while sparing processes in schizophrenia that are relatively unimpaired.

Prefrontal cortex

Deficits in prefrontal cortex (PFC)/executive processing have been extensively evaluated in schizophrenia, using measures such as the Wisconsin Card Sorting Test (WCST), Stroop, N-back, or AX-version of the Continuous Performance Test (AX-CPT) (Minzenberg et al., 2009). The NMDA receptor antagonists induce schizophrenia-like deficits on a large variety of executive processing tests when administered to normal volunteers, including Stroop (Bakker & Amini, 1961; Newcomer et al., 1999; Parwani et al., 2005; Rowland et al., 2005), digit symbol (Bakker & Amini, 1961); WCST (Krystal et al., 1994, 1998, 1999), N-back (Adler et al., 1998; Honey et al., 2008; Lofwall et al., 2006; Morgan et al., 2004a,b), working memory (Krystal et al., 2005), and AX-CPT (Heekeren et al., 2008; Umbricht et al., 2000) tasks. Thus, NMDA dysfunction, of itself, appears sufficient to reproduce the pattern of prefrontal impairments observed in schizophrenia.

For these tasks, both regionalized (e.g., prefrontal) and NMDA-based models would predict similar effects. For other tasks, however, differential effects are predicted. Thus for example, in task-switching paradigms, individuals are generally slower and less accurate in trials immediately following a switch than they are on subsequent trials, with such switch costs being related to activation of prefrontal/parietal networks (Braver et al., 2003; Wylie et al., 2006). Subjects are also slower and less accurate in performing dual versus single tasks ("mixing costs") and in trials where tasks produce conflicting versus congruent responses ("congruence costs") (Wylie et al., 2003). Despite prefrontal contributions to task switching, a consistent finding in schizophrenia is that patients have no elevated switch costs compared to controls. In contrast, patients do show increases in both mixing and congruence costs (Wylie & Tregellas, 2010) (Figure 11.1A). Similar patterns of impairment are seen in ketamine-treated monkeys (Stoet & Snyder, 2006) (Figure 11.1B), reinforcing the view that first, not all frontal-dependent processes are impaired in schizophrenia, and second, what differentiates preserved versus impaired processes may be the degree to which NMDA-dependent processing is involved rather than the brain regions that are engaged.

Hippocampus

A second highly reproducible disturbance in schizophrenia involves learning and declarative memory systems. To the extent that schizophrenia is associated with preferential deficits across domains, greater impairments are seen in learning and declarative memory than in other neurocognitive domains (Bilder et al., 2000; Reichenberg & Harvey, 2007; Saykin et al., 1991). Learning, in general, is one of the most extensively studied processes relative to NMDA receptor function. The NMDA receptors serve as a trigger for processes of long-term potentiation (LTP) and long-term depression (LTD) in the brain, which are the primary brain mechanisms underlying learning and memory (for review, see Javitt & Zukin, 1991). As a result, in animal models, NMDA receptor blockade produces a failure to encode new information but intact retention of old information, similar to the pattern observed in schizophrenia.

The ability of NMDA receptor antagonists to induce schizophrenia-like associative memory deficits in normal volunteers has also been extensively studied. Initial studies were performed by Harris et al. (1975), who observed deficits in memory and attention during ketamine emergence. Subsequently, deficits in both immediate and delayed recall were evaluated during ketamine infusion and documented (Krystal et al., 1994). Similar deficits have since been reported by several additional groups (Harborne et al., 1996; Radant et al., 1998), making this one of the best replicated current findings in ketamine research. Deficits, moreover, are observed preferentially for stimuli presented during the infusion versus those presented earlier, suggesting that ketamine affects encoding more than retention, which is similar to the pattern observed in schizophrenia (Hetem et al., 2000; Newcomer et al., 1999; Parwani et al., 2005).

In contrast to its actions shown on tests of executive processing and declarative memory, ketamine has little effect on more general measures of cognition, such as observed with the Mini-Mental State Examination (MMSE) (Krystal et al., 1994; Suzuki, 2000), supporting the relative specificity of the ketamine response.

Glutamatergic contributions to impaired sensory processing

Although glutamatergic and dopaminergic/regionalized models of schizophrenia produce overlapping predictions with regard to processes such as executive function and memory, they produce different prediction patterns for sensory function. Thus, dopaminergic models, in general, predict relative preservation of sensory function, as do models of schizophrenia focusing on localized prefrontal or hippocampal impairment. In contrast, NMDA receptors play a significant role in sensory as well as higher cortical processing, so that glutamatergic models predict sensory as well as higher cognitive impairments in schizophrenia. Over recent years, there has been a resurgence of studies of sensory function in schizophrenia, particularly of auditory and visual dysfunction, in order to test hypotheses stemming from glutamatergic conceptualizations.

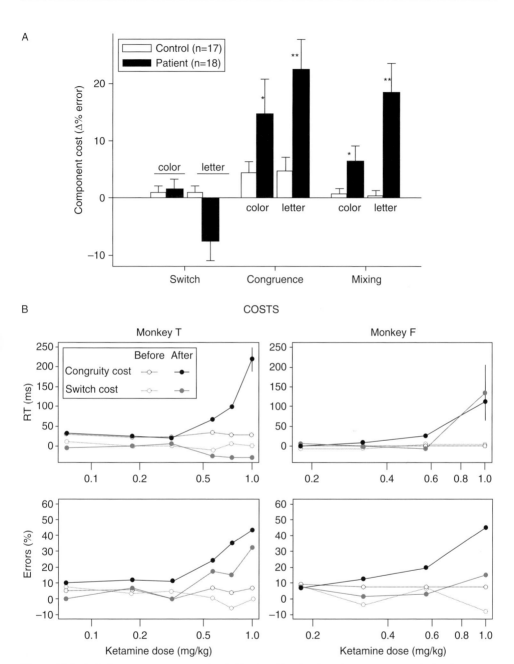

Figure 11.1. A. Performance pattern on task switching in schizophrenia patients versus controls, showing an absence of switch cost deficits, despite significant impairments in congruence and mixing costs (Wylie et al., 2010). B. Performance of monkeys on a similar task before and after ketamine, showing an increase in congruity but not switch costs (Stoet & Snyder, 2003). (Used with kind permission from Nature Publishing Group.)

Auditory function

Auditory functions in schizophrenia have been historically understudied, in part because no deficits are observed in simple audiometric screening tests. Nevertheless, auditory cortical function is not limited to simple tone detection. In particular, the auditory cortex plays a critical role in the matching of stimuli following delay. Specifically, in primates, lesions of the auditory cortex lead to an increase in the frequency difference (Δf) needed to differentiate tones, whether or not distractor stimuli are present. In contrast, prefrontal lesions affect the ability to ignore distractors but do not affect basic tone matching ability (Chao & Knight, 1995; Iversen & Mishkin, 1973), permitting differentiation of sensory-based versus attention-based deficits in auditory function.

Behavioral studies of auditory function

In one of the first studies conducted to evaluate tone matching performance in schizophrenia, it was found that controls required only about a 5% difference in frequency to differentiate tones following a brief (300 ms) delay; patients needed approximately a 20% difference. The degree of between-group separation on this task was highly reliable and as robust ($d=1.25$) as the deficit typically seen on more complex tasks, such as those involving executive processing or working memory (Strous et al., 1995). Subsequent studies demonstrated that deficits were due to impaired encoding, rather than impaired retention across delay (Javitt et al., 1997), and could not be accounted for by failures in either attention (March et al., 1999; Javitt et al., 1997) or increased distractibility (Rabinowicz et al., 2000). Deficits in tone discrimination, moreover, appear to differentiate schizophrenia patients from those with other psychotic illness as well as biological relatives (Force et al., 2008). Finally, similar deficits are also observed in other attributes such as temporal duration (Todd et al., 2003) or spatial ability (Perrin et al., 2010).

Prosodic-level impairments

Given impairments in simple tone matching in schizophrenia, a critical issue becomes how low-level deficits of this type may contribute to more general patterns of cognitive dysfunction in schizophrenia. In Western languages, tone-of-voice ("prosody") is used primarily to convey emotion or attitude. Thus, for example, when people are happy they tend to increase both the base pitch of their voice and the degree of voice modulation, whereas when they are sad, both parameters are decreased (Juslin & Laukka, 2003). Other emotions like fear and disgust may lead to alterations in features such as pitch contour. Whether a statement is sincere or sarcastic may also be conveyed by relatively subtle alterations in tonal feature.

During social interaction, individuals are required to pick up on these often subtle cues and to modulate their behavior accordingly. The ability to distinguish emotions is a critical component of the social cognition construct which, in turn, is a crucial determinant of social function in schizophrenia (Brekke et al., 2005; Harvey & Penn, 2010). Although such deficits are often assumed to reflect dysfunction within higher brain regions, recent studies have begun to evaluate the relationship with sensory-level dysfunction.

In an initial study, patients were evaluated in parallel on auditory and visual emotion discrimination tasks, along with assessments of tone matching ability. As expected, patients showed significant deficits in both auditory and visual emotion discrimination, along with tone matching. However, correlations were observed only within and not across the modality, suggesting significant bottom-up sensory contributions (Leitman et al., 2005).

Subsequently, deficits were also observed on other forms of prosody, such as interrogative and semantic prosody, and were found to be correlated with both impaired tone matching and impaired structural connectivity within auditory regions, as well as impaired sensory–limbic connectivity (Leitman et al., 2007, 2011).

Most recently, deficits have been demonstrated to involve features communicated primarily by modulation of pitch versus intensity, and to correlate with basic deficits in pitch discrimination (Figure 11.2A). Moreover, correlations between tone matching and auditory emotion recognition ability (Figure 11.2B) remained highly significant, even following consideration of other emotional or cognitive factors (Figure 11.2C), suggesting significant bottom-up contributions (Gold et al., 2011). Similar deficits contribute to impaired perception of sarcasm (Kern et al., 2009; Leitman et al., 2006) and to phonological reading impairments (Revheim et al., 2006), suggesting additional paths from impaired sensory function to impaired functional outcome in schizophrenia.

Neurophysiological approaches

Along with behavioral findings, auditory deficits are also documented using neurophysio-logical (e.g., event-related potentials, ERP) and functional magnetic resonance imaging (fMRI)-based approaches. Initial studies showing auditory neurophysiological dysfunction

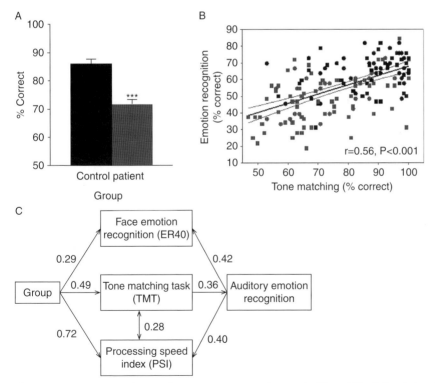

Figure 11.2. A. Tone matching performance in patients with controls. ***, p<0.001. B. Correlations between impairments in tone matching and auditory emotion recognition across patients (light circles) and controls (dark squares). C. Path analysis showing significant contributions of tone matching to auditory recognition deficits even following control for effects of general emotion deficits (face recognition) and general cognitive impairment (PSI). (Gold et al., 2011).

in schizophrenia were performed using the auditory N1 potential, which is a long-latency sensory evoked potential that is thought to reflect sensory registration within the auditory cortex (for review, see Rosburg et al., 2008). Deficits in N1 generation are more apparent at long versus short interstimulus intervals (Rosburg et al., 2008; Shelley et al., 1999), providing a specific pattern that can be evaluated in NMDA receptor antagonist studies. A similar pattern is observed following administration of NMDA receptor antagonists to both rodents (Ehlers et al., 1992; Maxwell et al., 2005) and monkeys (Javitt et al., 2000), supporting underlying NMDA receptor involvement.

More recently, sensory function in schizophrenia has been probed using mismatch negativity (MMN). Mismatch negativity is elicited by infrequent changes in the nature or pattern of repetitive auditory stimulation. Deviant stimuli may differ from standards in a number of stimulus dimensions, including pitch, duration, intensity, or location. Generators for MMN have been mapped to the auditory sensory cortex in the region of Heschl's gyrus (Javitt, 2000; Naatanen, 1995). Deficits in MMN generation were first demonstrated in schizophrenia over 20 years ago and currently represent one of the best replicated neurophysiological findings in schizophrenia (Javitt et al., 2008; Naatanen & Kahkonen, 2009; Umbricht & Krljes, 2005).

Schizophrenia-like deficits in MMN generation can be induced by local infusion of NMDA antagonists into primate auditory cortex (Javitt et al., 1996) and by systemic administration of NMDA antagonists in healthy volunteers (Gunduz-Bruce et al., 2011; Heekeren et al., 2008; Kreitschmann-Andermahr et al., 2001; Schmidt et al., 2011; Umbricht et al., 2000). In contrast, MMN is not modulated via a variety of other psychoactive agents, including the 5-HT2A agonist psilocybin (Heekeren et al., 2008; Schmidt et al., 2011; Umbricht et al., 2003), the D1/D2 agonists bromocriptine and pergolide (Leung et al., 2007, 2010), or stimulants such as methylphenidate (Korostenskaja et al., 2008), and is increased in amplitude by cannabis extract but not delta9-tetrahydrocannabinol (Juckel et al., 2007). In addition, MMN is not affected by either typical or atypical antipsychotics (Umbricht et al., 1998, 1999), shows no significant relationship with neuroendocrine indicators of the catecholamine state (Hansenne et al., 2003), and is not affected by acute dopamine or serotonin depletion (Leung et al., 2010), suggesting relative specificity of the NMDA antagonist psychotomimetic effect.

Finally, deficits in schizophrenia have also been associated with the impaired generation of the auditory steady-state response (Hong et al., 2004; Krishnan et al., 2009; Light et al., 2006; Spencer et al., 2008). Like MMN, the auditory steady-state response (ASSR) is generated within the primary auditory cortex and thus indexes sensory level dysfunction. In contrast to MMN, however, ASSR reflects altered temporal dynamics primarily of the parvalbumin (PV)-type GABA interneurons (Gonzalez-Burgos & Lewis, 2008; Vohs et al., 2010). Furthermore, acute ketamine increases the ASSR (Plourde et al., 1997), suggesting that PV downregulation may be an adaptation to chronic NMDA receptor underactivity and resultant oxidative stress (Behrens & Sejnowski, 2009). Thus, cognitive deficits in schizophrenia may reflect not only current NMDA receptor dysfunction but also consequences of developmental NMDA disturbances.

Visual dysfunction

Given the severe deficits observed in auditory function in schizophrenia, similar studies have now been performed investigating consequences of NMDA dysfunction in the early visual system (for review, see Javitt, 2009). The early visual system consists of discrete magnocellular and parvocellular pathways that differ in characteristics and function. The magnocellular pathway provides rapid transmission of low-resolution information to the cortex, in order to prime attentional systems and "frame" the overall visual scene. The parvocellular pathway, in contrast, provides slower, higher-resolution information to fill in scene details (Chen et al., 2007; Kveraga et al., 2007). The magnocellular system projects preferentially to the dorsal stream ("where") visual pathway, which is involved particularly in perception for action. In contrast, the parvocellular system projects preferentially to the ventral stream ("what") pathway, which is involved primarily in perception for identification.

Although no stimuli are entirely selective for the magnocellular versus parvocellular systems, stimuli can be biased toward these systems by manipulation of features including absolute luminance, contrast, spatial frequency, and duration. In general, magnocellular neurons are best isolated through the use of low luminance, low contrast, and brief, low spatial frequency stimuli. In contrast, parvocellular contributions can be observed when stimuli are presented at high versus low contrast, and at high spatial frequency (for review, see Javitt, 2009).

The NMDA receptors are located at multiple levels of the early visual system, including the retina, lateral geniculate nucleus (LGN), and primary cortex. The magnocellular system, in particular, functions in a nonlinear gain mode that is dependent upon NMDA receptor-mediated neurotransmission (Javitt, 2009), suggesting that magnocellular function in general, and nonlinear gain functions in particular, should be significantly impaired in schizophrenia, with secondary effects on processes such as visual recognition.

Behavioral, neurophysiological, and neuroimaging studies

Behaviorally, visual function deficits in schizophrenia have been documented using both backward masking and contrast sensitivity-type paradigms. In addition, patients show impaired generation of both steady-state and transient visual ERPs, with greater impairment when stimuli are biased toward the magnocellular versus the parvocellular pathway. In both pathways, however, deficits are most related to impairments in nonlinear gain processes, consistent with NMDA receptor-based theories (Javitt, 2009).

In addition to ERP, deficits in magnocellular function have been demonstrated using fMRI, with patients showing preferential activation deficits of visual subregions receiving magnocellular-mediated input (Martinez et al., 2008, 2011). Finally, in addition to showing deficits in detection of static stimuli, patients have severe deficits in detection of motion (Chen et al., 2005; Kim et al., 2006). Moreover, motion detection deficits correlate with impairments in contrast sensitivity to magnocellular-biased stimuli (Kim et al., 2006), suggesting significant bottom-up contribution. As with other features of magnocellular function, motion detection is critically dependent upon NMDA receptor function (Javitt, 2009), and thus may serve as a selective biomarker for NMDA receptor function within the early visual system.

Cognitive consequences of early visual dysfunction

As in the auditory system, failures of low-level visual function produce profound consequences on higher-order function. Furthermore, as in the auditory system, deficits are not readily apparent on routine screening (e.g., Snellen eye chart), and hence have typically been undetected. This is particularly the case with the "frame" function of the magnocellular system, which generates a low-resolution representation of an object that is projected rapidly to the prefrontal cortex even while more detailed object identification processes are occurring within the ventral stream visual pathway.

In many instances, the magnocellular/dorsal stream visual information is sufficient for response selection even in advance of full object identification. It may also contribute to the formation of "first impressions" of which a person is not consciously aware but which nevertheless may guide subsequent behavior (Bar et al., 2006). Because individuals are not necessarily consciously aware of processing occurring within the dorsal visual stream, they may also be unable to articulate disturbances in these processes, so that deficits may remain unobserved unless appropriate paradigms are used.

One process that has been particularly informative in both evaluating visual function in schizophrenia and in illustrating the relationship between dorsal and ventral stream function is the Perceptual Closure Task. In this task, patients are shown fragmented versions of line drawings and asked to identify the object. Given sufficient information, the brain automatically "closes" the object to permit object identification. Object closure has been shown to depend upon network operation of the visual system in which a low-resolution representation of the object fragment is projected rapidly to the frontal cortex and hippocampus, and activates representations of objects that could correspond to the object being depicted. Synchronous activity between the hippocampus and ventral stream visual regions then allows a match between the fine details of the represented object and the activated hippocampal representations. A successful match leads to generation of an ERP component, termed closure negativity (Ncl), which localizes to the ventral stream visual cortex (Javitt, 2009; Sehatpour et al., 2006, 2008).

Closure processes can be assisted by giving a literal prime (i.e., a hint as to what the object might be), which presumably assists the hippocampus in generating potential matches, or by repeating stimuli, which allows explicit identification without requiring hippocampal/visual synchrony (Doniger et al., 2001). Study of this process in schizophrenia thus permits assessment of the pattern of dysfunction relative to predictions of bottom-up versus top-down models in this illness.

In an initial study in schizophrenia, as predicted patients were shown to require more information (less fragmented images) in order to identify ("close") fragmented objects. Nevertheless, patients showed normal effects of both word and repetition priming, suggesting that while visual, bottom-up components of the circuit were impaired, portions of the circuit responsible for top-down priming remained relatively intact (Doniger et al., 2001). A subsequent ERP study demonstrated impaired Ncl component generation in schizophrenia, along with impaired generation of the visual P1 potential (Doniger et al., 2002), reflecting impaired dorsal stream function.

Finally, a recent combined ERP/fMRI study analyzed both frontal and hippocampal activation, along with dorsal and ventral stream activity. Reduced activity was seen in all nodes involved in the task, which may be viewed from either a bottom-up or top-down perspective. However, when a path analysis was performed to assess the relative contributions of each node within the network to impaired performance in schizophrenia, deficits in prefrontal/hippocampal activation were accounted for primarily by failure of input from the dorsal visual stream rather than from intrinsic dysfunction. Moreover, ventral stream dysfunction was accounted for entirely by failure of recurrent activation via the dorsal stream/frontal/hippocampal loop. Thus, while top-down deficits were observed, they were driven primarily by an initial failure of activation within the dorsal stream visual system, leading to input failure within higher brain regions.

Another informative paradigm is the AX-CPT task. This task is considered a paradigmatic executive processing/working memory task, and is reliably associated with reduced frontal activity in schizophrenia (e.g., Minzenberg et al., 2009). However, few studies have evaluated sensory-level function involved in the task. Most specifically, letters, like other visual stimuli, are processed simultaneously by both magnocellular and parvocellular visual systems. Moreover, explicit letter identification within the ventral stream is not required before the stimuli can be used to guide action within the dorsal stream. Patients with schizophrenia show a particular pattern of deficits in this task, characterized by increased errors to incorrectly cued ("BX") trials, as well as a decreased hit rate to correctly cued, correct target ("AX") trials (Minzenberg et al., 2009), giving rise to a reduced signal detection for contextually cued responses (d' context). Similar deficits are observed following ketamine administration to normal volunteers (Umbricht et al., 2000), suggesting NMDA receptor dysfunction as a parsimonious explanation.

In an ERP study designed to investigate the relative contributions of sensory-level versus higher cognitive contributions to impaired performance in schizophrenia (Dias et al., 2011), deficits were seen in both frontally generated ERP, such as the N2 and P3 components, and visual P1, which reflects dysfunction of dorsal stream visual regions. Moreover, as in the Perceptual Closure Task, deficits in frontal activation in the AX-CPT were driven primarily by earlier failures of sensory activation (Figure 11.3A). Performance deficits, as reflected in d' context scores, were also driven primarily by sensory-level dysfunction. In addition, consistent with the findings of this study, meta-analytic studies of AX-CPT show impaired activation of the visual along with the frontal cortices in schizophrenia, in regions that are implicated as well, based upon fMRI of sensory processing (Minzenberg et al., 2009). Along with deficits in AX-CPT function, patients showed reductions in contrast sensitivity to low but not high spatial frequency stimuli, consistent with a deficit primarily in magnocellular visual function (Figure 11.3B). Finally, deficits in contrast sensitivity correlated strongly with deficits in AX-CPT. Correlations remained significant even after controlling for effects of group membership (Figure 11.3C), highlighting the importance of early visual function to the performance of complex neurocognitive tasks such as the AX-CPT.

Early visual deficits may also contribute to several additional domains of cognitive dysfunction in schizophrenia. For example, magnocellular function is known to play a critical role in passage reading (Levy et al., 2010; Stein, 2001; Vidyasagar, 2004). Although reading was once considered to be intact in schizophrenia, based upon single word reading tests such as the Wide Range Achievement Test (WRAT), specific tests of paragraph reading have now shown severe deficits in schizophrenia, related to underlying magnocellular system dysfunction (Revheim et al., 2006).

Deficits in early visual processing may also contribute to impairments in face emotion recognition (Butler et al., 2009). Other visual paradigms, such as visual contour integration (Silverstein et al., 2009, 2010) also point to deficits in visual processing that may contribute significantly to higher cortical impairments. Interestingly, reduced contour integration is seen in recreational ketamine abusers during acute intoxication, again supporting a role for NMDA receptor dysfunction (Uhlhaas et al., 2007).

A general caveat to be drawn from these studies is that the fact that patients with schizophrenia can identify an object (e.g., read letters or words) cannot be taken as evidence that visual processing of the stimuli is normal. In general, relatively little attention is paid to

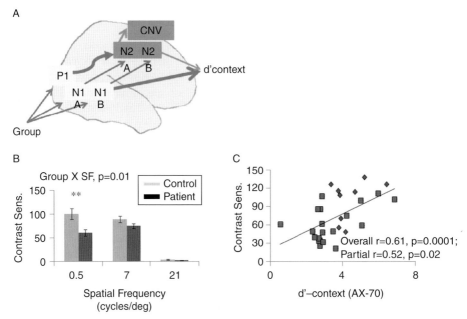

Figure 11.3. A. Path analysis of contributions of regional brain dysfunction to performance deficits on the AX-Continuous Performance Task (AX-CPT) in patients, showing that impaired generation of early plus sensory components such as P1 and N1 drives subsequent impairments in later potentials, as well as performance deficits as reflected by d'-context scores. B. Visual contrast sensitivity performance in patients versus controls showing preferential deficit in processing of magnocellular-biased, low (0.5 cycle/deg) spatial frequency stimuli. C. Correlation between impaired AX-CPT performance and impaired contrast sensitivity to low spatial frequency stimuli (Dias et al., 2011).

the specific physical characteristics of visual stimuli used in cognitive tasks. However, small differences in a stimulus characteristic may lead to major differences in the way stimuli are processed within the magnocellular versus parvocellular systems. As a result, patterns of cognitive impairment in schizophrenia may depend upon not only the tasks, but also the underlying stimuli (e.g., Javitt et al., 2007; Lee & Park, 2006).

Summary

Traditional studies of schizophrenia have focused heavily on processes such as executive function or working memory that localize to frontotemporal brain regions while focusing less on distributed dysfunction throughout the brain. Based upon emerging glutamatergic models, there is increasing focus on dysfunction within widespread networks, including both associational and sensory brain regions. Within each brain region, however, only a subset of functions is affected, involving primarily NMDA receptor-mediated processes. This recent focus on early sensory dysfunction has uncovered deficits in processes that were once thought to be relatively intact in schizophrenia, such as auditory function or reading, and provides new insights into mechanisms underlying specific patterns of cognitive dysfunction in this illness. Further progress in understanding neurobiological determinants of schizophrenia will depend upon considering both the bottom-up and the top-down aspects of information processing that are needed to navigate daily occupational and interpersonal challenges.

References

Adler, C. M., Goldberg, T. E., Malhotra, A. K., et al. (1998). Effects of ketamine on thought disorder, working memory, and semantic memory in healthy volunteers. *Biological Psychiatry*, **43**, 811–816.

Bakker, C. B. & Amini, F. B. (1961). Observations on the psychotomimetic effects of Sernyl. *Comprehensive Psychiatry*, **2**, 269–280.

Bar, M., Neta, M., & Linz, H. (2006). Very first impressions. *Emotion*, **6**, 269–278.

Barch, D. M. (2005). The cognitive neuroscience of schizophrenia. *Annual Review of Clinical Psychology*, **1**, 321–353.

Behrens, M. M. & Sejnowski, T. J. (2009). Does schizophrenia arise from oxidative dysregulation of parvalbumin-interneurons in the developing cortex? *Neuropharmacology*, **57**, 193–200.

Bilder, R. M., Goldman, R. S., Robinson, D., et al. (2000). Neuropsychology of first-episode schizophrenia: initial characterization and clinical correlates. *American Journal of Psychiatry*, **157**, 549–559.

Braver, T. S., Reynolds, J. R., & Donaldson, D. I. (2003). Neural mechanisms of transient and sustained cognitive control during task switching. *Neuron*, **39**, 713–726.

Brekke, J., Kay, D. D., Lee, K. S., et al. (2005). Biosocial pathways to functional outcome in schizophrenia. *Schizophrenia Research*, **80**, 213–225.

Butler, P. D., Abeles, I. Y., Weiskopf, N. G., et al. (2009). Sensory contributions to impaired emotion processing in schizophrenia. *Schizophrenia Bulletin*, **35**, 1095–1107.

Chao, L. L. & Knight, R. T. (1995). Human prefrontal lesions increase distractability to irrelevant sensory inputs. *Neuroreport*, **6**, 1605–1610.

Chen, C. M., Lakatos, P., Shah, A. S., et al. (2007). Functional anatomy and interaction of fast and slow visual pathways in macaque monkeys. *Cerebral Cortex*, **17**, 1561–1569.

Chen, Y., Bidwell, L., & Holzman, P. (2005). Visual motion integration in schizophrenia patients, their first-degree relatives, and patients with bipolar disorder. *Schizophrenia Research*, **74**, 271–281.

Coyle, J. T. (1996). The glutamatergic dysfunction hypothesis for schizophrenia. *Harvard Review of Psychiatry*, **3**, 241–253.

Dias, E. C., Butler, P. D., Hoptman, M. J., et al. (2011). Early sensory contributions to contextual encoding deficits in schizophrenia. *Archives of General Psychiatry*, **68**, 654–664.

Doniger, G. M., Foxe, J. J., Murray, M. M., et al. (2002). Impaired visual object recognition and dorsal/ventral stream interaction in schizophrenia. *Archives of General Psychiatry*, **59**, 1011–1020.

Doniger, G. M., Foxe, J. J., Schroeder, C. E., et al. (2001). Visual perceptual learning in human object recognition areas: a repetition priming study using high-density electrical mapping. *NeuroImage*, **13**, 305–313.

Ehlers, C. L., Kaneko, W. M., Wall, T. L., et al. (1992). Effects of dizocilpine (MK-801) and ethanol on the EEG and event-related potentials (ERPS) in rats. *Neuropharmacology*, **31**, 369–378.

Force, R. B., Venables, N. C., & Sponheim, S. R. (2008). An auditory processing abnormality specific to liability for schizophrenia. *Schizophrenia Research*, **103**, 298–310.

Gold, R., Butler, P. D., Revheim, N., et al. (2011). Auditory emotion recognition impairments in schizophrenia: relationship to acoustic features and cognition. *American Journal of Psychiatry*, **169**, 424–432.

Gonzalez-Burgos, G. & Lewis, D. A. (2008). GABA neurons and the mechanisms of network oscillations: implications for understanding cortical dysfunction in schizophrenia. *Schizophrenia Bulletin*, **34**, 944–961.

Gunduz-Bruce, H., Reinhart, R. M., Roach, B. J., et al. (2011). Glutamatergic modulation of auditory information processing in the human brain. *Biological Psychiatry*, **71**, 969–977.

Hansenne, M., Pinto, E., Scantamburlo, G., et al. (2003). Mismatch negativity is not correlated with neuroendocrine indicators of catecholaminergic activity in healthy subjects. *Human Psychopharmacology*, **18**, 201–205.

Harborne, G. C., Watson, F. L., Healy, D. T., et al. (1996). The effects of sub-anaesthetic doses of ketamine on memory, cognitive performance and subjective experience in healthy volunteers. *Journal of Psychopharmacology*, **10**, 134–140.

Harris, J. A., Biersner, R. J., Edwards, D., et al. (1975). Attention, learning, and personality during ketamine emergence: a pilot study. *Anesthesia and Analgesia*, **54**, 169–172.

Harvey, P. D. & Penn, D. (2010). Social cognition: the key factor predicting social outcome in people with schizophrenia? *Psychiatry (Edgmont)*, **7**, 41–44.

Heekeren, K., Daumann, J., Neukirch, A., et al. (2008). Mismatch negativity generation in the human 5HT2A agonist and NMDA antagonist model of psychosis. *Psychopharmacology (Berl)*, **199**, 77–88.

Hetem, L. A., Danion, J. M., Diemunsch, P., et al. (2000). Effect of a subanesthetic dose of ketamine on memory and conscious awareness in healthy volunteers. *Psychopharmacology (Berl)*, **152**, 283–288.

Honey, G. D., Corlett, P. R., Absalom, A. R., et al. (2008). Individual differences in psychotic effects of ketamine are predicted by brain function measured under placebo. *Journal of Neuroscience*, **28**, 6295–6303.

Hong, L. E., Summerfelt, A., McMahon, R., et al. (2004). Evoked gamma band synchronization and the liability for schizophrenia. *Schizophrenia Research*, **70**, 293–302.

Howes, O. D. & Kapur, S. (2009). The dopamine hypothesis of schizophrenia: version III – the final common pathway. *Schizophrenia Bulletin*, **35**, 549–562.

Iversen, S. D. & Mishkin, M. (1973). Comparison of superior temporal and inferior prefrontal lesions on auditory and non-auditory tasks in rhesus monkeys. *Brain Research*, **55**, 355–367.

Javitt, D. C. (1987). Negative schizophrenic symptomatology and the PCP (phencyclidine) model of schizophrenia. *Hillside Journal of Clinical Psychiatry*, **9**, 12–35.

Javitt, D. C. (2000). Intracortical mechanisms of mismatch negativity dysfunction in schizophrenia. *Audiology and Neurotology*, **5**, 207–215.

Javitt, D. C. (2009). When doors of perception close: bottom-up models of disrupted cognition in schizophrenia. *Annual Review of Clinical Psychology*, **5**, 249–275.

Javitt, D. C., Jayachandra, M., Lindsley, R. W., et al. (2000). Schizophrenia-like deficits in auditory P1 and N1 refractoriness induced by the psychomimetic agent phencyclidine (PCP). *Clinical Neurophysiology*, **111**, 833–836.

Javitt, D. C., Rabinowicz, E., Silipo, G., et al. (2007). Encoding vs. retention: differential effects of cue manipulation on working memory performance in schizophrenia. *Schizophrenia Research*, **91**, 159–168.

Javitt, D. C., Spencer, K. M., Thaker, G. K., et al. (2008). Neurophysiological biomarkers for drug development in schizophrenia. *Nature Reviews Drug Discovery*, **7**, 68–83.

Javitt, D. C., Steinschneider, M., Schroeder, C. E., et al. (1996). Role of cortical N-methyl-D-aspartate receptors in auditory sensory memory and mismatch negativity generation: implications for schizophrenia. *Proceedings of the National Academy of Sciences of the United States of America*, **93**, 11962–11967.

Javitt, D. C., Strous, R. D., Grochowski, S., et al. (1997). Impaired precision, but normal retention, of auditory sensory ("echoic") memory information in schizophrenia. *Journal of Abnormal Psychology*, **106**, 315–324.

Javitt, D. C. & Zukin, S. R. (1991). Recent advances in the phencyclidine model of schizophrenia. *American Journal of Psychiatry*, **148**, 1301–1308.

Juckel, G., Roser, P., Nadulski, T., et al. (2007). Acute effects of delta9-tetrahydrocannabinol and standardized cannabis extract on the auditory evoked mismatch negativity. *Schizophrenia Research*, **97**, 109–117.

Juslin, P. N. & Laukka, P. (2003). Communication of emotions in vocal expression and music performance: different channels, same code? *Psychological Bulletin*, **129**, 770–814.

Kern, R. S., Green, M. F., Fiske, A. P., et al. (2009). Theory of mind deficits for processing counterfactual information in persons with chronic schizophrenia. *Psychological Medicine*, **39**, 645–654.

Kim, D., Wylie, G., Pasternak, R., et al. (2006). Magnocellular contributions to impaired motion processing in schizophrenia. *Schizophrenia Research*, **82**, 1–8.

Korostenskaja, M., Kicic, D., & Kahkonen, S. (2008). The effect of methylphenidate on auditory information processing in healthy volunteers: a combined EEG/MEG study. *Psychopharmacology (Berl)*, **197**, 475–486.

Kreitschmann-Andermahr, I., Rosburg, T., Demme, U., et al. (2001). Effect of ketamine on the neuromagnetic mismatch field in healthy humans. *Brain Research. Cognitive Brain Research*, **12**, 109–116.

Krishnan, G. P., Hetrick, W. P., Brenner, C. A., et al. (2009). Steady state and induced auditory gamma deficits in schizophrenia. *NeuroImage*, **47**, 1711–1719.

Krystal, J. H., D'Souza, D. C., Karper, L. P., et al. (1999). Interactive effects of subanesthetic ketamine and haloperidol in healthy humans. *Psychopharmacology (Berl)*, **145**, 193–204.

Krystal, J. H., Karper, L. P., Bennett, A., et al. (1998). Interactive effects of subanesthetic ketamine and subhypnotic lorazepam in humans. *Psychopharmacology (Berl)*, **135**, 213–229.

Krystal, J. H., Karper, L. P., Seibyl, J. P., et al. (1994). Subanesthetic effects of the noncompetitive NMDA antagonist, ketamine, in humans. Psychotomimetic, perceptual, cognitive, and neuroendocrine responses. *Archives of General Psychiatry*, **51**, 199–214.

Krystal, J. H., Perry, E. B. Jr., Gueorguieva, R., et al. (2005). Comparative and interactive human psychopharmacologic effects of ketamine and amphetamine: implications for glutamatergic and dopaminergic model psychoses and cognitive function. *Archives of General Psychiatry*, **62**, 985–994.

Kveraga, K., Boshyan, J., & Bar, M. (2007). Magnocellular projections as the trigger of top-down facilitation in recognition. *Journal of Neuroscience*, **27**, 13232–13240.

Lee, J. & Park, S. (2006). The role of stimulus salience in CPT-AX performance of schizophrenia patients. *Schizophrenia Research*, **81**, 191–197.

Leitman, D. I., Foxe, J. J., Butler, P. D., et al. (2005). Sensory contributions to impaired prosodic processing in schizophrenia. *Biological Psychiatry*, **58**, 56–61.

Leitman, D. I., Hoptman, M. J., Foxe, J. J., et al. (2007). The neural substrates of impaired prosodic detection in schizophrenia and its sensorial antecedents. *American Journal of Psychiatry*, **164**, 474–482.

Leitman, D. I., Wolf, D. H., Laukka, P., et al. (2011). Not pitch perfect: sensory contributions to affective communication impairment in schizophrenia. *Biological Psychiatry*, **70**, 611–618.

Leitman, D. I., Ziwich, R., Pasternak, R., et al. (2006). Theory of Mind (ToM) and counterfactuality deficits in schizophrenia: misperception or misinterpretation? *Psychological Medicine*, **36**, 1075–1083.

Leung, S., Croft, R. J., Baldeweg, T., et al. (2007). Acute dopamine D(1) and D(2) receptor stimulation does not modulate mismatch negativity (MMN) in healthy human subjects. *Psychopharmacology (Berl)*, **194**, 443–451.

Leung, S., Croft, R. J., Guille, V., et al. (2010). Acute dopamine and/or serotonin depletion does not modulate mismatch negativity (MMN) in healthy human participants. *Psychopharmacology (Berl)*, **208**, 233–244.

Levy, T., Walsh, V., & Lavidor, M. (2010). Dorsal stream modulation of visual word recognition in skilled readers. *Vision Research*, **50**, 883–888.

Light, G. A., Hsu, J. L., Hsieh, M. H., et al. (2006). Gamma band oscillations reveal neural network cortical coherence dysfunction in schizophrenia patients. *Biological Psychiatry*, **60**, 1231–1240.

Lofwall, M. R., Griffiths, R. R., & Mintzer, M. Z. (2006). Cognitive and subjective acute dose effects of intramuscular ketamine in healthy adults. *Experimental and Clinical Psychopharmacology*, **14**, 439–449.

March, L., Cienfuegos, A., Goldbloom, L., et al. (1999). Normal time course of auditory recognition in schizophrenia, despite impaired precision of the auditory sensory ("echoic") memory code. *Journal of Abnormal Psychology*, **108**, 69–75.

Martinez, A., Hillyard, S. A., Bickel, S., et al. (2011). Consequences of magnocellular dysfunction on processing attended information in schizophrenia. *Cerebral Cortex*, **22**, 1282–1293.

Martinez, A., Hillyard, S. A., Dias, E. C., et al. (2008). Magnocellular pathway impairment in schizophrenia: evidence from functional magnetic resonance imaging. *Journal of Neuroscience*, **28**, 7492–7500.

Maxwell, C. R., Ehrlichman, R. S., Liang, Y., et al. (2005). Ketamine produces lasting disruptions in encoding of sensory stimuli. *Journal of Pharmacology and Experimental Therapeutics*, **316**, 315–324.

Minzenberg, M. J., Laird, A. R., Thelen, S., et al. (2009). Meta-analysis of 41 functional neuroimaging studies of executive function in schizophrenia. *Archives of General Psychiatry*, **66**, 811–822.

Morgan, C. J., Mofeez, A., Brandner, B., et al. (2004a). Acute effects of ketamine on memory systems and psychotic symptoms in healthy volunteers. *Neuropsychopharmacology*, **29**, 208–218.

Morgan, C. J., Mofeez, A., Brandner, B., et al. (2004b). Ketamine impairs response inhibition and is positively reinforcing in healthy volunteers: a dose-response study. *Psychopharmacology (Berl)*, **172**, 298–308.

Naatanen, R. (1995). The mismatch negativity: a powerful tool for cognitive neuroscience. *Ear and Hearing*, **16**, 6–18.

Naatanen, R. & Kahkonen, S. (2009). Central auditory dysfunction in schizophrenia as revealed by the mismatch negativity (MMN) and its magnetic equivalent MMNm: a review. *Int J Neuropsychopharmacology*, **12**, 125–135.

Newcomer, J. W., Farber, N. B., Jevtovic-Todorovic, V., et al. (1999). Ketamine-induced NMDA receptor hypofunction as a model of memory impairment and psychosis. *Neuropsychopharmacology*, **20**, 106–118.

Parwani, A., Weiler, M. A., Blaxton, T. A., et al. (2005). The effects of a subanesthetic dose of ketamine on verbal memory in normal volunteers. *Psychopharmacology (Berl)*, **183**, 265–274.

Perrin, M. A., Butler, P. D., Dicostanzo, J., et al. (2010). Spatial localization deficits and auditory cortical dysfunction in schizophrenia. *Schizophrenia Research*, **124**, 161–168.

Plourde, G., Baribeau, J., & Bonhomme, V. (1997). Ketamine increases the amplitude of the 40-Hz auditory steady-state response in humans. *British Journal of Anaesthesia*, **78**, 524–529.

Rabinowicz, E. F., Silipo, G., Goldman, R., et al. (2000). Auditory sensory dysfunction in schizophrenia: imprecision or distractibility? *Archives of General Psychiatry*, **57**, 1149–1155.

Radant, A. D., Bowdle, T. A., Cowley, D. S., et al. (1998). Does ketamine-mediated N-methyl-D-aspartate receptor antagonism cause schizophrenia-like oculomotor abnormalities? *Neuropsychopharmacology*, **19**, 434–444.

Reichenberg, A. & Harvey, P. D. (2007). Neuropsychological impairments in schizophrenia: integration of performance-based and brain imaging findings. *Psychological Bulletin*, **133**, 833–858.

Revheim, N., Butler, P. D., Schechter, I., et al. (2006). Reading impairment and visual processing deficits in schizophrenia. *Schizophrenia Research*, **87**, 238–245.

Rosburg, T., Boutros, N. N., & Ford, J. M. (2008). Reduced auditory evoked potential component N100 in schizophrenia – a critical review. *Psychiatry Research*, **161**, 259–274.

Rowland, L. M., Bustillo, J. R., Mullins, P. G., et al. (2005). Effects of ketamine on anterior cingulate glutamate metabolism in healthy humans: a 4-T proton MRS study. *American Journal of Psychiatry*, **162**, 394–396.

Saykin, A. J., Gur, R. C., Gur, R. E., et al. (1991). Neuropsychological function in schizophrenia. Selective impairment in memory and learning. *Archives of General Psychiatry*, **48**, 618–624.

Schmidt, A., Bachmann, R., Kometer, M., et al. (2011). Mismatch negativity encoding of prediction errors predicts S-ketamine-induced cognitive impairments. *Neuropsychopharmacology*, 37, 865–875.

Sehatpour, P., Molholm, S., Javitt, D. C., et al. (2006). Spatiotemporal dynamics of human object recognition processing: an integrated high-density electrical mapping and functional imaging study of "closure" processes. *NeuroImage*, 29, 605–618.

Sehatpour, P., Molholm, S., Schwartz, T. H., et al. (2008). A human intracranial study of long-range oscillatory coherence across a frontal-occipital-hippocampal brain network during visual object processing. *Proceedings of the National Academy of Sciences of the United States of America*, 105, 4399–4404.

Shelley, A. M., Silipo, G., & Javitt, D. C. (1999). Diminished responsiveness of ERPs in schizophrenic subjects to changes in auditory stimulation parameters: implications for theories of cortical dysfunction. *Schizophrenia Research*, 37, 65–79.

Silverstein, S. M., Berten, S., Essex, B., et al. (2009). An fMRI examination of visual integration in schizophrenia. *Journal of Integrative Neuroscience*, 8, 175–202.

Silverstein, S. M., Berten, S., Essex, B., et al. (2010). Perceptual organization and visual search processes during target detection task performance in schizophrenia, as revealed by fMRI. *Neuropsychologia*, 48, 2886–2893.

Spencer, K. M., Salisbury, D. F., Shenton, M. E., et al. (2008). Gamma-band auditory steady-state responses are impaired in first episode psychosis. *Biological Psychiatry*, 64, 369–375.

Stein, J. (2001). The magnocellular theory of developmental dyslexia. *Dyslexia*, 7, 12–36.

Stoet, G. & Snyder, L. H. (2006). Effects of the NMDA antagonist ketamine on task-switching performance: evidence for specific impairments of executive control. *Neuropsychopharmacology*, 31, 1675–1681.

Strous, R. D., Cowan, N., Ritter, W., et al. (1995). Auditory sensory ("echoic") memory dysfunction in schizophrenia. *American Journal of Psychiatry*, 152, 1517–1519.

Suzuki, M., Tsueda, K., Lansing, P.S., et al. (2000). Midazolam attenuates ketamine-induced abnormal perception and thought process but not mood changes. *Canadian Journal of Anaesthesia*, 47, 866–874.

Todd, J., Michie, P. T., & Jablensky, A. V. (2003). Association between reduced duration mismatch negativity (MMN) and raised temporal discrimination thresholds in schizophrenia. *Clinical Neurophysiology*, 114, 2061–2070.

Uhlhaas, P. J., Millard, I., Muetzelfeldt, L., et al. (2007). Perceptual organization in ketamine users: preliminary evidence of deficits on night of drug use but not 3 days later. *Journal of Psychopharmacology*, 21, 347–352.

Umbricht, D., Javitt, D., Novak, G., et al. (1998). Effects of clozapine on auditory event-related potentials in schizophrenia. *Biological Psychiatry*, 44, 716–725.

Umbricht, D., Javitt, D., Novak, G., et al. (1999). Effects of risperidone on auditory event-related potentials in schizophrenia. *International Journal of Neuropsychopharmacology*, 2, 299–304.

Umbricht, D. & Krljes, S. (2005). Mismatch negativity in schizophrenia: a meta-analysis. *Schizophrenia Research*, 76, 1–23.

Umbricht, D., Schmid, L., Koller, R., et al. (2000). Ketamine-induced deficits in auditory and visual context-dependent processing in healthy volunteers: implications for models of cognitive deficits in schizophrenia. *Archives of General Psychiatry*, 57, 1139–1147.

Umbricht, D., Vollenweider, F. X., Schmid, L., et al. (2003). Effects of the 5-HT2A agonist psilocybin on mismatch negativity generation and AX-continuous performance task: implications for the neuropharmacology of cognitive deficits in schizophrenia. *Neuropsychopharmacology*, 28, 170–181.

Vidyasagar, T. R. (2004). Neural underpinnings of dyslexia as a disorder of visuo-spatial attention. *Clinical and Experimental Optometry*, 87, 4–10.

Vohs, J. L., Chambers, R. A., Krishnan, G. P., et al. (2010). GABAergic modulation of the 40 Hz auditory steady-state response in a rat model of schizophrenia. *International*

Journal of Neuropsychopharmacology, **13**, 487–497.

Wylie, G. R., Javitt, D. C., & Foxe, J. J. (2003). Task switching: a high-density electrical mapping study. *NeuroImage*, **20**, 2322–2342.

Wylie, G. R., Javitt, D. C., & Foxe, J. J. (2006). Jumping the gun: is effective preparation contingent upon anticipatory activation in task-relevant neural circuitry? *Cerebral Cortex*, **16**, 394–404.

Wylie, K. P & Tregellas, J. R. (2010). The role of the insula in schizophrenia. *Schizophrenia Research*, **123**, 93–104.

Chapter

12

Translational cognitive neuroscience of schizophrenia: bridging neurocognitive and computational approaches toward understanding cognitive deficits

Alan Anticevic, John H. Krystal, and Deanna M. Barch

Overview

Schizophrenia is a complex neuropsychiatric syndrome presenting with a constellation of symptoms, including positive symptoms (delusions and hallucinations), negative symptoms, affective symptoms, and cognitive deficits. While delusions and hallucinations are considered the hallmark symptoms of the illness, cognitive deficits and affective dysfunction in patients with schizophrenia are increasingly receiving research focus–primarily due to growing consensus that these deficits are a substantial source of disability and loss of functional capacity for patients. The present chapter will focus on recent evidence for cognitive deficits in schizophrenia. First, we will review the behavioral and cognitive neuroscience evidence for dysfunction across different cardinal domains of cognition. In this component of the chapter we will emphasize evidence for abnormalities in working memory (WM), episodic memory (EM), and cognitive control (CC). Second, given the emerging wealth of knowledge from animal studies and computational models, we focus on WM as an example to understand cognitive deficits in schizophrenia from a translational perspective. Such a translational framework has the capacity to confer a mechanistic framework for understanding cognitive dysfunction in schizophrenia. To that end, we will discuss evidence across levels of analysis spanning from cells to circuits to systems, which offer clues for better understanding of cognitive dysfunction and developing putative treatment targets in schizophrenia. Building on pharmacological findings in humans, we will outline how such deficits may arise due to abnormalities in N-methyl-D-aspartate (NMDA) glutamate receptor dysfunction, as one hypothesis about the source of at least some cognitive deficits in schizophrenia. In this component of the chapter we will also discuss the critical utility of computational modeling in allowing us to test mechanistically derived translational hypotheses regarding WM abnormalities in schizophrenia derived at the level of cells.

General overview of cognitive dysfunction in schizophrenia

Schizophrenia is a complex and highly heterogeneous syndrome (Walker et al., 2004). Patients exhibit diverse symptoms encompassing distorted beliefs (delusions), aberrant internal visual/auditory percepts (hallucinations), as well as loss of affective expression and motivational drive (negative symptoms). One additional area of pervasive dysfunction for patients suffering from schizophrenia involves cognitive deficits. Cognitive abnormalities are consistently implicated in functional outcome (Green, 2006; Kee et al., 2003), exhibit onset prior to the emergence of the full syndrome (Cornblatt et al., 1999; Niendam et al., 2003), are relatively stable across the lifespan of the individual (Heaton et al., 2001; Irani et al., 2011), and–perhaps most importantly–are not ameliorated by current pharmacotherapy for psychosis (Buchanan et al., 2007). In fact, since the earliest theories of schizophrenia, cognitive deficits have played a central theme in the clinical character- ization of this illness (Kraeplin, 1950). Therefore, understanding the underlying neuro- pathology, which may give rise to disturbances in cognition, is a crucial challenge for the field of schizophrenia research.

There is clearly evidence for a generalized cognitive deficit in patients with schizophre- nia (Dickinson et al., 2008; Gur et al., 2001), as patients suffering from schizophrenia are impaired across virtually all cognitive measures relative to healthy controls. However, a critical question concerns what aspects of cognition reflect a specific deficit embedded in the context of such a generalized deficit, and which may be impaired in schizophrenia even when one accounts for a range of confounding factors that may be associated with psychosis, such as medication status and other disease-related phenomena. A growing body of work implicates WM, EM, and CC as such core deficits in cognition (Elevåg & Goldberg, 2000), which exhibit a specific pattern of impairment that is present even in unmedicated individuals with schizophrenia (Barch et al., 2001) and individuals thought to be at risk for the development of schizophrenia (e.g., first-degree relatives) (Delawalla et al., 2006). In the following sections we focus more specifically on these regions of cognitive dysfunction in schizophrenia.

However, prior to discussing these broad areas of the literature, it is important to briefly set the stage for the conceptual framework of cognitive neuroscience, which we will use as a platform for understanding cognitive dysfunction in schizophrenia. The past two decades have witnessed an explosive growth of knowledge regarding the neural correlates of various cognitive processes in healthy individuals. This burgeoning field of cognitive neuroscience has generated an increasingly robust platform for interpreting clinical neuropsychiatric phenomena (Barch, 2005a). This is primarily accomplished by garnering an increased understanding of neural systems known to be involved in various cognitive operations in healthy individuals. This understanding in turn constrains our search for what aspects of brain circuitry may be abnormal in clinical populations exhibiting deficits in these same cognitive operations. Therefore, we contend that using a cognitive neuroscience framework offers a promising tool for elucidating and ultimately treating cognitive impairment in schizophrenia by delineating abnormalities in neural circuits, the function of which is increasingly understood in healthy populations. We will review evidence within this cognitive neuroscience framework across cognitive domains– WM, CC, and EM–all of which may be linked by abnormalities in shared neural circuits in schizophrenia. Furthermore, in subsequent sections we will argue that it is precisely this cognitive neuroscience framework that provides great potential for establishing links with translational findings from basic preclinical, pharmacological, and computational neuro- science work. In this context, we will focus on WM specifically, as one domain of cognition that has particular promise for translation.

Working memory in schizophrenia
Cognitive neuroscience models of working memory

Before we proceed with a discussion of WM in the context of schizophrenia, it is important to discuss some of the leading cognitive models of WM to provide conceptual bearings on findings in schizophrenia. Working memory traditionally refers to temporary storage and manipulating information "online," typically in the service of some goal (Baddeley, 2000; Baddeley & Hitch, 1974). According to one prominent cognitive model, WM is thought to be composed of a central executive resource system, and two slave subsidiary systems: the phonological loop and the visuospatial sketchpad (Baddeley & Hitch, 1974); that is, WM is conceptualized as a multi-store process relying on distinct components. This cognitive model was later updated to include a fourth component: the episodic buffer (Baddeley, 2000). Such a conceptual delineation of WM processes has provided one platform from which we can begin to examine deficits in schizophrenia. Besides dividing the WM process into cognitive modules, one can consider WM as comprising distinct stages in time. In that sense, the WM process can be roughly subdivided into three distinct temporal components (Jonides et al., 2008): encoding of novel information and forming an internal representation; active maintenance of this information (i.e., refreshing the memory trace, which is synonymous with the function of two slave subsystems) over some period; as well as manipulation of maintained information in the service of some goal (which is synonymous with the central executive). In other words, the central executive is thought to be a system responsible for orchestrating the interplay between the various short-term buffers, long-term memory, and control processes that modify and integrate information in WM (Jonides et al., 2008).

It is important to note that there are additional models of WM function, which differ in some aspects from the one outlined here (Cowan, 2001, 2008) (for a detailed treatment of this topic, please refer to prior reviews (Jonides et al., 2008). The present review is not intended to arbitrate between cognitive models of WM, but rather to focus on critical shared aspects across models; namely, representation of information over time in the absence of a stimulus, and manipulation of internal representations in the service of some goal. Importantly, these different aspects of WM are supported by a distributed network-level neural architecture spanning both cortical and subcortical regions (Jonides et al., 2008; Owen et al., 2005). In fact, recent advances in functional neuroimaging support the notion that a distributed network of brain regions, which includes dorsal frontoparietal cortical regions, is involved in WM (Curtis et al., 2004; D'Esposito, 2007; D'Esposito et al., 1998; Miller & D'Esposito, 2005). It is this growing understanding of the distributed neural circuits involved in WM that has allowed clinical researchers to anchor their findings. For instance, our growing knowledge of the critical role of the prefrontal cortex in WM has offered some constraints on what specific circuits may exhibit dysfunction in schizophrenia. Furthermore, cognitive neuroscience paradigms have created a framework within which WM dysfunction can now be probed in neuropsychiatric illness.

Behavioral findings in schizophrenia

To date, the evidence suggests that patients with schizophrenia display deficits in WM, marked by less accurate and slower performance on a variety of tasks irrespective of WM modality (Barch, 2005a; Barch & Smith, 2008; Barch et al., 2001, 2003; Park & Holzman, 1992; Reichenberg & Harvey 2007). Additionally, studies have documented WM deficits when examining medicated and unmedicated patients, first-degree relatives, as well as individuals with schizotypal personality, suggesting that WM is a critical abnormality manifesting along the schizophrenia spectrum (Horan et al., 2008; MacDonald et al., 2003; Snitz et al., 2006). In recent years, a number of meta-analyses have quantified these findings and reported strong evidence for WM impairments in schizophrenia patients as compared to healthy controls. The meta-analytic findings reported effect sizes from 0.61 to 1.18 evident in both verbal and nonverbal WM tasks (Aleman et al., 1999; Dickinson et al., 2007; Heinrichs & Zakzanis, 1998; Lee & Park, 2005; Zakzanis & Heinrichs, 1999).

Even though the presence of WM deficits in schizophrenia is clear, it is critical to understand at which stage of the WM process the breakdown may be occurring. As noted previously, given that WM is not a unitary concept (and is not instantiated in a single neural structure), it is important to pinpoint which aspects of WM functioning are compromised. As noted earlier, in addition to focusing on domain-specific functions (i.e., verbal vs. visuospatial), WM can be further subdivided into distinct temporal components that are required for successful operation: (1) selection of stimuli for entry into WM and encoding of these representations; (2) maintenance of the representation in conjunction with pro-tecting the information by inhibiting irrelevant stimuli; and (3) successful retrieval of memoranda when needed (Baddeley, 2000; Baddeley et al., 1974; Jonides et al., 2008; Lee & Park, 2005). Breakdown in any of these components may compromise the overall WM process and produce abnormalities in patients. However, breakdowns in different components may have drastically different implications for understanding the neurobio-logical underpinning of WM malfunction, as they may be supported by different neurobio-logical mechanisms. At the risk of oversimplification, consider for instance that WM deficits in schizophrenia are purely a product of encoding abnormalities, which could be a manifestation of lower-level, early visual cortical malfunction (i.e., the incoming information is simply not accurately represented at the lower level of the visual hierarchy). This would imply that information being represented in WM might be degraded even in the absence of maintenance deficits. In contrast, consider that encoding is intact, but that deficits manifest at the maintenance stage of the WM process, which may implicate a completely different neural mechanism; namely, the frontoparietal cortical system (Leung et al., 2002; Wager & Smith, 2003) responsible for keeping real-time mnemonic representa-tions once the physical stimuli are no longer available. Therefore, to best understand WM abnormalities in schizophrenia, it is critical to determine at which stage (or stages) the breakdown in the WM process may be occurring.

Working memory: encoding deficits or maintenance deficits in schizophrenia?

An influential meta-analysis suggested that patients with schizophrenia exhibit deficits in all phases of WM and that the degree of impairment is fairly constant even when extending the maintenance period (Lee & Park, 2005). Specifically, Lee and Park found that the effect size of the observed impairment across studies did not change as a function of the delay period used. This may imply that breakdowns in WM may be occurring as early as the encoding stage; that is, when internal representations are still forming. Consistent with this framing, studies examining encoding deficits have demonstrated that patients with schizophrenia exhibit short-term memory deficits even in the absence of a delay (Hartman et al., 2003; Tek et al., 2002). However, other work has qualified these findings. Specifically, two studies have shown that encoding impairments can be minimized if patients are allotted more time to complete the encoding process, which suggests a speed-of-processing deficit rather than a pure encoding process deficit per se (Badcock et al., 2008; Hartman et al., 2003). Nevertheless, speed-of-processing reductions at encoding may still be interpreted as an encoding deficit in that the speed with which the information can be encoded robustly will degrade the quality of internal representations. Badcock and colleagues conducted a study that highlights this issue. They employed a spatial WM task during which they presented small circles located on a hidden radial grid. Subjects were required to identify the location of the circle using a touch screen following a zero-second and a four-second delay. This allowed the authors to examine encoding and maintenance components of WM as well as two components of encoding accuracy: (1) general direction on the radial grid (i.e., global features); and (2) precise distance from the target location (fine-grained detail). First, they focused on the zero-second delay, which allows a more pure assessment of encoding deficits. They demonstrated that using fixed- and short-target durations (<500 ms) resulted in only a small fraction of the patient sample (<50%) performing at a high level of accuracy (~80%). In other words, when patients were not given very much time to encode the stimuli, most of the sample performed poorly. In contrast, when given the same brief encoding duration, a much larger fraction of the control sample (73%) performed well (~80% accuracy). However, when equating for processing speed at encoding using an adaptive staircase procedure, there were no significant differences between patient and control subjects in general direction and overall precision accuracy, even though the patient group still demonstrated numerically lower performance. In other words, when patients were allowed more time to represent the stimuli in WM, their performance following a zero-second delay performance was not significantly different than that of control subjects. Nevertheless, it should be noted that other studies demonstrated that encoding deficits exist even after controlling for perceptual processing differences (Tek et al., 2002) (although not the time necessary to encode the stimulus). A complementary study in the verbal WM domain by Javitt and colleagues (Javitt et al., 1997) demonstrated that patients with schizophrenia show similar tone discrimination at short delays when the difficulty of the task was taken into account. Therefore, while encoding deficits may be reduced in the presence of more time to encode, these findings still argue that speed of processing can impact precision of WM representations. Taken together, these studies suggest that inefficiencies in the encoding process could certainly be a contributing factor to the overall profile of WM deficits in schizophrenia.

At the same time, Badcock and colleagues as well as other researchers have shown that patients demonstrate WM deficits when a delay period is introduced (i.e., maintenance component is added), which persist even when controlling for encoding differences (Badcock et al., 2008; Lee & Park, 2005; Tek et al., 2002). For instance, Badcock et al. showed that even after equating for the time needed to encode the stimuli, there were significant differences between the groups following a four-second delay, suggesting a persistent maintenance deficit (although delays longer than 4 s also raise the issue of active vs. passive maintenance). An elegant study by Lencz et al. (2003) demonstrated the presence of both encoding and maintenance deficits in a visual delayed match-to-sample task. Specifically, they showed that when performance at encoding (i.e., no delay) was titrated at the single-subject level, maintenance deficits persisted (i.e., 4-s 8-s delay). Additional work in the visuospatial domain further suggests the presence of WM deficits in schizophrenia during the delay phase. For instance, Fleming and colleagues examined WM and basic perceptual processing (no memory component required) in schizophrenia (Fleming et al., 1997). Specifically, they used a delayed response task with a seven-second and zero-second (no) delay in addition to the Judgment of Line Orientation Test (a simple visual perception task) (Treccani et al., 2005). Their findings suggested relatively spared visuospatial processing in patients (i.e., when no memory demands were required), but deficits on tasks with a mnemonic component. Of note, there are other findings suggesting basic perceptual deficits in patients with schizophrenia (Blanchard & Neale, 1994; Buchanan et al., 1994; Hardoy et al., 2004). However, these studies did not include a spatial WM task in the same sample, thus making it difficult to examine if the patient samples in these studies would have demonstrated more severe differential deficits when performing a WM task. Another investigation by Dreher and colleagues further characterized WM deficits using tasks tapping into either spatial recall (item) or temporal recall (order) in schizophrenia (Dreher et al., 2001). Specifically, they employed a computerized version of the Corsi Block Task typically employed in neuropsychological testing (Lezak, 1995), where they manipulated set size and the delay period thus allowing examination of different difficulty levels, as well as deficits related to encoding and maintenance components of WM. In summary, patients demonstrated overall worse performance across all four tasks and both delay periods. However, patients performed significantly worse as the delay period increased, in contrast to controls whose performance did not differ significantly as a function of delay. In addition, unlike controls, patients with schizophrenia performed worse at longer delays as a function of increasing WM set size. Other studies have replicated these core findings, confirming the presence of spatial WM deficits in schizophrenia (Pukrop et al., 2003; Saperstein et al., 2006).

Taken together, the reviewed evidence suggests that there are abnormalities evident across both encoding and maintenance phases of WM in schizophrenia. Results indicate that encoding deficits may manifest in part due to the time necessary to form an accurate internal representation rapidly (Badcock et al., 2008; Hartman et al., 2003), and/or to reflect a deficit in the ability to represent the sensory properties of the stimulus, irrespective of time (Tek et al., 2002). While the precise nature of encoding abnormalities has yet to be ascertained, some authors have argued that these deficits do not represent pure sensory abnormalities in patients, but may also encompass an attentional component (Lencz et al., 2003). Therefore, it is likely that abnormalities in early formation of internal representations interact with subsequent deficits in ongoing maintenance of this information once the physical stimulus is absent. However, maintenance abnormalities could be taking place due to separate or joint malfunctions in two very different mechanisms: (1) deficiencies in cognitive and neural systems responsible for maintaining information, resulting in more rapid information decay regardless of external influences; and/or (2) deficiencies in neural systems responsible for protection of internal WM stores from external/internal sources of interference. Importantly, the abnormalities in these separate aspects of WM function may implicate distinct neurobiological mechanisms contributing to maintenance deficits in schizophrenia; namely, dorsal and ventrolateral prefrontal executive regions shielding information from distraction (Thompson-Schill et al., 2002) or superior frontoparietal regions that seem to be involved in representing information over extended periods of time (Curtis et al., 2004). We briefly review behavioral evidence for these possibilities.

Working memory maintenance: interference control or decay deficits in schizophrenia?

To elucidate the source of WM maintenance deficits in schizophrenia, several researchers sought to establish which mechanisms may be contributing to maintenance abnormalities. In their classic studies, Oltmanns and Neale demonstrated that patients with schizophrenia perform more poorly on digit span tests containing distraction when compared to healthy controls (Oltmanns & Neale, 1975). More specifically, they used four different tasks of varying digit span lengths, two of which contained distraction. This yielded two sets of tasks (distractor and no distractor) that were equated on difficulty. Oltmanns and Neale demonstrated that patients show a more precipitous drop in performance as a function of distraction when using the longer digit length task. Critically, Otlmanns and Neale carefully equated the digit span tasks for psychometric properties (i.e., task difficulty, distribution parameters, and reliability), which allowed detection of differential and not generalized deficits (Chapman & Chapman, 1978). Oltmanns and Neale's overall findings suggest that patients with schizophrenia may exhibit interference control deficits. A series of studies replicated this general pattern of results (Addington et al., 1997; Finkelstein et al., 1997; Harvey & Pedley, 1989; Oltmanns et al., 1978). Furthermore, a recent elegant behavioral study by Hahn and colleagues demonstrated WM filtering deficits, although when focusing on the encoding period. They manipulated spatial WM encoding by rendering specific encoding items more salient (by surrounding them with a flicker). Their results demonstrated that patients and controls benefit from bottom-up effects on attention during WM encoding. However, when the bottom-up manipulation was distracting (by flickering around items not required to be encoded), patients were unable to override prepotent bottom-up visual distraction during WM encoding and bias their attention away from such distraction. In fact, individuals with schizophrenia encoded items that co-occurred with salient distractors more robustly, whereas such distraction was successfully filtered by control participants (Hahn et al., 2010).

Other recent behavioral experiments conducted by Cellard and colleagues demonstrated that effects of interference in schizophrenia extend to the maintenance phase in the visuospatial domain (Cellard et al., 2007). They employed a spatial WM task that required subjects to reconstruct a sequence of dots presented at random locations. Interference trials contained a centrally presented dot that subjects were instructed to ignore. The results indicated that patients performed worse than controls on both the interference-free and distractor versions of the tasks; however, the effect of distraction on patients' performance was significantly greater than that for healthy controls. In addition, Leiderman and colleagues employed a WM task that included a single (object or spatial WM alone) or dual task component (object and spatial combined, which the authors suggested taps into the central executive component of the WM process) (Leiderman & Strejilevich, 2004). They also used two delay periods (5 sec and 30 sec) and introduced a distractor task (counting) during all conditions. Leiderman and colleagues demonstrated that patients performed worse in the dual task condition (spatial-object task) when compared to single task conditions (object or spatial). In contrast, control subjects did not show the additional performance drop as a function of dual task demands as did schizophrenia patients. This suggests that the added task demands introduced during the maintenance period (as a function of the dual task) impacted schizophrenia patients' performance more than that of healthy controls. Patients' performance degraded even further on the dual task once a longer temporal delay was introduced (30 sec). Javitt and colleagues (Javitt et al., 1997) reported similar results in the context of echoic WM. We briefly reviewed earlier that their findings suggested similar group results across extended delays when matched for performance. However, their experiment also contained a condition with distraction, which was presented across all difficulty levels. These findings are in concert with those in the visuospatial domain–patients' performance across increasing delays degraded more extensively when faced with distraction even in the easier condition (patients' performance was virtually at floor during the more difficult condition; thus making it difficult to test distractor effects).

Taken together, these results argue that deficits exist not only in the maintenance mechanisms but also in the ability to resist external sources of interference, and that these abnormalities are present in both visuospatial and verbal domains. That is, there are certainly problems evident with the decay of WM information across increasing temporal delays (although such deficits may not have been assessed under optimal psychophysiological conditions; e.g., complete darkness and silence). However, there is also clear evidence for a major problem in interference control in schizophrenia. Most recently, we have extended this work to show that patients exhibit increased distractibility during object WM even when matched for performance in the absence of distraction on a single-subject level (Anticevic et al., 2011b). This work also points to specific neural abnormalities present in schizophrenia that are associated with distractor filtering, which we discuss more extensively in the next sections.

Neuroimaging findings during working memory in schizophrenia

In addition to the behavioral evidence of WM deficits, there is growing functional neuroimaging literature demonstrating the presence of brain abnormalities associated with WM dysfunction in schizophrenia. The majority of findings suggest that regions comprising the dorsal frontoparietal network are affected in patients and may be contributing to WM abnormalities (Manoach, 2003). Specifically, reductions in the dorsolateral prefrontal cortex (DLPFC) (Brodmann's area 9/46) activations have been documented while patients perform WM tasks, suggesting that patients exhibit task-related "hypo-frontality" (Barch et al., 2001; Callicott et al., 1998). These findings have also been confirmed through quantitative meta-analytic studies (Glahn et al., 2005; van Snellenberg et al., 2006), both of which point to the DLPFC as playing a key role in WM deficits present in schizophrenia.

Prefrontal recruitment during working memory: the inverted-U hypothesis

The emerging evidence has generated a controversy regarding the precise pattern of cortical blood oxygenation level-dependent (BOLD) signal abnormalities associated with WM dysfunction in patients with schizophrenia (Manoach, 2003). Specifically, there are discrepant findings with regard to over- or under-recruitment of dorsal prefrontal regions during WM (Callicot et al., 2003). A number of findings have suggested that WM capacity in healthy subjects may be dependent on the level of recruitment of the DLPFC, which is thought to operate according to an inverted-"U" model of WM capacity (Driesen et al., 2008; Goldman-Rakic et al., 2000; Johnson et al., 2006; Potkin et al., 2009). In other words, the model suggests that with increasing WM demands, there is a concomitant parametric DLPFC BOLD signal increase (Braver et al., 1997). However, as WM load demands reach and exceed capacity limitations, DLPFC signals begin to drop, presumably due to information load exceeding available computational resources (Braver et al., 1997; Goldman-Rakic et al., 2000). In line with this hypothesis, recent evidence suggests that patients with schizophrenia may exhibit a shifted inverted-U function, such that capacity limitations are reached faster (i.e., with lower WM load levels), which may result in over- or under-recruitment when compared to healthy controls, depending on the level of WM load at which the groups are compared (Johnson et al., 2006). For instance, the hypothesis states that at low difficulty levels patients may find performance more effortful and may have to recruit more prefrontal computational resources to accomplish the task. Evidence for this framework was advanced by studies demonstrating that patients activated the DLPFC more when performing above chance (but slightly worse than controls) (Callicott et al., 2000; Monoach, 2003; Monoach et al., 1999, 2000, 2003). Comparing the two groups at such a difficulty level has resulted in findings of DLPFC "hyper-frontality" in the patient group when compared to controls. Conversely, as the difficulty of the task exceeds capacity limits in the patient group (which happens at lower task difficulty when compared to controls), the observed DLPFC signals may show a drop if patients cannot sustain task engagement (Monoach, 2003; Monoach et al., 1999, 2000, 2003). This may result in findings of DLPFC "hypo-frontality" in patients with schizophrenia at higher WM difficulty levels when compared to controls. In contrast, when WM performance is matched across patients and controls, such that both patients and controls perform the task at similar levels of accuracy, both groups can demonstrate relatively similar levels of prefrontal recruitment (Monoach et al., 2000; Callicott et al., 2000; Honey et al., 2002) (however, see Anticevic et al., 2011a). Taken together, this evidence suggests that some studies investigating DLPFC abnormalities associated with WM function may not have adequately matched the groups on performance, which may in turn result in either findings of hypo- or hyper-frontality, depending on specific task parameters employed (i.e., overall difficulty level). Indeed, in line with this hypothesis, a meta-analysis by Van Snellenberg and colleagues demonstrated that the magnitude of WM performance differences between patients and healthy controls was positively correlated with magnitude of activation differences in dorsolateral prefrontal regions (van Snellenberg et al., 2006). In other words, Van Snellenberg and colleagues showed that studies with the largest difference in WM performance between patients and controls (such that patients performed worse) are the ones documenting the largest evidence for DLPFC hypo-frontality in patients – between-group differences in WM performance significantly moderated between-group DLPFC findings. This finding implies that different studies may be examining different locations of the inverted-U curve, thus showing evidence of hyper- or hypo-frontality in patients with schizophrenia, depending on task parameters. To this end, it is crucial to ensure careful performance matching for valid interpretation of brain activation differences between patients and controls.

In summary, even though the controversy surrounding the precise pattern of lateral prefrontal signals during WM may not be fully resolved (and the proposed inverted-U model may be an oversimplification of the underlying pathophysiology involved in WM), there is still considerable evidence from functional neuroimaging studies that patients show aberrant patterns of brain activity while performing WM tasks (Glahn et al., 2005; Ragland et al., 2007; Reichenberg & Harvey, 2007). Importantly, recent investigations are adding evidence in support of the shifted inverted-U model of DLPFC functioning in schizophrenia, suggesting that there may be inefficient prefrontal recruitment that is manifested differently depending on WM demands (Callicott et al., 2003; Glahn et al., 2005; Manaoch, 2003; Potkin et al., 2009). Even though most studies examining prefrontal cortex dysfunction in schizophrenia have typically studied patients on psychotropic medication, there is also evidence that medication-naïve patients exhibit abnormalities in prefrontal activation (Barch et al., 2001).

Neural evidence for abnormalities across phases of working memory in schizophrenia

Most studies reviewed in the previous sections have employed a variety of continuous performance tasks (e.g., N-back) (Glahn et al., 2005), which blend different WM processes. However, as noted, WM is not composed of a single operation (Jonides et al., 2008) and both cognitive (Baddeley, 2000) and neurobiological (Goldman-Rakic, 1994) models have identified different WM processes: (1) encoding of novel information; (2) maintenance, manipulation, and updating; and (3) retrieval of information. Thus to fully understand WM dysfunction in schizophrenia, it is critical to employ tasks that assay distinct WM processes because dysfunction of each process may contribute unique sources of deficit in this illness (Neufeld, 2007). As described earlier, behavioral studies have reported both encoding and maintenance abnormalities in schizophrenia (Lee & Park, 2005). Therefore, it is critical to parse the temporal aspects of brain activation in schizophrenia more carefully by using WM tasks that temporally dissociate encoding, maintenance, and response periods, which we will refer to as "delayed" WM tasks (Driesen et al., 2008). The use of delayed WM tasks allows examination of different components of WM to determine whether schizophrenia is associated with abnormal WM signal patterns during the encoding, maintenance, or response phase (or any combination of these three possibilities). It should be noted here that the limited temporal resolution of functional magnetic resonance imaging (fMRI) may, to a certain extent, prevent one from drawing clear lines between encoding and "early maintenance." This can be a very important distinction from a neurobiological perspective as distinct mechanisms have been implicated in encoding versus early maintenance of WM (Durstewitz & Seamans, 2002, 2008; Durstewitz et al., 1999, 2000). Nevertheless, fMRI work has offered some clues regarding phase-specific WM deficits in schizophrenia.

To address such questions, Driesen and colleagues (2008) used a delayed spatial WM task, which was an adaptation of tasks typically employed in neurophysiological studies of nonhuman primates and has been used as a reliable probe of prefrontal maintenance signals in healthy controls (Leung et al., 2002). Importantly, this task included a long delay interval (16 s) that allowed the separate investigation of encoding and maintenance activity. Driesen and co-workers specifically focused on three right-lateralized prefrontal regions of interest (ROI) previously implicated in WM processes (i.e., superior middle frontal gyrus, middle frontal gyrus, and inferior frontal gyrus) (Leung et al., 2002). Overall, Driesen et al. demonstrated that, even in the absence of between-group accuracy differences, patients showed little decay in prefrontal signal levels at encoding, but demonstrated marked BOLD signal loss in frontal regions during maintenance. In addition, at probe onset, patients did not show the same level of BOLD signal recovery as did controls. These results suggested that patients demonstrated abnormalities in sustained prefrontal signal during the maintenance phase of WM (although in specific isolated prefrontal ROIs), which is consistent with behavioral studies documenting increased WM decay in the absence of interference, as well as possible concomitant deficits in retrieval-related processes.

Another study examining delayed WM in the verbal domain was conducted by Johnston et al. (2006). They examined between-group differences during WM encoding and retrieval (they omitted maintenance from the analysis as they argue that signals during maintenance and encoding are highly collinear, possibly due to the resolution of the fMRI signal). Furthermore, they examined differences as a function of a WM load, such that performance was comparable between groups at different load levels. When focusing on the encoding phase, they identified a distributed network of regions including both frontal and parietal components that patients failed to recruit to the same level as controls, even when comparing conditions that resulted in similar performance levels. Interestingly, they found that patients also failed to recruit certain regions to the same extent as controls did during the retrieval phase – but this was only true when examining performance matched conditions. That is, when comparing patients and controls at the same lower load condition, patients over-recruited a wide network of regions encompassing frontal, parietal, and hippocampus clusters. This complex pattern of group differences across WM phases, modulated by load/difficulty, only highlights the importance of considering all phases of WM when making inferences regarding deficits in schizophrenia.

It should be noted, however, that Johnson and colleagues could not offer additional evidence regarding maintenance deficits in the verbal domain. Nevertheless, somewhat in contrast to results reported by Driesen et al., work in the verbal domain did not find the most prominent group activation differences during WM maintenance (Schlösser et al., 2008); Schlösser and colleagues found more prominent group differences when examining conditions requiring manipulation of verbal information (i.e., alphabetizing the remembered letters). This reflected mainly over-recruitment of executive regions in the patient group relative to healthy subjects. One possibility is that this activation difference reflected task demands; that is, Schlösser and co-workers employed a task that was substantially more challenging for patients and, as noted, performance has been shown to be a critical moderating variable of group activation differences (Van Snellenberg et al., 2006). Another possibility may be that there are critical neural activation differences between maintenance of *verbal* versus *spatial* WM representations in schizophrenia – a hypothesis that awaits direct and systematic prospective testing.

Our subsequent work has replicated and extended the aforementioned findings using a comparable nonverbal delayed WM task that employed ambiguous polygon shapes as memoranda. We showed that, when examining a broader network of regions involved in WM, patients indeed exhibited encoding abnormalities, but there was clear evidence for maintenance deficits as well, primarily centered on the prefrontal cortex. Importantly, we ensured careful performance matching to rule out performance-related confounds related to differences in DLPFC signals (Van Snellenberg et al., 2006). Our findings suggest that the profile of WM deficits across phases of WM is in line with behavioral findings; that is, patients exhibit *both* encoding and maintenance activation abnormalities even when matched for performance.

Interestingly, our results also revealed abnormalities in regional deactivation in areas mainly overlapping with what is termed the default mode network (DMN), a finding consistent with other studies on DMN activity during WM in schizophrenia (Metzak et al., 2011; Whitfield-Gabrieli et al., 2009). Specifically, control participants showed suppression during the encoding phase on WM trials in a superior frontal cortical region as well as around the right angular gyrus cortex, whereas patients failed to exhibit this deactivation. Furthermore, for healthy controls there was a significant inverse linear relationship between prefrontal activation and regional suppression at encoding; however, patients showed a breakdown in this relationship, which was highly consistent with a prior report showing a similar effect (Metzak et al., 2011). Taken together, these findings suggest that there may be a malfunction in reciprocal communication between brain networks involved in active task engagement and passive mental states – a function attributed to the DMN (Andrews-Hanna et al., 2010). That is, DMN activation is typically associated with self-referential and spontaneous cognition, in contrast to regions associated with active engagement in effortful mental tasks such as the frontoparietal networks (Dosenbach et al., 2008). It is now widely accepted, based on evidence from both task-based and connectivity findings, that in healthy adults there exists an inverse/anti-correlated relationship between these distributed neural systems purportedly supporting these broad, but different aspects of cognition (Fox et al., 2005; Shulman et al., 1997). In fact, our previous work in healthy adults has clearly demonstrated that the degree of DMN suppression is directly related to accurate WM performance (Anticevic et al., 2010). Thus, only focusing on deficits in task-based activation, while important, may not provide the complete picture of neural deficits that may compromise WM function in schizophrenia. Related to this point, in the preceding sections on behavioral deficits we have discussed that filtering and interference resolution is a critical component of WM function and that there is clear evidence for breakdowns in WM filtering during the WM maintenance phase. In that sense, one can conceptualize the lack of suppression in patients as possibly contributing additional sources of unwanted signals during WM. In other words, if there is a breakdown of such distributed regional suppression during WM in patients, superfluous activation of regions involved in passive mentation may contribute an additional source of noise during WM and render the ongoing task representations more susceptible to interference.

While this framework argues that lack of task-based suppression may be interpreted in part as contributing additional noise to WM, understanding neural deficits in suppressing external interference during WM is equally critical. Despite strong behavioral evidence, there have been very few attempts to date to understand the neural basis of putative filtering deficits during WM in schizophrenia, either during encoding or maintenance. To that end, in a parallel investigation, we examined the neural correlates of deficits associated with WM interference (Anticevic et al., 2011b). Using the same delayed WM task framework described earlier, we presented various types of distraction during the maintenance period of WM. We found that patients fail to recruit a right lateralized DLPFC region previously implicated in distractor resistance (Postle, 2005), a region that control participants clearly activated in response to distraction (Figure 12.A). Moreover, the degree of DLPFC recruitment in our study predicted correct WM performance for control participants such that higher BOLD signals correlated with better WM performance, specifically during distraction (Figure 12.B). In contrast, patients not only failed to activate this region but also did not show a relationship between regional BOLD signals and performance, suggesting a breakdown in the ability to filter distraction.

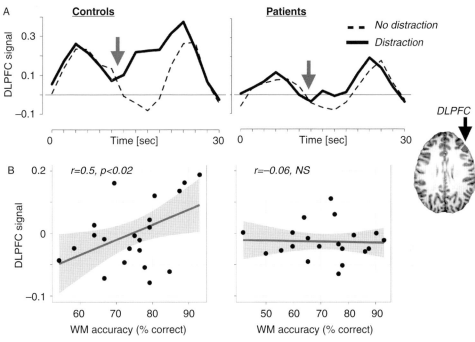

Figure 12.1. Prefrontal filtering deficits in schizophrenia. A. Our recent fMRI findings showed that schizophrenia patients fail to recruit a region of the right dorsolateral prefrontal cortex (DLPFC) specifically in response to distraction during delayed working memory (WM) (gray arrows mark distractor onset) (Anticevic et al., 2011b). B. The degree of DLPFC recruitment correlated significantly with WM accuracy for controls, specifically during the distractor condition, illustrating the functional relevance of the DLPFC response. No such relationship was observed for patients, supporting the hypothesis of a failure in distractor filtering. This is one example of the advances that can be made with our state-of-the-art fMRI tools, illustrating specific neural correlates of cognitive deficits in schizophrenia and their link to behavior. However, this approach alone is limited in elucidating deficits at the cellular level – critical for targeted treatment development (see Figure 12.2).

Taken together, our recent findings suggest that, while it is critical to examine abnormalities in WM signals across regions showing activation in response to cognitive probes, it is also important to consider deactivation abnormalities present during WM, as well as breakdowns in protection of WM stores (i.e., filtering deficits). In fact, at present it is unclear to what extent neural abnormalities in resisting external interference independently contribute to breakdown in WM functioning in schizophrenia, be it from lack of suppression of task-irrelevant internal signal or excessive external interference. Such deficits may also arise from proactive interference suppression (Sakai et al., 2002) (i.e., failure of preparatory filtering signals in the face of upcoming distraction) or from resolving interference once distraction actually occurred (reactive interference resolution). It will be important for future work to adjudicate to what extent there are neural deficits in these possibly separate mechanisms of distractor resistance in schizophrenia (Fletcher, 2011).

Summary of working memory findings in schizophrenia

In summary, both behavioral and functional neuroimaging evidence points to WM abnormalities in schizophrenia, which extend across both encoding and the maintenance phases.

These deficits are also associated with abnormalities in brain signals, which may involve distributed cortical frontoparietal, striatal, and thalamic interactions. Such deficits may involve not only abnormalities in sustaining activation across a delay, but also breakdowns in interference resolution from incoming distraction. While the reviewed cognitive neuroscience literature has undoubtedly advanced our understanding of WM pathology in schizophrenia and constrained our search for neural markers of such deficits, we have yet to form a mechanistic understanding of WM dysfunction. Only such an understanding, grounded in cellular mechanisms, offers the possibility for targeted treatment of cognitive abnormalities in schizophrenia. In the following sections, we discuss a translational cognitive neuroscience framework within the context of WM, which offers the promise of linking our levels of understanding from cells to circuits to symptoms. Prior to proceeding to our discussion of translational cognitive neuroscience of WM, it is critical to revisit our initial arguments concerning broader aspects of cognitive deficits in schizophrenia. In that sense, WM is one cognitive probe showing deficits in schizophrenia, which offers promising translational potential, but breakdowns in circuits that may confer WM deficits may also result in abnormal functioning in other cognitive domains; namely, CC and EM. Therefore, we offer a brief treatment of these additional domains of dysfunction.

Episodic memory in schizophrenia
Cognitive neuroscience models of episodic memory

As with trying to understand the nature of WM deficits in schizophrenia, it is useful to review briefly the cognitive neuroscience literature on the processing and brain regions involved in EM as a means of organizing the research pertaining to EM deficits in schizophrenia. A key place to start is work on the specific role that the hippocampal formation plays in EM. For many years we have known that the hippocampus plays a critical role in the formation of long-term memories, based in part on studies with amnesic patients such as H.M., who have had lesions to the hippocampus and/or surrounding medial temporal areas (Scoville & Milner, 1957). Following such lesions, these patients exhibit profound deficits in the ability to learn and/or retrieve new episodic memories, despite relatively intact cognitive functioning in other domains (Corkin, 1984; Scoville & Milner, 1957; Squire, 1987). Nonhuman primate models also demonstrate that lesions within the hippocampus and adjacent medial temporal cortex lead to impairments in the ability to retrieve newly learned information successfully (Murray, 1996). Furthermore, these animal studies have highlighted the importance between the function of the hippocampus proper and surrounding medial temporal cortex, as the severity and nature of EM deficits in nonhuman primates varies as a function of the amount of medial temporal cortex involvement.

A common theme running through theories regarding the role of the hippocampal formation in EM is the idea that it is critical for the rapid binding of novel configurations of information (Cohen & Eichenbaum, 2001; Konkel & Cohen, 2009; McClelland et al., 1995; Shimamura, 2010; Squire & Knowlton, 1995). Consistent with this hypothesis, a number of human neuroimaging studies have shown activation of the hippocampus during the encoding or retrieval of novel relational information (Davachi, 2006; Giovanello et al., 2004; Heckers et al., 2004; Sperling et al., 2001; Wendelken & Bunge, 2010), and work in amnestic patients emphasizes the importance of hippocampal structures in relational processing (Bowles et al., 2010; Ryan & Cohen, 2004). Moreover, a number of functional neuroimaging studies in healthy humans have demonstrated that enhanced hippocampal/parahippocampal activity at the time of encoding predicts subsequent successful retrieval of that information (Brewer et al., 1998a,b; Kirchoff et al., 2000; Otten et al., 2001; Wagner et al., 1998). In addition, work with depth electrodes implanted in humans undergoing epilepsy surgery has also demonstrated that hippocampal activity at the time of encoding predicted subsequent memory for verbal stimuli (Cameron et al., 2001). Although more recent models of EM suggest differential roles for hippocampal versus perirhinal regions of the medial temporal lobes in encoding of item versus relational memory (Davachi, 2006), there is still a strong consensus on the importance of the hippocampus for relational encoding of a range of information types.

At the same time that we are gaining a better understanding of the specific EM functions subserved by the hippocampus, we have garnered information about the fact that prefrontal structures also make important contributions to EM. Damage to the prefrontal cortex can lead to EM deficits, although EM is not the only cognitive function impaired in these individuals (Janowsky et al., 1989). Such findings have contributed to the hypothesis that prefrontal cortex damage alters EM by impairing strategic contributions to memory formation and retrieval (Janowsky et al., 1989). For example, studies have shown activation of ventral prefrontal regions, such as Brodmann's areas 45 and 47, when participants are asked to process verbal information using semantic elaboration strategies (Wagner et al., 1998) that promote subsequent memory. In addition, a compelling finding supporting a critical role for such prefrontal structures in EM is results showing that the increased activation during encoding in frontal regions such as BA 45 and 47 is highly predictive of subsequent memory performance (Alkire et al., 1998; Baker et al., 2001; Brewer et al., 1998a,b; Kirchoff et al., 2000; Otten et al., 2001; Wagner et al., 1998). For a recent meta-analysis, see Spaniol et al. (2009). Furthermore, there is recent work suggesting that the DLPFC may contribute specifically to successful relational memory formation and retrieval (Blumenfeld et al., 2011; Murray & Ranganath, 2007).

Episodic memory impairments in schizophrenia

As described in the previous section, most theories of hippocampal function posit that it plays a key role in binding together novel configurations of information. One way to examine whether individuals with schizophrenia have binding deficits is to determine if they are more impaired on memory for associative information (e.g., the association of previously unrelated words or items) as compared to memory for individual items. To address this question, Achim and Lepage conducted a meta-analysis comparing performance on associative and item memory tests in individuals with schizophrenia, and concluded that there was evidence for a 20% greater impairment in associative as compared to item memory in individuals with schizophrenia (Achim & Lepage, 2003). However, a number of the associative memory studies included in this meta-analysis were tests of source memory rather than associations of novel pairs of items, and the human neuropsychological and imaging literature suggests that prefrontal function may make important contributions to source memory (Mitchell & Johnson, 2009). In addition, few of the studies that have compared item and associative memory have dealt with the ubiquitous problems of discriminating power. Associative memory tests are often more difficult than item memory tests. Greater task difficulty by itself does not necessarily indicate higher discriminating power, but it does raise the question regarding whether a pattern of greater impairment on associative versus item memory is truly indicative of a selective deficit in binding of novel information. More recently, clinical researchers have begun to use tasks derived from the animal literature on hippocampal function, such as the Transitive Inference Test, which measures the ability to learn the relationships among hierarchically arranged stimulus pairs, as well as the Transitive Patterning Test in which individuals have to learn about the relationship between items for correct selection. Individuals with schizophrenia are impaired on critical conditions of this task requiring relational processing, but not on conditions that require simpler associative reinforcement mappings (Coleman et al., 2010; Titone et al., 2004) or other control conditions (Hanlon et al., 2005, 2011). Other work has used eye-movement measures of relational memory, shown to be impaired in patients with hippocampal lesions (Hannula & Ranganath, 2008, 2009), to identify relational memory impairments in schizophrenia (Hannula et al., 2010; Williams et al., 2010). There is also work indicating impairments in both item and relational retrieval for information that was relationally encoded in schizophrenia (Ragland et al., 2012). Still other work has provided evidence for greater deficits in recollection than familiarity in schizophrenia, which have also been interpreted as reflecting relational memory impairments (Danion et al., 2005; van Erp et al., 2008).

Many researchers have taken this body of work to suggest that EM impairments in schizophrenia reflect medial temporal lobe deficits, with a specific focus on the hippocampus (Heckers & Konradi, 2010). However, the findings in healthy individuals about the role of the prefrontal cortex in EM raise the possibility that at least some EM impairments among individuals with schizophrenia also reflect deficits in prefrontally mediated cognitive functions that contribute to successful memory encoding and retrieval, including strategic mechanisms that may facilitate memory formation. Consistent with this hypothesis, a number of studies suggest that individuals with schizophrenia are impaired in their ability to generate effective mnemonic strategies (for review, see Barch, 2005a). However, when provided with strategies that promote successful episodic encoding, individuals with schizophrenia are typically able to benefit as much as controls from these strategies (Bonner-Jackson & Barch, 2011; Bonner-Jackson et al., 2008; Heckers et al., 1998; Koh & Peterson, 1978; Ragland et al., 2003, 2005; Weiss et al., 2003), and can even show intact item recognition when provided with support for effective encoding (Mathews & Barch, 2004). Furthermore, a meta-analysis of brain activity alterations during EM performance in schizophrenia showed consistent evidence for reduced activation in both the ventrolateral prefrontal cortex and the DLPFC, but did not find consistent evidence for altered hippocampal activity (Ragland et al., 2009). Recent work on relational memory encoding and retrieval has shown evidence for impaired DLPFC function associated with impaired relational memory function in schizophrenia (Ragland et al., 2011), although other recent work has also implicated hippocampal function (Hanlon et al., 2005, 2011; Luck et al., 2010; Ongur et al., 2006). These findings do suggest a need to take into account a role for prefrontally mediated cognitive functions as well as hippocampal-mediated functions in understanding the source and nature of EM deficits in schizophrenia. Furthermore, the findings on strategic changes in schizophrenia and the role of the DLPFC in EM suggest that examining the role of executive control deficits and effective encoding manipulations may be a fruitful avenue for future research on enhancing EM in schizophrenia.

Executive control in schizophrenia

The previously discussed reviews of WM and EM function in schizophrenia posit a potentially central role for impairments in prefrontal cortex function, although it is clear that prefrontal deficits cannot account for all WM and EM impairments in schizophrenia. In adddition, numerous other studies suggest impairments on a range of tasks designed to measure various aspects of executive function in schizophrenia, a cognitive domain also thought to rely heavily on prefrontal functions. However, despite this wealth of empirical evidence on the existence of executive function deficits in schizophrenia, there is relatively little agreement on the precise nature or causes of executive control impairments in schizophrenia. Again, the basic cognitive neuroscience literature provides several theories or hypotheses as to what the nature of executive control dysfunction in schizophrenia might be. We will briefly review several of these theories, including the hypotheses regarding the role of the DLPFC and dopamine-mediated context processing disturbances and/or pro-active control as well as the hypotheses regarding anterior cingulate/dopamine-mediated disturbances in conflict/error detection.

Context processing in schizophrenia

In previous work based in part upon computational modeling, Cohen and colleagues put forth the hypothesis that the intact function of dopamine in the DLPFC was responsible for the processing of context, and that a disturbance in this mechanism was responsible for a range of cognitive deficits in schizophrenia (Barch et al., 2001; Braver et al., 1999; Braver & Cohen, 1999; Cohen & Servan-Schreiber, 1992; Cohen et al., 1999). Context refers to prior task-relevant information that is represented in such a form that it can bias selection of the appropriate behavioral response. Because context representations are maintained online, in an active state, they are continually accessible and available to influence processing. Consequently, context can be viewed as the subset of representations within WM that govern how other representations are used. One important insight that has emerged from this work is a single deficit in one aspect of executive control can contribute to deficits in cognitive domains often treated as independent. As such, this theory argues that deficits in WM, attention, and inhibition in schizophrenia can all be understood in terms of a deficit in context processing (Barch et al., 2001; Braver et al., 1999; Braver & Cohen, 1999; Cohen & Servan-Schreiber, 1992; Cohen et al., 1999). When a task involves competing, task-irrelevant processes (as in the Stroop task), context representations serve to inhibit such task-irrelevant processes by providing top-down support for task-relevant processes. When a task involves a delay between a cue and a later contingent response, the mechanism employed to represent context information can be used to maintain task-relevant information against the interfering and cumulative effects of noise over time. Additionally, in both inhibition and WM conditions, context representations serve an attentional function, by selecting task-relevant information for processing over other potentially competing sources of information. Thus, the context hypothesis can explain why patients with schizophrenia demonstrate deficits on at least some tasks thought to tap WM, as well as deficits on other executive control tasks that may not involve a high WM load (e.g., Stroop) (Barch et al., 1999). Furthermore, the context-processing hypothesis explains why patients show deficits on tasks in which context information needs to be determined and maintained, even if this context information constitutes a low WM load (Barch et al., 2003; Cohen et al., 1999). Numerous prior studies have provided support for these hypotheses concerning context-processing deficits in schizophrenia (for a review, see Barch & Braver, 2007), as well as evidence for impairments in individuals at risk for schizophrenia (MacDonald et al., 2005, 2006; Snitz et al., 2006), suggesting that such deficits may be associated with liability to schizophrenia as well as manifest illness.

Proactive and reactive control in schizophrenia

In more recent years, the key role of context processing in cognition and in schizophrenia has been re-conceptualized somewhat more broadly as the function of proactive CC (Barch & Braver, 2007; Braver et al., 2009; Edwards et al., 2010; Haddon & Killcross, 2007). This conceptualization builds upon earlier ideas of context processing to argue for flexible mechanisms of CC that allow humans to deal with the diversity of challenges that we face in everyday life. In this theory, termed dual mechanisms of control (Braver et al., 2007, 2009; Edwards et al., 2010), a distinction is made between proactive and reactive modes of CC. The proactive control model can be thought of as a form of "early selection," in which goal-relevant information is actively maintained in a sustained or anticipatory manner, before the occurrence of cognitively demanding events. This allows for optimal biasing of attention, perception, and action systems in a goal-driven manner. In this context, goals refer to the information one needs to accomplish in a particular task situation or the intended outcome of a series of actions or mental operations. In real life, such goal information may include the main points one wishes to communicate in a conversation, or the need to organize a shopping trip so that one can make sure to get everything that is needed. In contrast, in the reactive mode, attentional control is recruited as a "late correction" mechanism that is mobilized only when needed, such as after a high-interference event is detected (e.g., an unexpected distracting stimulus is encountered and there is a need to retrieve the topic of conversation). Thus, proactive control relies on the anticipation and prevention of interference before it occurs, whereas reactive control relies on the detection and resolution of interference after its onset.

This theory postulates that proactive control depends on actively representing information in the lateral prefrontal cortex, and that the updating and maintenance of such information depends on precise inputs from neurotransmitter systems such as dopamine into the prefrontal cortex. However, as discussed in more detail later, it is clear that other neurotransmitter mechanisms are critical for active maintenance of information in the prefrontal cortex, and that deficits in NMDA receptor function may underlie impaired delay-related activity during WM in schizophrenia. As outlined in detail in Braver (in press), proactive and reactive control functions are not mutually exclusive, and some balance between the two modes is necessary to meet most ongoing cognitive demands successfully. However, Braver (in press) has argued that the two control modes can be distinguished based on their temporal characteristics (e.g., *when* they are engaged in the course of cognitive processing) and the requirement to actively maintain control representations over time for proactive control. In addition, Braver has suggested that there may be biases to favor one processing mode over the other, which may be dependent on task demands (e.g., high conflict situations may push toward a proactive control mode) and individual differences like WM capacity, fluid intelligence, and even personality traits such as reward sensitivity. Proactive control may also be particularly vulnerable to disruption, given that it is resource demanding and dependent upon temporally precise active maintenance mechanisms. Thus, populations characterized by disordered prefrontal function (such as schizophrenia) may rely more heavily on reactive control, as it may be more robust in the face of such dysfunction (Edwards et al., 2010). Consistent with this hypothesis, there is ample evidence for an association between impairments in DLPFC activity and deficits of proactive control in schizophrenia (Barbalat et al., 2009; Minzenberg et al., 2009), for both medicated (Holmes et al., 2005) and unmedicated patients (Barch et al., 2001; MacDonald et al., 2005) as well as those at risk for the development of schizophrenia (Fusar-Poli et al., 2007; MacDonald et al., 2009). For example, a recent comprehensive meta-analysis of imaging studies of executive control and proactive control conducted by Minzenberg and colleagues (Minzenberg et al., 2009) provided clear evidence for reduced activity in the DLPFC in schizophrenia.

Conflict detection/error monitoring

The reviews of WM and EM discussed earlier, and the description of context processing and proactive control in schizophrenia, placed a heavy emphasis on the function of the prefrontal cortex, especially the dorsolateral regions. However, it is very clear that regions other than the DLPFC play a role in executive control, and that mechanisms other than just active maintenance or proactive control influence executive function. Thus, an alternative (or perhaps complementary) hypothesis about the specific nature of executive control deficits in schizophrenia suggests that disturbances in the ability to detect conflict or errors in ongoing processing emerge at least in part due to dysfunction of the anterior cingulate cortex (ACC). Such ACC abnormalities may lead to deficits in the ability to regulate and control a range of other components of executive control in schizophrenia. This hypothesis builds on models of ACC function that postulate a critical role for this brain region in either detecting conflict or errors and signaling the prefrontal regions to enhance CC (Botvinik et al., 2001), predicting conditions likely to elicit errors (Alexander & Brown, 2011; Brown & Braver, 2005), or detecting mismatches between "correct" or intended output (Holroyd & Coles, 2002).

At the behavioral level, there is very mixed evidence in schizophrenia regarding impairments on indices thought to reflect the ability to detect or respond to conflict or errors. For example, some studies have found that individuals with schizophrenia detect and/or correct errors as frequently as do healthy controls (Kopp & Rist, 1994), while other studies have found reduced rates of error correction among individuals with schizophrenia (Turken et al., 2003). In addition, some studies have found that individuals with schizophrenia show an intact "Rabbit" effect, which is the slowing of responses on trials following errors (Laurens et al., 2003; Mathalon et al., 2002; Morris et al., 2006; Polli et al., 2006, 2008), while other studies have found that this effect is reduced in patients with schizophrenia (Alain et al., 2002; Becerril et al., 2011; Carter et al., 2001; Enticott et al., 2011; Kerns et al., 2005; Kopp & Rist, 1999). In contrast, evoked response potential (ERP), fMRI, and positron emission tomography (PET) studies have provided more consistent evidence for altered conflict/error processing. For example, a number of studies have shown reduced error-related negativity (ERN) amplitudes or ACC activity in patients with schizophrenia on error trials (Alain et al., 2002; Bates et al., 2002, 2004; Becerril et al., 2011; Carter et al., 2001; Kerns et al., 2005; Kopp & Rist, 1994, 1999; Laurens et al., 2003; Mathalon et al., 2002, 2009; Perez et al., 2011; Polli et al., 2008), even when these same individuals show intact behavioral indices or error detection (Kopp & Rist, 1994, 1999; Laurens et al., 2003). Furthermore, there is also some evidence of reduced ACC responses to error likelihood prediction in schizophrenia (Krawitz et al., 2011). Interestingly however, there is some evidence that individuals with schizophrenia may show intact feedback-related negativity (FRN) responses to explicit external feedback, even in the context of impaired ERN responses (Horan et al., 2011). This may reflect a difference between externally provided information about accuracy (indexed by the FRN) versus internal representations of accuracy that must be generated by the individuals (and potentially better indexed by the ERN).

At the same time that there is consistent evidence for reduced ACC activity in responses to errors in schizophrenia, it is interesting to note that many imaging studies of WM and executive control in schizophrenia have shown robust activation of the ACC among individuals with schizophrenia (Barch, 2005b), with even some evidence for increased ACC activity (Minzenberg et al., 2009). Any of the theories of ACC function described would predict that ACC activity should be increased in individuals with schizophrenia if they were actually experiencing greater conflict or errors, which is the typical behavioral result for WM and executive control studies in schizophrenia. Such findings raise interesting questions about the relationship between deficits in ACC and DLPFC function in schizophrenia, in that theories about primary deficits in either area would also predict deficits in the function of the other region as a consequence. If ACC activity is important for the recruitment of control processes supported by the DLPFC, one would predict abnormal DLPFC activity in individuals with schizophrenia who have such ACC deficits. In contrast, impaired DLPFC function leading to increased conflict and errors would predict increased ACC function in individuals with schizophrenia according to the conflict monitoring theory (if they experience more conflict and errors that would elicit ACC activity), but might predict reduced ACC activity according to the error-detection theory (if reduced DLPFC activity reflects degraded representations of the predictive information needed to drive an error correcting dopamine signal that in turn elicits ACC activity). Of course, individuals with schizophrenia may experience deficits in both ACC and DLPFC activity that are of equal relevance to understanding cognition, and potentially reflect the common importance of dopaminergic inputs to both the DLPFC and ACC. Clearly more research is needed that focuses on the relationship between conflict/error detection and the engagement of control processing in individuals with schizophrenia, in order to help provide a better understanding of the dynamic processes that give rise to WM and executive control deficits in schizophrenia.

The preceding sections summarize our evolving understanding of cognitive impairment in schizophrenia from the perspective of cognitive neuroscience. However, in order to ultimately treat cognitive deficits, we need to move toward understanding the mechanisms underlying observed deficits. To achieve this goal, we need a mechanistic framework. In the final section we will discuss a path forward, which involves combining several leading neuroscientific methodologies, which may allow us to understand cellular-level mechanisms of cognitive deficits in this illness.

Toward translational cognitive neuroscience of working memory

As reviewed earlier, cognitive neuroscience has established the tools to probe the underlying circuitry that may be affected in schizophrenia in relationship to disrupted cognition, such as WM, EM, and executive control. Such findings have provided guidance as to the neurobiological and psychological mechanisms that may be contributing to impairments in these cognitive domains. However, these approaches have had less success in addressing the underlying cellular mechanisms – which is where pharmacological therapies are ultimately applied. Therefore, understanding of cognitive dysfunction at this level is critical to move toward targeted and rationally designed treatment. A way to close this existing explanatory gap is to directly align two leading methodologies with our clinical case-control studies: namely pharmacological neuroimaging (ph-fMRI) (Honey & Bullmore, 2004) and computational modeling (Montague et al., 2012). Testing hypotheses regarding neural dysfunction in schizophrenia via pharmacological manipulations in healthy adults allows mechanistic perturbations of the underlying circuitry thought to be compromised in individuals suffering from the illness. In turn, such manipulations may reveal clues regarding specific links between disruptions in neurotransmitter systems, which can in turn be connected to system-level deficits and ultimately behavior. A powerful approach is to design such investigations to directly test predictions from computational models of neural function. Specifically, we propose that biophysically realistic computational modeling holds tremendous promise for accomplishing this goal and for generating predictions regarding development of future therapies. In the subsequent section we will argue for the critical utility of blending cognitive neuroscience with pharmacological manipulations that transiently and safely mimic the cardinal symptoms of the illness. We will focus specifically on WM as one candidate neurocognitive probe, motivated by recent development of biophysically realistic models of WM function (Brunel & Wang, 2001; Compte et al., 2000; Wang, 2001, 2010; Wang et al., 2004) and the arguments that spatial WM may be a powerful endophenotype for understanding cognitive deficits in schizophrenia (Glahn et al., 2003). We will conclude by articulating how this approach offers a potential experimental framework for understanding mechanisms that ultimately may lead to rational treatment development for cognitive deficits in schizophrenia.

Pharmacological models of psychosis: evolving use in human neuroimaging

As noted, schizophrenia is a highly heterogeneous illness and patients often present with diverse symptoms and differing illness trajectories. Furthermore, most patients in case-control studies are under long-term medication regimens. All of these variables obscure our ability to make inferences regarding specific neural mechanisms (Barch et al., 2001). An alternative approach, which circumvents these confounds, involves transiently and safely modeling the full spectrum of symptoms in healthy volunteers using pharmacological manipulations (Krystal et al., 1994). There are currently two leading pharmacological models of psychosis used to invoke cardinal symptoms of schizophrenia in healthy volunteers; namely, ketamine and delta-9-tetrahydrocannabinol (THC) (D'Souza et al., 2004; Krystal et al., 1994). Here we will focus specifically on the translational potential of ketamine as an example, given the evolving understanding of the NMDA glutamate receptor dysfunction in psychosis and their critical importance for WM functions (Krystal et al., 2002, 2003; Wang et al., 2008) (discussed later). Before proceeding to the translational potential of the ketamine model in the context of WM specifically, we briefly discuss: (1) evidence for behavioral effects of ketamine; (2) neurobiological effects of ketamine particularly in relation to the NMDA hypofunction hypothesis in schizophrenia. We specifically argue that linking such pharmacological models of cognitive dysfunction with neurocognitive probes of WM offers the promise for mechanistically testing hypotheses of cognitive disturbances in schizophrenia derived from formal computational models.

Behavioral effects of ketamine

Ketamine is a well-established pharmacological model of psychosis and its psychotomimetic effects have been replicated extensively both in human (Krystal et al., 2003) and animal studies (Moghaddam & Javitt, 2011). The seminal investigation conducted in healthy human volunteers by Krystal and colleagues (Krystal et al., 1994) provided evidence that transient administration of ketamine produced transient symptoms with striking resemblance to schizophrenia, including positive, negative, disorganized symptoms and cognitive deficits – effects that have been replicated across a number of studies (Krystal et al., 1998; Malhotra et al., 1997; Newcomer et al., 1999; Oye et al., 1992; Vollenweider et al., 1997). Ketamine effects on thought disorder symptoms mimic those found in patients (Adler et al., 1998) and ketamine exacerbates symptoms in patients diagnosed with the illness (Lahti et al., 1995b, 2001). Transient ketamine administration also produces disturbances in cognition, including effects on attention, WM, declarative memory, abstract reasoning, mental flexibility, insight, planning, and judgment (Krystal et al., 1994, 1998, 1999; Malhotra et al., 1997; Morgan & Curran, 2006; Newcomer et al., 1999)–all deficits present in patients diagnosed with schizophrenia (Reichenberg & Harvey, 2007). We do not extensively review the large literature examining ketamine effects on WM (for a more comprehensive review, see Morgan & Curran, 2006); however, it is important to note that ketamine administration induces reductions in WM performance in humans (Morgan & Curran, 2006) and other species (Neill et al., 2010). Taken together, this converging evidence suggests that the behavioral effect of ketamine resembles the schizophrenia syndrome and mimics cognitive disturbance in particular, providing a powerful platform to examine cognitive deficits in psychosis from a mechanistic perspective (i.e., the NMDA glutamate receptor hypofunction hypothesis, discussed in the next section).

Neurobiological effects of ketamine: NMDA hypofunction hypothesis

Optimal cortical function depends on the balanced interaction of pyramidal excitatory (glutamatergic) and inhibitory (GABAergic) neurons (Shadlen & Newsome, 1994). Disruptions of this balance can have drastic behavioral consequences (Marin, 2012; Yizhar et al., 2011) relevant to serious mental illness. Building on the rich behavioral evidence of ketamine's effects, there is a growing understanding of its underlying mechanisms of action from preclinical neuroscience studies that point to ketamine disrupting excitatory and inhibitory cortical balance. Interestingly, an emerging hypothesis of cellular-level disturbances in schizophrenia suggests a similar mechanism; namely, a deficit in the interaction between excitatory and inhibitory cortical neurons (Benes et al., 1991; Lewis & Moghaddam, 2006; Lewis et al., 2004, 2005, 2012; Marin, 2012). Specifically, this hypothesis is based on the disrupted mechanism of cortical inhibition; that is, a lack of inhibitory drive from GABA interneurons onto pyramidal neurons resulting in disinhibition of pyramidal cells (Lewis et al., 2012; Marin, 2012). One line of evidence for abnormalities in this mechanism comes from postmortem investigations of the DLPFC in patients with schizophrenia. These postmortem studies consistently show reduced levels of the mRNA for the 67-kilodalton isoform of glutamic acid decarboxylase (GAD67, encoded by *GAD1*), a key factor in optimal GABA levels, in the DLPFC of patients with schizophrenia (for review, see Lewis et al., 2005). Furthermore, proper functioning of GABA neurons has been linked to optimal WM function, purportedly by virtue of GABA's role in exerting lateral inhibition and synchronizing persistent firing of pyramidal cells in the DLPFC (Rao et al., 2000). Therefore, it is hypothesized that a disruption of the excitation/inhibitory balance between pyramidal and GABA neurons may be one crucial pathophysiological mechanism operating in schizophrenia, relevant to observed cognitive deficits.

Importantly, as alluded to earlier, the leading hypothesis regarding ketamine's effects on cortical function proposes precisely such a disinhibition of the cortical microcircuit (Greene, 2001; Homayoun & Moghaddam, 2007; Kotermanski & Johnson, 2009; Krystal et al., 2002, 2003). Specifically, it is hypothesized that ketamine, and possibly other NMDA antagonists, exert their effects via preferential blockade of NMDA receptors on GABAergic interneurons in the cortical microcircuit (Kotermanski & Johnson, 2009) (for a discussion of mechanisms behind this preferential blockade, see Greene, 2001). In turn, this may result in excessive pyramidal cell activity and a hyper-glutamatergic state of cortical disinhibition (Homayoun & Moghaddam, 2007), which may induce excessive activation and hyper-synchrony of cortical circuits, as well as possible "hyper-frontality" (Moghaddon & Javitt, 2011). These hypothesized effects are supported by evidence from human neuroimaging literature, as a number of PET and bloodBOLD fMRI imaging studies have suggested excessive cortical activation during acute administration of ketamine to healthy volunteers (Breier et al., 1997; Lahti et al., 1995a, 2002; Vollenweider et al., 1997, 2000). Extensive treatment of the hypothesized mechanisms behind these observations is beyond the scope of the present review and has received attention in prior reviews (Adell et al., 2011). Importantly, possible disruptions of cortical inhibition – due to disruptions of GABAergic signaling–may underlie acute effects of ketamine. Through this mechanistic link between ketamine's effects and hypothesized neuropathology in schizophrenia, we can adapt existing computational models of WM to perturb this very mechanism, balance of excitation and inhibition, allowing a bridge between pharmacology, and cognition and computational modeling.

Computational models of working memory function: promise for integration with pharmacological neuroimaging

Although a number of neuroimaging studies have demonstrated that acute ketamine administration alters cortical function and cognition in humans (Corlett et al., 2006; Honey et al., 2008), very few studies have extended this to cognitive deficits and specifically WM function (Honey et al., 2004). A number of elegant ph-fMRI investigations have successfully employed the ketamine model to examine the neural correlates of positive schizophrenia symptoms – specifically delusion formation – but this has not been fully extended to the domain of cognitive deficits. We argue that this is critical not only from a clinical standpoint but also because WM offers the ideal opportunity for a translational cognitive neuroscience marker that is compromised in schizophrenia (Glahn et al., 2003). To date, only a single ph-fMRI study has examined the effects of ketamine on WM, but did so using a verbal N-back cognitive task that does not allow for clear translation to animal physiology (Honey et al., 2004). We suggest an approach using spatial WM as a translational neuropsychiatry endophenotype. Due to the shared neural substrates, both human neuroimaging and primate neurophysiology have provided increasingly better characterization of visuospatial WM mechanisms (Driesen et al., 2008; Goldman-Rakic,

1984, 1987, 1995, 1996; Goldman-Rakic et al., 2000, 2004; Leung et al., 2002). A series of seminal electrophysiological studies with nonhuman primates conducted by Patricia Goldman-Rakic and colleagues (Funahashi et al., 1989; Goldman-Rakic, 1988, 1995) have shown that the persistent firing of DLPFC pyramidal cells underlie computations necessary for robust and stable internal representations in the face of competing external stimuli (Rao et al., 2000). Furthermore, it is widely understood that optimal WM function depends on the slow NMDA receptors at the recurrent synapses and the balance between synaptic excitation and inhibition between pyramidal and GABAergic interneurons, respectively (Constantinidis & Wang, 2004; Goldman-Rakic & Friedman, 1991; Rao et al., 2000; Wang, 2001, 2010; Wang et al., 2004, 2008). It follows directly that acute antagonism of the NMDA glutamate receptors via ketamine – targeting GABA cells – would disrupt cortical signals critical for spatial WM, a hypothesis supported by behavioral evidence (Morgan & Curran, 2006).

Based on such an understanding of the basic cellular properties of spatial WM function derived from primate physiology experiments, Wang and colleagues have developed a biophysically constrained and realistic spatial WM network model of spiking neurons (Compte et al., 2000; Wang, 2001; Wang et al., 2004). The model is based on a Mexican-hat architecture (Camperi & Wang, 1998), with a critical interplay between excitatory and inhibitory cells in a cortical circuit that underlies the persistence of pyramidal cell activity. The model incorporates local recurrent excitation (E-E) between pyramidal cells with similar spatial preferences and broad synaptic feedback inhibition (E-I) from GABAergic cells. When local excitatory synapses are sufficiently activated, the network exhibits robust firing that follows a bell-shaped pattern (or "bump" attractor state), which stores the memory of a spatial location as an analog quantity. Furthermore, consistent with experimental data, prior simulations have found that in this model, WM function depends on the slow NMDA receptors at the recurrent synapses and the balance between synaptic excitation and inhibition (Constantinidis & Wang, 2004; Wang, 2001, 2006), thought to be disrupted in schizophrenia (Marin, 2012). This computational model of WM – grounded in primate physiology – offers a unique possibility to explore the effects of neuromodulation (Brunel & Wang, 2001) and cell-type specific virtual lesions or impairments, as recently accomplished in vivo in rodents (Yizhar et al., 2011). Because the model contains the same basic cellular architecture present in the human cortex, namely E-E and E-I NMDA conductance, hypothesized aspects of schizophrenia neuropathology can be represented within the model itself, as done with dopamine (Brunel & Wang, 2001). This is a unique advantage of biophysically based WM models: while computational modeling of cognition in psychiatry has guided our predictions conceptually (Montague et al., 2012), this framework is distinguished by its foundation in a computational model rooted in neurophysiological data and building on assumptions based on molecular and systems neuroscience. However, the ultimate potential of this framework is to represent hypothesized aspects of schizophrenia neuropathology, articulated earlier (namely NMDA hypofunction on GABA cells), within the model itself and test model predictions via a feasible pharmacological framework that allows for direct and safe experimental comparison in humans. Ketamine administration offers an exciting opportunity in this regard, as it transiently, reversibly, and safely induces some of the characteristic positive, negative, and cognitive symptoms of schizophrenia in healthy volunteers (Krystal et al., 2003) via a mechanism that can be implemented in the model.

While this combination of approaches can generate powerful behavioral predictions, some might argue that biophysical realism at the level of cells may offer little explanatory power when combined with fMRI (Montague et al., 2012) (as the fMRI signal averages over millions of neurons). While this is a reasonable concern, recent work with L-Dopa has already begun to put these concerns to rest and nicely illustrates the power of computational modeling at the level of synapses when combined with human neuroimaging (Moran et al., 2011). Using magnetoencephalographic (MEG) measurement in the context of a WM task, Moran and colleagues have shown that the DLPFC signal tracks specific predictions from a synaptic-level model of cortical functions following L-Dopa pharmacological manipulation. They found that the degree of NMDA and α-amino-3-hydroxy-5-methyl-4-isoxazole propionic acid (AMPA) signaling change in the model indeed predicted both MEG and behavioral effects. This study highlights the potential of uncovering hidden cellular mechanisms, invisible with our state-of-the-art human neuroimaging (Figure 12.2), yet critical for our understanding of emergent system-level neural activity and behavior.

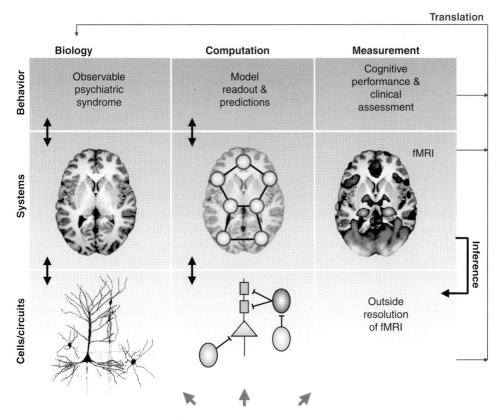

Figure 12.2. Framework for translational cognitive neuroscience of schizophrenia. The proposed framework combines pharmacological manipulation and cellular-level computational modeling with behavioral measurement and neural system read-out with state-of-the-art fMRI. This allows direct mechanism examination through manipulation of the underlying circuitry and comparing results with deficits observed in schizophrenia patients. This computational neuropsychiatry approach allows us to traverse levels of scientific explanation by establishing mechanistic links between cells, neural systems, and psychiatric symptoms. (See color plate section for colored image.)

We propose that the same approach can and needs to be harnessed in the service of characterizing cognitive deficits in schizophrenia, in this case through understanding of spatial WM deficits specifically. Through the combination of the aforementioned computational models of WM and NMDA glutamate receptor antagonism via ketamine, there is a path forward for a mechanistic understanding of cognitive deficits in schizophrenia. We contend that this approach provides a testable experimental framework using behavior and ph-fMRI, and allows for the iterative implementation of possible cognitive treatments in the model itself in future work. This in turn will generate predictions regarding behavior and neuronal activity that can be tested experimentally using novel compounds that the model predicts to be effective in improving cognitive deficits in schizophrenia. This is critical because most psychiatric treatment regimens, particularly those that are used to treat schizophrenia, have evolved without a rational framework motivating their design and do not alleviate cognitive deficits. Therefore, the articulated translational cognitive neuroscience approach holds promise for defining mechanisms that may help focus our treatments of cognitive dysfunction in individuals suffering from this illness.

Summary and conclusions

In this chapter, we have reviewed the extensive evidence that individuals with schizophrenia experience deficits in WM function and that these deficits extend across both encoding and the maintenance phases of WM. Further, we have also reviewed evidence that WM deficits in schizophrenia are associated with disturbances in a distributed cortical frontoparietal, striatal, and thalamic circuit, although impairments in DLPFC function may play a particular key role. Such impairments may involve not only abnormalities in sustaining activation across a delay, but also breakdowns in interference resolution from incoming distraction. Further, we have reviewed additional evidence suggesting that individuals with schizophrenia also experience deficits in several domains of executive function, including context processing, proactive control, and conflict detection, that may depend – at least in part – on the same neural circuits that support WM function. We have also discussed evidence suggesting that individuals with schizophrenia have deficits in EM function that involve impairments in relational integration and retrieval. These deficits in relational processing of components of EM appear to reflect impairments in both binding processes supported by the hippocampus and the types of beneficial encoding strategies supported by regions of prefrontal cortex. We have also suggested that in order to understand better and thus develop effective treatments for such impairing cognitive deficits in schizophrenia, we may need to adopt a translational cognitive neuroscience approach that uses biophysically plausible computational models and pharmacological challenge approaches that would allow us to test specific mechanistic hypotheses about the sources of cognitive impairment in schizophrenia. We have articulated the use of such a framework to understand the potential role of NMDA receptor dysfunction and excitatory/inhibitory circuits in WM deficits in schizophrenia. However, this is just one potential example and this approach can be extended to model different cognitive deficits (e.g., proactive control, EM) and different potential pathophysiological mechanisms. Regardless of the specific mechanisms tested, it is our belief that the use of such a framework will help move forward the search for effective treatments for cognitive impairment in schizophrenia, given the central role of such deficits in constraining life function for individuals with this illness.

References

Achim, A. M. & Lepage, M. (2003). Is associative recognition more impaired than item recognition memory in schizophrenia? A meta-analysis. *Brain and Cognition*, **53**, 121–124.

Addington, J., Addington, D., & Gasbarre, L. (1997). Distractibility and symptoms in schizophrenia. *Journal of Psychiatry and Neuroscience*, **22**, 180–184.

Adell, A., Jiménez-Sánchez, L., López-Gil, X., et al. (2011). Is the acute NMDA receptor hypofunction a valid model of schizophrenia? *Schizophrenia Bulletin*, **38**, 9–14.

Adler, C. M., Malhotra, A. K., Goldberg, T., et al. (1998). *A Comparison of Ketamine-induced and Schizophrenic Thought Disorder.* 53rd Annual Convention, Society of Biological Psychiatry, Toronto: Canada.

Alain, C., McNeely, H. E., & Yu, H., et al. (2002). Neurophysiological evidence of error monitoring deficits in patients with schizophrenia. *Cerebral Cortex*, **12**, 840–846.

Aleman, A., Hijman, R., de Haan, E. H., et al. (1999). Memory impairment in schizophrenia: a meta-analysis. *American Journal of Psychiatry*, **156**, 1358–1366.

Alexander, W. H. & Brown, J. W. (2011). Medial prefrontal cortex as an action-outcome predictor. *Nature Neuroscience*, **14**, 1338–1344.

Alkire, M. T., Haier, R. J., Fallon, J. H., et al. (1998). Hippocampal, but not amygdala, activity at encoding correlates with long-term, free recall of nonemotional information. *Proceedings of the National Academy of Sciences of the United States of America*, **95**, 14506–14510.

Andrews-Hanna, J. R., Reidler, J. S., Huang, C., et al. (2010). Evidence for the default network's role in spontaneous cognition. *Journal of Neurophysiology*, **104**, 322–335.

Anticevic, A., Repovs, G., & Barch, D. M. (2011a). Working memory encoding and maintenance deficits in schizophrenia: neural evidence for activation and deactivation abnormalities. *Schizophrenia Bulletin* [Epub ahead of print].

Anticevic, A., Repovs, G., Shulman, G. L., et al. (2010). When less is more: TPJ and default network deactivation during encoding predicts working memory performance. *NeuroImage*, **49**, 2638–2648.

Anticevic, A., Repovs, G., Corlett, P. R., et al. (2011b). Negative and non-emotional interference with visual working memory in schizophrenia. *Biological Psychiatry*, **70**, 1159–1168.

Badcock, J. C., Badcock, D. R., Read, C., et al. (2008). Examining encoding imprecision in spatial working memory in schizophrenia. *Schizophrenia Research*, **100**, 144–152.

Baddeley, A. D. (2000). The episodic buffer: a new component of working memory? *Trends in Cognitive Sciences*, **4**, 417–423.

Baddeley, A. D. & Hitch, G. J. (1974). Working memory. In G. Bower (ed.), *The Psychology of Learning and Motivation*. New York, NY: Academic Press, pp. 47–89.

Baker, J. T., Sanders, A. L., Maccotta, L., et al. (2001). Neural correlates of verbal memory encoding during semantic and structural processing tasks. *Neuroreport*, **12**, 1251–1256.

Barbalat, G., Chambon, V., Franck, N., et al. (2009). Organization of cognitive control within the lateral prefrontal cortex in schizophrenia. *Archives of General Psychiatry*, **66**, 377–386.

Barch, D. M. (2005a). The cognitive neuroscience of schizophrenia. In T. Cannon & S. Mineka (eds.), *Annual Review of Clinical Psychology*. Washington, DC: American Psychological Association, pp. 321–353.

Barch, D. M. (2005b). The relationships among cognition, motivation, and emotion in schizophrenia: how much and how little we know. *Schizophrenia Bulletin*, **31**, 875–881.

Barch, D. M. & Braver, T. S. (2007). Cognitive control in schizophrenia: psychological and neural mechanisms. In R. W. Engle, G. Sedek, U. von Hecker, et al. (eds.), *Cognitive Limitations in Aging and Psychopathology*. Cambridge: Cambridge University Press, pp. 122–159.

Barch, D. M., Carter, C. S., Braver, T. S., et al. (2001). Selective deficits in prefrontal cortex regions in medication naive schizophrenia patients. *Archives of General Psychiatry*, 50, 280–288.

Barch, D. M., Carter, C. S., & Cohen, J. D. (2003). Context processing deficit in schizophrenia: diagnostic specificity, 4-week course, and relationships to clinical symptoms. *Journal of Abnormal Psychology*, 112, 132–143.

Barch, D. M., Carter, C., Perlstein, W., et al. (1999). Increased Stroop facilitation effects in schizophrenia are not due to increased automatic spreading activation. *Schizophrenia Research*, 39, 51–64.

Barch, D. M., Sheline, Y. I., Csernansky, J. G., et al. (2003). Working memory and prefrontal cortex dysfunction: specificity to schizophrenia compared with major depression. *Biological Psychiatry*, 53, 376–384.

Barch, D. M. & Smith, E. (2008). The cognitive neuroscience of working memory: relevance to CNTRICS and schizophrenia. *Biological Psychiatry*, 64, 11–17.

Bates, A. T., Kiehl, K. A., Laurens, K. R., et al. (2002). Error-related negativity and correct response negativity in schizophrenia. *Clinical Neurophysiology*, 113, 1454–1463.

Bates, A. T., Liddle, P. F., Kiehl, K. A., et al. (2004). State dependent changes in error monitoring in schizophrenia. *Journal of Psychiatric Research*, 38, 347–356.

Becerril, K. E., Repovs, G., & Barch, D. M. (2011). Error processing network dynamics in schizophrenia. *NeuroImage*, 54, 1495–1505.

Benes, F. M., McSparren, J., Bird, E. D., et al. (1991). Deficits in small interneurons in prefrontal and cingulate cortices of schizophrenic and schizoaffective patients. *Archives of General Psychiatry*, 48, 996–1001.

Blanchard, J. J. & Neale, J. M. (1994). The neuropsychological signature of schizophrenia: generalized or differential deficit. *American Journal of Psychiatry*, 151, 40–48.

Blumenfeld, R. S., Parks, C. M., Yonelinas, A. P., et al. (2011). Putting the pieces together: the role of dorsolateral prefrontal cortex in relational memory encoding. *Journal of Cognitive Neuroscience*, 23, 257–265.

Bonner-Jackson, A. & Barch, D. M. (2011). Strategic manipulations for associative memory and the role of verbal processing abilities in schizophrenia. *Journal of the International Neuropsychological Society*, 17, 796–806.

Bonner-Jackson, A., Yodkovik, N., Csernansky, J. G., et al. (2008). Episodic memory in schizophrenia: the influence of strategy use on behavior and brain activation. *Psychiatry Research*, 164, 1–15.

Botvinick, M. M., Braver, T. S., Barch, D. M., et al. (2001). Conflict monitoring and cognitive control. *Psychological Review*, 108, 624–652.

Bowles, B., Crupi, C., Pigott, S., et al. (2010). Double dissociation of selective recollection and familiarity impairments following two different surgical treatments for temporal-lobe epilepsy. *Neuropsychologia*, 48, 2640–2647.

Braver, T. S. (2012). The variable nature of cognitive control: a dual-mechanisms framework. *Trends in Cognitive Sciences*, 16, 106–113.

Braver, T. S., Barch, D. M., & Cohen, J. D. (1999). Cognition and control in schizophrenia: a computational model of dopamine and prefrontal function. *Biological Psychiatry*, 46, 312–328.

Braver, T. S. & Cohen, J. D. (1999). Dopamine, cognitive control, and schizophrenia: the gating model. *Progress in Brain Research*, 121, 327–349.

Braver, T. S., Cohen, J. D., Nystrom, L. E., et al. (1997). A parametric study of prefrontal cortex involvement in human working memory. *NeuroImage*, 5, 49–62.

Braver, T. S., Gray, J. R., & Burgess, G. C. (2007). Explaining the many varieties of working memory variation: dual mechanisms of cognitive control. In A. R. Conway, C. Jarrold, M. J. Kane, et al. (eds.), *Variation in Working Memory*. Oxford: Oxford University Press, pp. 76–106.

Braver, T. S., Paxton, J. L., Locke, H. S., et al. (2009). Flexible neural mechanisms of cognitive control within human prefrontal cortex. *Proceedings of the National Academy of Sciences of the United States of America*, 106, 7351–7356.

Breier, A., Malhotra, A. K., Pinals, D. A., et al. (1997). Association of ketamine-induced psychosis with focal activation of the prefrontal cortex in healthy volunteers. *American Journal of Psychiatry*, **154**, 805–811.

Brewer, J., Zhao, Z. H., & Gabrieli, J. D. E. (1998a). Parahippocampal and frontal responses to single events predict whether those events are remembered or forgotten. *Science*, **281**, 1185–1187.

Brewer, J. B., Zhao, Z., Glover, G. H., et al. (1998b). Making memories: brain activity that predicts how well visual experience will be remembered. *Science*, **281**, 1185–1187.

Brown, J. W. & Braver, T. S. (2005). Learned predictions of error likelihood in the anterior cingulate cortex. *Science*, **307**, 1118–1121.

Brunel, N. & Wang, X. J. (2001). Effects of neuromodulation in a cortical network model of object working memory dominated by recurrent inhibition. *Journal of Computational Neuroscience*, **11**, 63–85.

Buchanan, R. W., Javitt, D. C., Marder, S. R., et al. (2007). The Cognitive and Negative Symptoms in Schizophrenia Trial (CONSIST): the efficacy of glutamatergic agents for negative symptoms and cognitive impairments. *American Journal of Psychiatry*, **164**, 1593–1602.

Buchanan, R. W., Strauss, M. E., Kirkpatrick, B., et al. (1994). Neuropsychological impairments in deficit vs nondeficit forms of schizophrenia. *Archives of General Psychiatry*, **51**, 804–811.

Callicott, J. H., Bertolino, A., Mattay, V. S., et al. (2000). Physiological dysfunction of the dorsolateral prefrontal cortex in schizophrenia revisited. *Cerebral Cortex*, **10**, 1078–1092.

Callicott, J. H., Mattay, V. S., Verchinski, B. A., et al. (2003). Complexity of prefrontal cortical dysfunction in schizophrenia: more than up or down. *American Journal of Psychiatry*, **160**, 2209–2215.

Callicott, J. H., Ramsey, N. F., Tallent, K., et al. (1998). Functional magnetic resonance imaging brain mapping in psychiatry: methodological issues illustrated in a study of working memory in schizophrenia. *Neuropsychopharmacology*, **18**, 186–196.

Cameron, K. A., Yashar, S., Wilson, C. L., et al. (2001). Human hippocampal neurons predict how well word pairs will be remembered. *Neuron*, **30**, 289–298.

Camperi, M. & Wang, X. J. (1998). A model of visuospatial working memory in prefrontal cortex: recurrent network and cellular bistability. *Journal of Computational Neuroscience*, **5**, 383–405.

Carter, C. S., MacDonald, A. W. 3rd., Ross, L.L., et al. (2001). Anterior cingulate cortex activity and impaired self-monitoring of performance in patients with schizophrenia: an event-related fMRI study. *American Journal of Psychiatry*, **158**, 1423–1428.

Cellard, C., Tremblay, S., Lehoux, C., et al. (2007). Processing spatial-temporal information in recent-onset schizophrenia: the study of short-term memory and its susceptibility to distraction. *Brain and Cognition*, **64**, 201–207.

Chapman, L. J. & Chapman, J. P. (1978). The measurement of differential deficit. *Journal of Psychiatric Research*, **14**, 303–311.

Cohen, J. D., Barch, D. M., Carter, C., et al. (1999). Context-processing deficits in schizophrenia: Converging evidence from three theoretically motivated cognitive tasks. *Journal of Abnormal Psychology*, **108**, 120–133.

Cohen, N. J. & Eichenbaum, H. (2001). *From Conditioning to Conscious Recollection*. New York: Oxford University Press.

Cohen, J. D. & Servan-Schreiber, D. (1992). Context, cortex and dopamine: a connectionist approach to behavior and biology in schizophrenia. *Psychological Review*, **99**, 45–77.

Coleman, M. J., Titone, D., Krastoshevsky, O., et al. (2010). Reinforcement ambiguity and novelty do not account for transitive inference deficits in schizophrenia. *Schizophrenia Bulletin*, **36**, 1187–1200.

Compte, A., Brunel, N., Goldman-Rakic, P. S., et al. (2000). Synaptic mechanisms and network dynamics underlying spatial working memory in a cortical network model. *Cerebral Cortex*, **10**, 910–923.

Constantinidis, C. & Wang, X.-J. (2004). A neural circuit basis for spatial working memory. *Neuroscientist*, **10**, 553–565.

Corkin, S. (1984). Lasting consequences of bilateral medial temporal lobectomy: clinical course and experimental findings in H. M. *Seminars in Neurology*, **4**, 249–259.

Corlett, P. R., Honey, G. D., Aitken, M. R. F., et al. (2006). Frontal responses during learning predict vulnerability to the psychotogenic effects of ketamine: linking cognition, brain activity, and psychosis. *Archives of General Psychiatry*, **63**, 611–621.

Cornblatt, B., Obuchowski M., Roberts S., et al. (1999) Cognitive and behavioral precursors of schizophrenia. *Developmental Psychopathology*, **11**, 487–508.

Cowan, N. (2001). The magical number 4 in short-term memory: a reconsideration of mental storage capacity. *Behavioral and Brain Sciences*, **24**, 87–185.

Cowan, N. (2008) What are the differences between long-term, short-term, and working memory? In W. S. Sossin, J.-C. Lacaille, V. F. Castellucci, et al. (eds.), *Progress in Brain Research, Vol. 169. Essence of Memory.* Amsterdam: Elsevier, pp. 323–338.

Curtis, C. E., Rao, V. Y., & D'Esposito, M. (2004). Maintenance of spatial and motor codes during oculomotor delayed response tasks. *Journal of Neuroscience*, **24**, 3944–3952.

Danion, J. M., Cuervo, C., Piolino, P., et al. (2005). Conscious recollection in autobiographical memory: an investigation in schizophrenia. *Consciousness and Cognition*, **14**, 535–547.

Davachi, L. (2006). Item, context and relational episodic encoding in humans. *Current Opinion in Neurobiology*, **16**, 693–700.

Delawalla, Z., Barch, D. M., Fisher-Eastep, J. L., et al. (2006). Factors mediating cognitive deficits and psychopathology among siblings of individuals with schizophrenia. *Schizophrenia Bulletin*, **32**, 525–537.

D'Esposito, M. (2007). From cognitive to neural models of working memory. *Philosophical Transactions of the Royal Society of London. Series B: Biological Sciences*, **362**, 761–772.

D'Esposito, M., Aguirre, G. K., Zarahn, E., et al. (1998). Functional MRI studies of spatial and nonspatial working memory. *Cognitive Brain Research*, **7**, 1–13.

Dickinson, D., Ragland, J. D., Gold, J. M., et al. (2008). General and specific cognitive deficits in schizophrenia: Goliath defeats David? *Biological Psychiatry*, **64**, 823–827.

Dickinson, D., Ramsey, M. E., & Gold, J. M. (2007). Overlooking the obvious: a meta-analytic comparison of digit symbol coding tasks and other cognitive measures in schizophrenia. *Archives of General Psychiatry*, **64**, 532–542.

Dosenbach, N. U., Fair, D. A., Cohen, A. L., et al. (2008). A dual-networks architecture of top-down control. *Trends in Cognitive Sciences*, **12**, 99–105.

Dreher, J. C., Banquet, J. P., Allilaire, J. F., et al. (2001). Temporal order and spatial memory in schizophrenia: a parametric study. *Schizophrenia Research*, **51**, 137–147.

Driesen, N. R., Leung, H. C., Calhoun, V. D., et al. (2008). Impairment of working memory maintenance and response in schizophrenia: functional magnetic resonance imaging evidence. *Biological Psychiatry*, **64**, 1026–1034.

D'Souza, D. C., Perry, E., MacDougall, L., et al., (2004). The psychotomimetic effects of intravenous delta-9-tetrahydrocannabinol in healthy individuals: implications for psychosis. *Neuropsychopharmacology*, **29**, 1558–1572.

Durstewitz, D., Kelc, M., & Gunturkun, O. (1999). A neurocomputational theory of the dopaminergic modulation of working memory functions. *Journal of Neuroscience*, **19**, 2807–2822.

Durstewitz, D. & Seamans, J. K. (2002). The computational role of dopamine D1 receptors in working memory. *Neural Networks*, **15**, 561–572.

Durstewitz, D. & Seamans, J. K. (2008). The dual-state theory of prefrontal cortex dopamine function with relevance to catechol-o-methyltransferase genotypes and schizophrenia. *Biological Psychiatry*, **64**, 739–749.

Durstewitz, D., Seamans, J. K., & Sejnowski, T. J. (2000). Dopamine-mediated stabilization of delay-period activity in a network model of prefrontal cortex. *Journal of Neurophysiology*, **83**, 1733–1750.

Edwards, B. G., Barch, D. M., & Braver, T. S. (2010). Improving prefrontal cortex function in schizophrenia through focused training of cognitive control. *Frontiers in Human Neuroscience*, **4**, 32.

Elvevåg, B. & Goldberg, T. E. (2000). Cognitive impairment in schizophrenia is the core of the disorder. *Critical Reviews in Neurobiology*, **14**, 1–21.

Enticott, P. G., Upton, D. J., Bradshaw, J. L., et al. (2011). Stop task after-effects in schizophrenia: behavioral control adjustments and repetition priming. *Neurocase* [Epub ahead of print].

Finkelstein, J. R., Cannon, T. D., Gur, R. E., et al. (1997). Attentional dysfunctions in neuroleptic-naive and neuroleptic-withdrawn schizophrenic patients and their siblings. *Journal of Abnormal Psychology*, **106**, 203–212.

Fleming, K., Goldberg, T. E., Binks, S., et al. (1997). Visuospatial working memory in patients with schizophrenia. *Biological Psychiatry*, **41**, 43–49.

Fletcher, P. C. (2011). Hurry up and wait: action, distraction, and inhibition in schizophrenia. *Biological Psychiatry*, **70**, 1104–1106.

Fox, M. D., Snyder, A. Z., Vincent, J. L., et al. (2005). The human brain is intrinsically organized into dynamic, anticorrelated functional networks. *Proceedings of the National Academy of Sciences of the United States of America*, **102**, 9673–9678.

Funahashi, S., Bruce, C. J., & Goldman-Rakic, P. S. (1989). Mnemonic coding of visual space in the monkey's dorsolateral prefrontal cortex. *Journal of Neurophysiology*, **61**, 331–349.

Fusar-Poli, P., Perez, J., Broome, M., et al. (2007). Neurofunctional correlates of vulnerability to psychosis: a systematic review and meta-analysis. *Neuroscience and Biobehavioral Reviews*, **31**, 465–484.

Giovanello, K. S., Schnyer, D. M., & Verfaellie, M. (2004). A critical role for the anterior hippocampus in relational memory: evidence from an fMRI study comparing associative and item recognition. *Hippocampus*, **14**, 5–8.

Glahn, D. C., Ragland, J. D., Abramoff, A., et al. (2005). Beyond hypofrontality: a quantitative meta-analysis of functional neuroimaging studies of working memory in schizophrenia. *Human Brain Mapping*, **25**, 60–69.

Glahn, D. C., Therman, S., Manninen, M., et al. (2003). Spatial working memory as an endophenotype for schizophrenia. *Biological Psychiatry*, **53**, 624–626.

Goldman-Rakic, P. S. (1984). Modular organization of prefrontal cortex. *Trends in Neurosciences*, **7**, 419–424.

Goldman-Rakic, P. S. (1987). Circuitry of primate prefrontal cortex and regulation of behavior by representational memory. In F. Plum & V. Mountcastle (eds.), *Handbook of Physiology: The Nervous System V*. Bethesda, MD: American Physiological Society, pp. 373–417.

Goldman-Rakic, P. S. (1988). Topography of cognition: parallel distributed networks in primate association cortex. *Annual Review of Neuroscience*, **11**, 137–156.

Goldman-Rakic, P. S. (1994). Working memory dysfunction in schizophrenia. *Journal of Neuropsychiatry*, **6**, 348–357.

Goldman-Rakic, P. S. (1995). Cellular basis of working memory. *Neuron*, **14**, 477–485.

Goldman-Rakic, P. S. (1996). The prefrontal landscape: implications of functional architecture for understanding human mentation and the central executive. In A. C. Roberts, T. W. Robbins, & L. Weiskrantz (eds.), *The Prefrontal Cortex: Executive and Cognitive Functions*. Oxford: Oxford University Press, pp. 87–103.

Goldman-Rakic, P. S., Castner, S. A., Svensson, T. H., et al. (2004). Targeting the dopamine D1 receptor in schizophrenia: insights for cognitive dysfunction. *Psychopharmacology (Berl)*, **174**, 3–16.

Goldman-Rakic, P. S. & Friedman, H. R. (1991). The circuitry of working memory revealed by anatomy and metabolic imaging. In H. S. Levin, H. M. Eisenberg, & A. L. Benton (eds.). *Frontal Lobe Function and Dysfunction*. New York, NY: Oxford University Press, pp. 72–91.

Goldman-Rakic, P. S., Muly, E. C., & Williams, G. V. (2000). D1 receptors in prefrontal cells and circuits. *Brain Research Reviews*, **31**, 295–301.

Green, M. F. (2006). Cognitive impairment and functional outcome in schizophrenia and bipolar disorder. *Journal of Clinical Psychiatry*, **67**, e12.

Greene, R. (2001). Circuit analysis of NMDAR hypofunction in the hippocampus, in vitro, and psychosis of schizophrenia. *Hippocampus*, **11**, 569–577.

Gur, R. C., Ragland, J. D., Moberg, P. J., et al. (2001). Computerized neurocognitive scanning: II. The profile of schizophrenia. *Neuropsychopharmacology*, **25**, 777–788.

Haddon, J. E. & Killcross, S. (2007). Contextual control of choice performance: behavioral, neurobiological, and neurochemical influences. *Annals of the New York Academy of Sciences*, **1104**, 250–269.

Hahn, B., Robinson, B. M., Kaiser, S. T., et al. (2010). Failure of schizophrenia patients to overcome salient distractors during working memory encoding. *Biological Psychiatry*, **68**, 603–609.

Hanlon, F. M., Houck, J. M., Pyeatt, C. J., et al. (2011). Bilateral hippocampal dysfunction in schizophrenia. *NeuroImage*, **58**, 1158–1168.

Hanlon, F. M., Weisend, M. P., Yeo, R. A., et al. (2005). A specific test of hippocampal deficit in schizophrenia. *Behavioral Neuroscience*, **119**, 863–875.

Hannula, D. E. & Ranganath, C. (2008). Medial temporal lobe activity predicts successful relational memory binding. *Journal of Neuroscience*, **28**, 116–124.

Hannula, D. E. & Ranganath, C. (2009). The eyes have it: hippocampal activity predicts expression of memory in eye movements. *Neuron*, **63**, 592–599.

Hannula, D. E., Ranganath, C., Ramsay, I. S., et al. (2010). Use of eye movement monitoring to examine item and relational memory in schizophrenia. *Biological Psychiatry*, **68**, 610–616.

Hardoy, M. C., Carta, M. G., Catena, M., et al. (2004). Impairment in visual and spatial perception in schizophrenia and delusional disorder. *Psychiatry Research*, **127**, 163–166.

Hartman, M., Steketee, M. C., Silva, S., et al. (2003). Working memory and schizophrenia: evidence for slowed encoding. *Schizophrenia Research*, **59**, 99–113.

Harvey, P. D. & Pedley, M. (1989). Auditory and visual distractibility in schizophrenia. Clinical and medication status correlations. *Schizophrenia Research*, **2**, 295–300.

Heaton, R., Gladsjo, V., Palmer, B. W., et al. (2001). Stability and course of neuropsychological deficits in schizophrenia. *Archives of General Psychiatry*, **58**, 24–32.

Heckers, S. & Konradi, C. (2010). Hippocampal pathology in schizophrenia. *Current Topics in Behavioral Neurosciences*, **4**, 529–553.

Heckers, S., Rauch, S. L., Goff, D., et al. (1998). Impaired recruitment of the hippocampus during conscious recollection in schizophrenia. *Nature Neuroscience*, **1**, 318–323.

Heckers, S., Zalesak, M., Weiss, A. P., et al. (2004). Hippocampal activation during transitive inference in humans. *Hippocampus*, **14**, 153–162.

Heinrichs, R. W. & Zakzanis, K. K. (1998). Neurocognitive deficit in schizophrenia: a quantitative review of the evidence. *Neuropsychology*, **12**, 426–445.

Holmes, A. J., MacDonald, A. 3rd., Carter, C.S., et al. (2005). Prefrontal functioning during context processing in schizophrenia and major depression: an event-related fMRI study. *Schizophrenia Research*, **76**, 199–206.

Holroyd, C. B. & Coles, M. G. (2002). The neural basis of human error processing: reinforcement learning, dopamine, and the error-related negativity. *Psychological Review*, **109**, 679–709.

Homayoun, H. & Moghaddam, B. (2007). NMDA receptor hypofunction produces opposite effects on prefrontal cortex interneurons and pyramidal neurons. *Journal of Neuroscience*, **27**, 11496–11500.

Honey, G. & Bullmore, E. (2004). Human pharmacological MRI. *Trends in Pharmacological Sciences*, **25**, 366–374.

Honey, G. D., Bullmore, E. T., & Sharma, T. (2002). De-coupling of cognitive performance and cerebral functional response during working memory in schizophrenia. *Schizophrenia Research*, **53**, 45–56.

Honey, G. D., Corlett, P. R., Absalom, A. R., et al. (2008). Individual differences in psychotic effects of ketamine are predicted by brain function measured under placebo. *Journal of Neuroscience*, **28**, 6295–6303.

Honey, R. A., Honey, G. D., O'Loughlin, C., et al. (2004). Acute ketamine administration alters the brain responses to executive demands in a verbal working memory task: an fMRI study. *Neuropsychopharmacology*, **29**, 1203–1204.

Horan, W. P., Braff, D. L., Nuechterlein, K. H., et al. (2008). Verbal working memory impairments in individuals with schizophrenia and their first-degree relatives: findings from the Consortium on the Genetics of Schizophrenia. *Schizophrenia Research*, **103**, 218–228.

Horan, W. P., Foti, D., Hajcak, G., et al. (2012). Impaired neural response to internal but not external feedback in schizophrenia. *Psychological Medicine*, **42**, 1637–1647.

Irani, F., Kalkstein, S., Moberg, E. A., et al. (2011). Neuropsychological performance in older patients with schizophrenia: a meta-analysis of cross-sectional and longitudinal studies. *Schizophrenia Bulletin*, **37**, 1318–1326.

Janowsky, J. S., Shimamura, A. P., Kritchevsky, M., et al. (1989). Cognitive impairment following frontal lobe damage and its relevance to human amnesia. *Behavioral Neuroscience*, **103**, 548–560.

Javitt, D. C., Strous, R. D., Grochowski, S., et al. (1997). Impaired precision, but normal retention, of auditory sensory ("echoic") memory information in schizophrenia. *Journal of Abnormal Psychology*, **106**, 315–324.

Johnson, M. R., Morris, N. A., Astur, R. S., et al. (2006). A functional magnetic resonance imaging study of working memory abnormalities in schizophrenia. *Biological Psychiatry*, **60**, 11–21.

Jonides, J., Lewis, R. L., Nee, D. E., et al. (2008). The mind and brain of short-term memory. *Annual Review of Psychology*, **59**, 193–224.

Kee, K. S., Green, M. F., Mintz, J., et al. (2003). Is emotion processing a predictor of functional outcome in schizophrenia? *Schizophrenia Bulletin*, **29**, 487–497.

Kerns, J. G., Cohen, J. D., MacDonald, A. W. 3rd., et al., (2005), Decreased conflict- and error-related activity in the anterior cingulate cortex in subjects with schizophrenia. *American Journal of Psychiatry*, **162**, 1833–1839.

Kirchhoff, B. A., Wagner, A. D., Maril, A., et al. (2000). Prefrontal-temporal circuitry for episodic encoding and subsequent memory. *Journal of Neuroscience*, **20**, 6173–6180.

Koh, S. D. & Peterson, R. A. (1978). Encoding orientation and the remembering of schizophrenic young adults. *Journal of Abnormal Psychology*, **87**, 303–313.

Konkel, A. & Cohen, N. J. (2009). Relational memory and the hippocampus: representations and methods. *Frontiers in Neuroscience*, **3**, 166–174.

Kopp, B. & Rist, F. (1994). Error-correcting behavior in schizophrenic patients. *Schizophrenia Research*, **13**, 11–22.

Kopp, B. & Rist, F. (1999). An event-related brain potential substrate of disturbed response monitoring in paranoid schizophrenic patients. *Journal of Abnormal Psychology*, **108**, 337–346.

Kotermanski, S. E. & Johnson, J. W. (2009). Mg2+ imparts NMDA receptor subtype selectivity to the Alzheimer's drug memantine. *Journal of Neuroscience*, **29**, 2774–2779.

Kraeplin, E. (1950). *Dementia Praecox and Paraphrenia*. New York, NY: International Universities Press.

Krawitz, A., Braver, T. S., Barch, D. M., et al. (2011). Impaired error-likelihood prediction in medial prefrontal cortex in schizophrenia. *NeuroImage*, **54**, 1506–1517.

Krystal, J. H., Anand, A., & Moghaddam, B. (2002). Effects of NMDA receptor antagonists: implications for the pathophysiology of schizophrenia. *Archives of General Psychiatry*, **59**, 663–664.

Krystal, J. H., D'Souza, D. C., Karper, L. P., et al. (1999). Interactive effects of subanesthetic ketamine and haloperidol. *Psychopharmacology (Berl)*, **145**, 193–204.

Krystal, J. H., D'Souza, D. C., Mathalon, D., et al. (2003). NMDA receptor antagonist effects, cortical glutamatergic function, and schizophrenia: toward a paradigm shift in medication development. *Psychopharmacology (Berl)*, **169**, 215–233.

Krystal, J. H., Karper, L. P., Bennett, A., et al. (1998). Interactive effects of subanesthetic ketamine and subhypnotic lorazepam in humans. *Psychopharmacology (Berl)*, **135**, 213–229.

Krystal, J. H., Karper, L. P., Seibyl, J. P., et al. (1994). Subanesthetic effects of the noncompetitive NMDA antagonist, ketamine, in humans. Psychotomimetic, perceptual, cognitive, and neuroendocrine responses. *Archives of General Psychiatry*, **51**, 199–214.

Lahti, A. C., Holcomb, H. H., Medoff, D. R., et al. (1995a). Ketamine activates psychosis and alters limbic blood flow in schizophrenia. *Neuroreport*, **6**, 869–872.

Lahti, A. C., Holcomb, H. H., Medoff, D. R., et al. (2002). Abnormal patterns of regional cerebral blood flow in schizophrenia with primary negative symptoms during an effortful auditory recognition task. *American Journal of Psychiatry*, **158**, 1797–1808.

Lahti, A. C., Koffel, B., LaPorte, D., et al. (1995b). Subanesthetic doses of ketamine stimulate psychosis in schizophrenia. *Neuropsychopharmacology*, **13**, 9–19.

Lahti, A. C., Weiler, M. A., Tamara Michaelidis, B. A., et al. (2001). Effects of ketamine in normal and schizophrenic volunteers. *Neuropsychopharmacology*, **25**, 455–467.

Laurens, K. R., Ngan, E. T., Bates, A. T., et al. (2003). Rostral anterior cingulate cortex dysfunction during error processing in schizophrenia. *Brain*, **126**, 610–622.

Lee, J. & Park, S. (2005). Working memory impairments in schizophrenia: a meta-analysis. *Journal of Abnormal Psychology*, **114**, 599–611.

Leiderman, E. A. & Strejilevich, S. A. (2004). Visuospatial deficits in schizophrenia: central executive and memory subsystems

impairments. *Schizophrenia Research*, **68**, 217–223.

Lencz, T., Bilder, R. M., Turkel, E., et al. (2003). Impairments in perceptual competency and maintenance on a visual delayed match-to-sample test in first-episode schizophrenia. *Archives of General Psychiatry*, **60**, 238–243.

Leung, H. -C., Gore, J. C., Goldman-Rakic, P. S. (2002). Sustained mnemonic response in the human middle frontal gyrus during on-line storage of spatial memoranda. *Journal of Cognitive Neuroscience*, **14**, 659–671.

Lewis, D. A., Curley, A. A., Glausier, J. R., et al. (2012). Cortical parvalbumin interneurons and cognitive dysfunction in schizophrenia. *Trends in Neurosciences*, **35**, 57–67.

Lewis, D. A., Hashimoto, T., & Volk, D. W. (2005). Cortical inhibitory neurons and schizophrenia. *Nature Reviews. Neuroscience*, **6**, 312–324.

Lewis, D. A. & Moghaddam, B. (2006). Cognitive dysfunction in schizophrenia: convergence of gamma-aminobutyric acid and glutamate alterations. *Archives of Neurology*, **63**, 1372–1376.

Lewis, D. A., Volk, D. W., Hashimoto, T. (2004). Selective alterations in prefrontal cortical GABA neurotransmission in schizophrenia: a novel target for the treatment of working memory dysfunction. *Psychopharmacology (Berl)*, **174**, 143–150.

Lezak, M. D. (1995). *Neuropsychological Assessment*. 3rd ed. New York, NY: Oxford University Press.

Luck, D., Danion, J. M., Marrer, C., et al. (2010). Abnormal medial temporal activity for bound information during working memory maintenance in patients with schizophrenia. *Hippocampus*, **20**, 936–948.

MacDonald, A. W. 3rd., Becker, T. M., & Carter, C.S. (2006). Functional magnetic resonance imaging study of cognitive control in the healthy relatives of schizophrenia patients. *Biological Psychiatry*, **60**, 1241–1249.

MacDonald, A., Carter, C. S., Kerns, J. G., et al. (2005). Specificity of prefrontal dysfunction and context processing deficits to schizophrenia in a never medicated first-episode psychotic sample. *American Journal of Psychiatry*, **162**, 475–484.

MacDonald, A. W. 3rd., Goghari, V. M., Hicks, B. M., et al. (2005). A convergent-divergent approach to context processing, general intellectual functioning, and the genetic liability to schizophrenia. *Neuropsychology*, **19**, 814–821.

MacDonald, A. W., Pogue-Geile, M. F., Johnson, M. K., et al. (2003). A specific deficit in context processing in the unaffected siblings of patients with schizophrenia. *Archives of General Psychiatry*, **60**, 57–65.

MacDonald, A. W. 3rd., Thermenos, H. W., Barch, D. M., et al. (2009). Imaging genetic liability to schizophrenia: systematic review of fMRI studies of patients' nonpsychotic relatives. *Schizophrenia Bulletin*, **35**, 1142–1162.

Malhotra, A. K., Pinals, D. A., Adler, C. M., et al. (1997). Ketamine-induced exacerbation of psychotic symptoms and cognitive impairment in neuroleptic-free schizophrenics. *Neuropsychopharmacology*, **17**, 141–150.

Manoach, D. S. (2003). Prefrontal cortex dysfunction during working memory performance in schizophrenia: reconciling discrepant findings. *Schizophrenia Research*, **60**, 285–298.

Manoach, D. S., Gollub, R. L., Benson, E. S., et al. (2000). Schizophrenic subjects show aberrant fMRI activation of dorsolateral prefrontal cortex and basal ganglia during working memory performance. *Biological Psychiatry*, **48**, 99–109.

Manoach, D. S., Greve, D. N., Lindgren, K. A., et al. (2003). Identifying regional activity associated with temporally separated components of working memory using event-related functional MRI. *NeuroImage*, **20**, 1670–1684.

Manoach, D. S., Press, D. Z., Thangaraj, V., et al. (1999). Schizophrenic subjects activate dorsolateral prefrontal cortex during a working memory task, as measured by fMRI. *Biological Psychiatry*, **45**, 1128–1137.

Marin, O. (2012). Interneuron dysfunction in psychiatric disorders. *Nature Reviews. Neuroscience*, **13**, 107–120.

Mathalon, D. H., Dedor, M., Faustman, W. O., et al. (2002). Response-monitoring dysfunction in schizophrenia: an event-related brain potential study. *Journal of Abnormal Psychology*, **111**, 22–41.

Mathalon, D. H., Jorgensen, K. W., Roach, B. J., et al. (2009). Error detection failures in schizophrenia: ERPs and FMRI. *International Journal of Psychophysiology*, **73**, 109–117.

Mathews, J. R. & Barch, D. M. (2004). Episodic memory for emotional and nonemotional words in schizophrenia. *Cognition and Emotion*, **18**, 721–740.

McClelland, J. L., McNaughton, B. L., O'Reilly, R. C. (1995). Why there are complementary learning systems in the hippocampus and neocortex: Insights from the successes and failures of connectionist models of learning and memory. *Psychological Review*, **102**, 419–457.

Metzak, P. D., Riley, J. D., Wang, L., et al. (2011). Decreased efficiency of task-positive and task-negative networks during working memory in schizophrenia. *Schizophrenia bulletin* [Epub ahead of print].

Miller, B. T. & D'Esposito, M. (2005). Searching for "the top" in top-down control. *Neuron*, **48**, 535–538.

Minzenberg, M. J., Laird, A. R., Thelen, S., et al. (2009). Meta-analysis of 41 functional neuroimaging studies of executive function in schizophrenia. *Archives of General Psychiatry*, **66**, 811–822.

Mitchell, K. J. & Johnson, M. K. (2009). Source monitoring 15 years later: what have we learned from fMRI about the neural mechanisms of source memory? *Psychological Bulletin*, **135**, 638–677.

Moghaddam, B. & Javitt, D. (2012). From revolution to evolution: the glutamate hypothesis of schizophrenia and its implication for treatment. *Neuropsychopharmacology*, **37**, 4–15.

Montague, P. R., Dolan, R. J., Friston, K. J., et al. (2012). Computational psychiatry. *Trends in Cognitive Sciences*, **16**, 72–80.

Moran, R. J., Symmonds, M., Stephan, K. E., et al. (2011). An in vivo assay of synaptic function mediating human cognition. *Current Biology*, **21**, 1320–1325.

Morgan, C. J. & Curran, H. V. (2006). Acute and chronic effects of ketamine upon human memory: a review. *Psychopharmacology (Berl)*, **188**, 408–424.

Morris, S. E., Yee, C. M., & Nuechterlein, K. H. (2006). Electrophysiological analysis of error monitoring in schizophrenia. *Journal of Abnormal Psychology*, **115**, 239–250.

Murray, E. A. (1996). What have ablation studies told us about neural substrates of stimulus memory? *Seminars in the Neurosciences*, **8**, 13–22.

Murray, L. J. & Ranganath, C. (2007). The dorsolateral prefrontal cortex contributes to successful relational memory encoding. *Journal of Neuroscience*, **27**, 5515–5522.

Neill, J. C., Barnes, S., Cook, S., et al. (2010). Animal models of cognitive dysfunction and negative symptoms of schizophrenia: focus on NMDA receptor antagonism. *Pharmacology and Therapeutics*, **128**, 419–432.

Neufeld, R. W. J. (2007). On the centrality and significance of stimulus-encoding deficit in schizophrenia. *Schizophrenia Bulletin*, **33**, 982–993.

Newcomer, J. W., Farber, N. B., Jevtovic-Todorovic, V., et al. (1999). Ketamine-induced NMDA receptor hypofunction as a model of memory impairment and psychosis. *Neuropsychopharmacology*, **20**, 106–118.

Niendam, T. A., Bearden, C. E., Rosso, I. M., et al. (2003). A prospective study of childhood neurocognitive functioning in schizophrenic patients and their siblings. *American Journal of Psychiatry*, **160**, 2060–2062.

Oltmanns, T. F. & Neale, J. M. (1975). Schizophrenic performance when distractors are present: attentional deficit or differential task difficulty? *Journal of Abnormal Psychology*, **84**, 205–209.

Oltmanns, T. F., Ohayon, J., & Neale, J. M. (1978). The effect of anti-psychotic medication and diagnostic criteria on distractibility in schizophrenia. *Journal of Psychiatric Research*, **14**, 81–91.

Ongur, D., Cullen, T. J., Wolf, D. H., et al. (2006). The neural basis of relational memory deficits in schizophrenia. *Archives of General Psychiatry*, **63**, 356–365.

Otten, L. J., Henson, R. N. A., & Rugg, M. D. (2001). Depth of processing effects on neural correlates of memory encoding. *Brain*, **124**, 399–412.

Owen, A. M., McMillan, K. M., Laird, A. R., et al. (2005). N-back working memory paradigm: a meta-analysis of normative functional neuroimaging studies. *Human Brain Mapping*, **25**, 46–59.

Oye, I., Paulsen, O., & Maurset, A. (1992). Effects of ketamine on sensory perception: evidence for a role of N-methyl-D-aspartate receptors. *Journal of Pharmacology and Experimental Therapeutics*, **260**, 1209–1213.

Park, S. & Holzman, P. S. (1992). Schizophrenics show spatial working memory deficits. *Archives of General Psychiatry*, **49**, 975–982.

Perez, V. B., Ford, J. M., Roach, B. J., et al. (2012). Error monitoring dysfunction across the illness course of schizophrenia. *Journal of Abnormal Psychology*, **121**, 372–387.

Polli, F. E., Barton, J. J., Thakkar, K. N., et al. (2008). Reduced error-related activation in two anterior cingulate circuits is related to impaired performance in schizophrenia. *Brain*, **131**, 971–986.

Polli, F. E., Barton, J. J., Vangel, M., et al. (2006). Schizophrenia patients show intact immediate error-related performance adjustments on an antisaccade task. *Schizophrenia Research*, **82**, 191–201.

Postle, B. R. (2005). Delay-period activity in the prefrontal cortex: one function is sensory gating. *Journal of Cognitive Neuroscience*, **17**, 1679–1690.

Potkin, S. G., Turner, J. A., Brown, G. G., et al. (2009). Working memory and DLPFC inefficiency in schizophrenia: The FBIRN study. *Schizophrenia Bulletin*, **35**, 19–31.

Pukrop, R., Matuschek, E., Ruhrmann, S., et al. (2003). Dimensions of working memory dysfunction in schizophrenia. *Schizophrenia Research*, **62**, 259–268.

Ragland, J. D., Blumenfeld, R. S., Ramsay, I. S., et al. (2012). Neural correlates of relational and item-specific encoding during working and long-term memory in schizophrenia. *NeuroImage*, **59**, 1719–1726.

Ragland, J. D., Gur, R. C., Valdez, J. N., et al. (2005). Levels-of-processing effect on frontotemporal function in schizophrenia during word encoding and recognition. *American Journal of Psychiatry*, **162**, 1840–1848.

Ragland, J. D., Laird, A. R., Ranganath, C., et al. (2009). Prefrontal activation deficits during episodic memory in schizophrenia. *American Journal of Psychiatry*, **166**, 863–874.

Ragland, J. D., Moelter, S. T., McGrath, C., et al. (2003). Levels-of-processing effect on word recognition in schizophrenia. *Biological Psychiatry*, **54**, 1154–1161.

Ragland, J. D., Ranganath, C., Barch, D. M., et al. (2012). Relational and Item-Specific Encoding (RISE): task development and psychometric characteristics. *Schizophrenia Bulletin*, **38**, 114–124.

Ragland, J. D., Yoon, J., Minzenberg, M. J., et al. (2007). Neuroimaging of cognitive disability in schizophrenia: search for a pathophysiological mechanism. *International Review of Psychiatry*, **19**, 417–427.

Rao, S. G., Williams, G. V., & Goldman-Rakic, P. S. (2000). Destruction and creation of spatial tuning by disinhibition: GABA(A) blockade of prefrontal cortical neurons engaged by working memory. *Journal of Neuroscience*, **20**, 485–494.

Reichenberg, A. & Harvey P. D. (2007). Neuropsychological impairments in schizophrenia: integration of performance-based and brain imaging findings. *Psychological Bulletin*, **133**, 833–858.

Ryan, J. D. & Cohen, N. J. (2004). Processing and short-term retention of relational information in amnesia. *Neuropsychologia*, **42**, 497–511.

Sakai, K., Rowe, J. B., & Passingham, R. E. (2002). Active maintenance in prefrontal area 46 creates distractor-resistant memory. *Nature Neuroscience*, **5**, 479–484.

Saperstein, A. M., Fuller, R. L., Avila, M. T., et al. (2006). Spatial working memory as a cognitive endophenotype of schizophrenia: assessing risk for pathophysiological dysfunction. *Schizophrenia Bulletin*, **32**, 498–506.

Schlösser, R. G. M., Koch, K., Wagner, G., et al. (2008). Inefficient executive cognitive control in schizophrenia is preceded by altered functional activation during information encoding: an fMRI study. *Neuropsychologia*, **46**, 336–347.

Scoville, W. B. & Milner, B. (1957). Loss of recent memory after bilateral hippocampal lesions. *Journal of Neurology, Neurosurgery, and Psychiatry*, **20**, 11–21.

Shadlen, M. N. & Newsome, W. T. (1994). Noise, neural codes and cortical organization. *Current Opinion in Neurobiology*, **4**, 569–579.

Shimamura, A. P. (2010). Hierarchical relational binding in the medial temporal lobe: the strong get stronger. *Hippocampus*, **20**, 1206–1216.

Shulman, G. L., Corbetta, M., Buckner, R. L., et al. (1997). Common blood flow changes across visual tasks: I. Increases in subcortical structures and cerebellum but not in nonvisual cortex. *Journal of Cognitive Neuroscience*, **9**, 624–647.

Snitz, B. E., Macdonald, A. W., & Carter, C. S. (2006). Cognitive deficits in unaffected first-degree relatives of schizophrenia patients: a meta-analytic review of putative endophenotypes. *Schizophrenia Bulletin*, **32**, 179–194.

Spaniol, J., Davidson, P. S., Kim, A. S., et al. (2009). Event-related fMRI studies of episodic encoding and retrieval: meta-analyses using activation likelihood estimation. *Neuropsychologia*, **47**, 1765–1779.

Sperling, R. A., Bates, J. F., Cocchiarella, A. J., et al. (2001). Encoding novel face-name associations: a functional MRI study. *Human Brain Mapping*, **14**, 129–139.

Squire, L. R. (1987). *Memory and Brain.* New York, NY: Oxford University Press.

Squire, L. R. & Knowlton, B. J. (1995). Memory, hippocampus, and brain systems. In M. Gazzaniga (ed.), *The Cognitive Neurosciences.* Cambridge, MA: MIT Press, pp. 825–837.

Tek, C., Gold, J., Blaxton, T., et al. (2002). Visual perceptual and working memory impairments in schizophrenia. *Archives of General Psychiatry*, **59**, 146–153.

Thompson-Schill, S. L., Jonides, J., Marshuetz, C., et al. (2002). Effects of frontal lobe damage on interference effects in working memory. *Cognitive, Affective and Behavioral Neuroscience*, **2**, 109–120.

Titone, D., Ditman, T., Holzman, P. S., et al. (2004). Transitive inference in schizophrenia: impairments in relational memory organization. *Schizophrenia Research*, **68**, 235–247.

Treccani, B., Torri, T., & Cubelli, R. (2005). Is judgment of line orientation selectively impaired in right brain damaged patients? *Neuropsychologia*, **43**, 598–608.

Turken, A. U., Vuilleumier, P., Mathalon, D. H., et al. (2003). Are impairments of action monitoring and executive control true dissociative dysfunctions in patients with schizophrenia? *American Journal of Psychiatry*, **160**, 1881–1883.

Van Erp, T. G., Lesh, T. A., Knowlton, B. J., et al. (2008). Remember and know judgments during recognition in chronic schizophrenia. *Schizophrenia Research*, **100**, 181–190.

Van Snellenberg, J. X., Torres, I. J., & Thornton, A. E. (2006). Functional neuroimaging of working memory in schizophrenia: task performance as a moderating variable. *Neuropsychology*, **20**, 497–510.

Vollenweider, F. X., Leenders, K. L., Scharfetter, C., et al. (1997). Metabolic hyperfrontality and psychopathology in the ketamine model of psychosis using positron emission tomography (PET) and [18F] fluorodeoxyglucose (FDG). *European Neuropsychopharmacology*, **7**, 9–24.

Vollenweider, F. X., Vontobel, P., Oye, I., et al. (2000). Effects of (S)-ketamine on striatal dopamine: a [11C]raclopride PET study of a model psychosis in humans. *Journal of Psychiatric Research*, **34**, 35–43.

Wagner, A. D., Schacter, D., Rotte, M., et al. (1998). Building memories: remembering and forgetting of verbal experiences as predicted by brain activity. *Science*, **281**, 1188–1191.

Wager, T. D. & Smith, E. E. (2003). Neuroimaging studies of working memory: a meta-analysis. *Cognitive, Affective and Behavioral Neuroscience*, **3**, 255–274.

Walker, E., Kestler, L., Bollini, A., et al. (2004). Schizophrenia: etiology and course. *Annual Review of Psychology*, **55**, 401–430.

Wang, X.-J. (2001). Synaptic reverberation underlying mnemonic persistent activity. *Trends in Neurosciences*, **24**, 455–463.

Wang, X.-J. (2006). Toward a prefrontal microcircuit model for cognitive deficits in schizophrenia. *Pharmacopsychiatry*, **39**, S80–S87.

Wang, X.-J. (2010). Neurophysiological and computational principles of cortical rhythms in cognition. *Physiological Review*, **90**, 1195–1268.

Wang, H., Stradtman, G. G., Wang, X.-J., et al. (2008). A specialized NMDA receptor function in layer 5 recurrent microcircuitry of the adult rat prefrontal cortex. *Proceedings of the National Academy of Sciences of the United States of America*, **105**, 16791–16796.

Wang, X.-J., Tegnér, J., Constantinidis, C., et al. (2004). Division of labor among distinct subtypes of inhibitory neurons in a cortical microcircuit of working memory. *Proceedings of the National Academy of Sciences of the United States of America*, **101**, 1368–1373.

Weiss, A. P., Schacter, D. L., Goff, D. C., et al. (2003). Impaired hippocampal recruitment during normal modulation of memory performance in schizophrenia. *Biological Psychiatry*, **53**, 48–55.

Wendelken, C. & Bunge, S. A. (2010). Transitive inference: distinct contributions of rostrolateral prefrontal cortex and the hippocampus. *Journal of Cognitive Neuroscience*, **22**, 837–847.

Whitfield-Gabrieli, S., Thermenos, H., Milanovic, S., et al. (2009). Hyperactivity and hyperconnectivity of the default network in schizophrenia and in first-degree relatives of persons with schizophrenia. *Proceedings of the National Academy of Sciences of the United States of America*, **106**, 1279–1284.

Williams, L. E., Must, A., Avery, S., et al. (2010). Eye-movement behavior reveals relational memory impairment in schizophrenia. *Biological Psychiatry*, **68**, 617–624.

Yizhar, O., Fenno, L. E., Prigge, M., et al. (2011). Neocortical excitation/inhibition balance in information processing and social dysfunction. *Nature*, **477**, 171–178.

Zakzanis, K. K. & Heinrichs, R. W. (1999). Schizophrenia and the frontal brain: a quantitative review. *Journal of the International Neuropsychological Society*, **5**, 556–566.

Chapter

13

Assessment of cognition in schizophrenia treatment studies

Richard Keefe

Introduction

The authors of other chapters in this book have made it very clear that cognition is a core part of schizophrenia, related to key genetic and biological mechanisms, and a prime driver of the dysfunction and disability that characterizes the course of schizophrenia. Yet, as of the printing of this book, there are no treatments for cognitive impairment in schizophrenia approved by the U.S. Food and Drug Administration (FDA). Antipsychotic medications have very little impact on cognitive impairment in chronic schizophrenia (Keefe et al., 2007), and their benefits in first-episode schizophrenia are small and related to the symptom improvement found in early-phase treatment (Davidson et al., 2009). Cognitive impairment in schizophrenia is thus a tremendous unmet need. Scores of pharmaceutical and device companies and government agencies have been involved in funding studies that may identify a treatment that can benefit cognition in patients with schizophrenia.

These efforts have been facilitated by an interdisciplinary consortium, originally funded by the National Institute of Mental Health, called the Measurement and Treatment Research to Improve Cognition in Schizophrenia (MATRICS) project. The MATRICS project identified tests that would best measure cognition in clinical trials (Nuechterlein et al., 2008) and outlined clinical trial designs believed to best test the treatment effects of a compound on cognition in patients with schizophrenia (Buchanan et al., 2005, 2011a).

The MATRICS group determined that the best design for testing the effects of pharmacological treatment on cognition in schizophrenia is a randomized, placebo-controlled trial in patients who are clinically stable and who are receiving stable doses of antipsychotic medication, the so-called "add-on" or "co-treatment" design (Buchanan et al. 2005, 2011a). Of course, a single treatment that could reduce symptoms and improve cognition would be ideal, but the regulatory path for this type of clinical trial was viewed as more complex and has presented a higher hurdle for development due to regulatory concerns that cognitive benefit in the context of symptom amelioration is likely a secondary effect of symptom reduction, referred to as a pseudospecific effect (Buchanan et al., 2005, 2011a).

Current status of clinical trials on cognition in schizophrenia

In order to assess the current state of research in this area, we compiled a description of all schizophrenia cognition studies available on the U.S. government website (clinicaltrials. gov) that met our search criteria (Keefe et al., 2011a). For double-blind, add-on trials we also assessed whether the study had sufficient statistical power (beta=0.80) to identify true treatment differences assuming a two-tailed alpha of 0.05, primary outcome test–retest reliability of intraclass correlation (ICC) = 0.90, and true effect size d=0.5 (medium effect). Our analysis showed that the add-on, placebo-controlled double-blind design is predominant across completed and ongoing trials and that the use of widely accepted standardized cognitive batteries is increasing. However, other critical methodological issues, such as sample sizes to achieve standard statistical power, appear to be suboptimal in many studies. The studies included pharmacological treatments with many diverse mechanisms of action, although agents acting at the NMDA receptor have been examined most frequently. The current absence of available results for many trials precludes any assessment of the most promising mechanisms of action.

In our review of the literature, most completed trials had a sample size of <100 subjects, with many enroling <50 subjects. Only one in 17 completed trials with available results had sufficient power to detect a medium (d=0.5) effect size, suggesting that many of these studies could have concluded incorrectly that a drug with true efficacy did not have a beneficial effect (Keefe & Harvey, 2008; Leon, 2008). Of course, some of the studies included in this analysis were conducted in the early phases of drug development and because they were exploratory, involved small sample sizes. Given the large investment in time and resources required to run larger trials, small-sample studies can contribute valuable evidence of efficacy and safety. These early-phase studies assist drug developers in making important decisions about whether to invest financial resources in a drug's development. The application of non-standard thresholds for statistical significance is reasonable in these circumstances, as is targeting patient populations that may be the most responsive to treatment. However, the results of underpowered studies, especially when negative, should be interpreted with caution (Kraemer et al., 2006; Leon et al., 2011). The fact that the overwhelming majority of studies have not had sufficient statistical power challenges the field to draw accurate general conclusions about the potential for drug development for cognitive impairment in schizophrenia. In fact, since our analysis of these trials, multiple positive results have been reported at conferences and press releases (Hilt et al., 2011; Hosford et al., 2011), but have not been published yet in the peer-reviewed literature.

The demographic and clinical characteristics of the patients in these studies may be important for future trial design. Most of the studies included clinically stable people with schizophrenia, with a lower age limit of 18 years, and an upper age limit ranging between 55 and 65 years (AstraZeneca & Targacept, 2008; Buchanan et al., 2007; Buchanan et al., 2008; Friedman et al., 2008; Goff et al., 2008a,b; Honer et al., 2006; Javitt et al., 2011; Kane et al., 2010; Kelly, 2009; Levkovitz et al., 2010; Lieberman et al., 2009; Memory Pharmaceuticals, 2008), and a mean age between 40 and 49 years. Although cognitive impairments are generally stable over relatively short periods of time in the longitudinal course of schizophrenia (Bonner-Jackson et al., 2010; Bowie et al., 2004; Rund, 1998), cognitive function is age-dependent in healthy controls and schizophrenia samples. Larger deficits in working memory have been shown to exist in elderly versus first-episode patients with schizophrenia, while worse recall of material in episodic memory, changes in select time-based measures of problem solving, and fine motor dexterity have all been associated with greater length of illness (Sponheim et al., 2010; Zanello et al., 2009). In some studies of behavioral interventions, as reviewed in Chapter 16 of the book, younger people with schizophrenia and those early in the course of illness appeared to benefit more from cognitive remediation than older people (Eack et al., 2009, 2010; Wykes et al., 2009). Although the sample of chronic, stable participants with schizophrenia may be relatively convenient to recruit, these individuals may not be those who are most likely to show improvements in cognition (Marder, 2011). A trial performed in younger subjects with recent illness onset (Buchanan et al., 2011b) may yield more positive results than those conducted in patients with an average illness duration of >20 years (AstraZeneca & Targacept, 2008; Buchanan et al., 2007; Buchanan et al., 2008; Friedman et al., 2008; Goff et al., 2008a,b; Honer et al., 2006; Javitt et al., 2011; Kane et al., 2010; Kelly 2009; Levkovitz et al., 2010; Lieberman et al., 2009; Memory Pharmaceuticals, 2008). It is reasonable to expect that younger patients with greater potential neuroplasticity may be optimal candidates for pharmacological intervention, but surprisingly few data are available that address this question empirically.

Compared with the add-on trials that have already been completed, the currently ongoing add-on trials are longer, have larger sample sizes, and are more likely to use a widely accepted standardized cognitive battery (e.g., MCCB) (Kern et al., 2008; Nuechterlein et al., 2008). These results suggest that the MATRICS recommendations are being implemented in the more recent trials. In addition, an increasing number of ongoing add-on studies are recruiting recent-onset subjects; their results may help to determine which subjects are most likely to have cognitive benefits (Marder, 2011). The MATRICS guidelines (Buchanan et al., 2005) noted that, in general, it is not necessary to exclude subjects with a high level of cognitive functioning in whom further improvement in cognition would not be expected to be demonstrated, because with a properly constructed cognitive test battery, this level of performance is very rare. However, the question remains whether severely cognitively impaired subjects should be enroled into schizophrenia cognition clinical trials. It is possible that the presence of a floor effect on a cognitive test, indicating that performance is so poor that it cannot get worse, indicates minimal capacity for cognitive improvement. One of the challenges is that because we do not have medications that are known to improve cognition in schizophrenia, we are unable to determine which demographic factors may predict a response. Future analyses on data sets that indicate some positive results may help address this methodological question, will have implications about future study designs as well, and may indicate which patients would most benefit from a cognitive enhancing compound.

Our analysis of the studies listed on the U.S. government website (clinicaltrials.gov) suggested that the currently ongoing trials have more statistical power, providing optimism that the concept of pharmacological improvement of cognition in schizophrenia will receive, in the near future, a more true test. Among the ongoing add-on trials, 30.7% estimated an expected enrolment of ≥100 subjects. Many of these larger studies are multi-site trials, which present investigators and sponsors with specific challenges, described later (for a review, see Keefe and Harvey, 2008). As these large-scale multisite studies are completed, it may be possible to determine whether specific recommendations for performing multisite trials with neurocognitive assessments have been successfully imple-mented, and how these recommendations may impact trial results. As some of these trials are global, it is also important to ensure the cross-cultural and linguistic adaptability of primary (Harvey et al., 2010) and co-primary outcome measures (Green et al., 2011). Early results suggest that good psychometric characteristics of cognitive outcome measures are possible in large multisite studies if sufficient care is given to training and data quality (Keefe et al., 2011b). Our results also show that the percentage of ongoing add-on trials with sufficient statistical power to detect medium effect sizes has doubled in comparison to the completed add-on trials. However, more than half of ongoing trials still may have an inadequate sample size. Although adequate sample size is an important determinant in the estimation of statistical power in each study, a key and under-appreciated component of statistical power calculations is that relatively small changes in the reliability of the neurocognitive endpoints can have a strong effect on the sample size needed, especially when the magnitude of the expected effect is small to medium (Keefe et al., 2011a).

Outcome measures and study designs

One of the crucial components of cognition clinical trial design is the choice of outcome measure. Previous authors in this volume have focused on the various aspects of cognition that are impaired in schizophrenia, including theories about whether global or specific aspects of cognition are the primary areas of concern. These varied perspectives should be accounted for in cognition clinical trial design. Later-phase trials, such as Phase III trials described later, are more likely to be designed to demonstrate efficacy of a compound in terms of its cognitive benefit and its capacity to improve cognition-related functioning. As such, more global measures like the FDA-recommended MATRICS Consensus Cognitive Battery (MCCB) composite scores are most appropriate. In earlier-phase work, when the concept of cognitive change with a compound needs to be proven before a drug can be moved along the development pathway, it may be more appropriate to use a cognitive outcome that has a more direct relationship to what is known about the pharmacological effects of the compound under study.

MATRICS Consensus Cognitive Battery

The MATRICS project focused primarily on later-phase trials that would satisfy regulatory requirements for product registration, and deriving a cognitive test battery that could be used to measure treatment effects consistently across clinical studies. More than 90 individual cognitive tests from seven domains of cognitive function (verbal learning and memory, visual learning and memory, vigilance, working memory, social cognition, processing speed, and reasoning and problem solving) were evaluated based upon criteria derived from a consensus of experts in various fields related to schizophrenia cognition clinical trials (Green et al., 2004). These criteria emphasized characteristics required for cognitive measures in the context of clinical trials: test–retest reliability; utility as a repeated measure; relationship to functional status; potential changeability in response to pharmacological agents; and practicality for clinical trials and tolerability for patients. The 10 tests that comprise the MCCB were chosen on the basis of their ability to demonstrate these characteristics (Nuechterlein et al., 2008), which are listed in Table 13.1. The MCCB requires approximately 75 minutes to administer and allows for measurement of cognition in seven different cognitive domains. The battery comes with a computerized scoring system that produces T-scores and percentiles for individual tests, cognitive domains, and composite scores, corrected for age and gender based on a 300-subject normative group (Kern et al., 2008).

A composite score on the MCCB was accepted by FDA leaders as the primary endpoint for registration trials of cognition in schizophrenia (Buchanan et al., 2005), and continues to be considered the gold standard measure for schizophrenia cognitive outcomes (Buchanan et al., 2011a). In multisite government and industry clinical trials, the MCCB has demonstrated sensitivity to cognitive deficits in all domains, excellent test–retest reliability, small

Table 13.1. Measurement and Treatment Research to Improve Cognition in Schizophrenia Consensus Cognitive Battery

Domain	Tests
Speed of processing	• Category fluency • BACS symbol coding • Trail making-A
Attention/vigilance	• Continuous Performance Test (identical pairs version)
Working memory	• Letter–number span • WMS-III spatial span
Verbal learning	• Hopkins Verbal Learning Test-R
Visual learning	• Brief Visuospatial Memory Test-R
Reasoning and problem solving	• NAB mazes
Social cognition	• MSCEIT managing emotions

BACS, Brief Assessment of Cognition in Schizophrenia; WMS, Wechsler Memory Test; NAB, Neuropsychological Assessment Battery; MSCEIT, Mayer–Salovey–Caruso emotional intelligence test.

practice effects, and is strongly correlated with measures of functional capacity (Buchanan et al., 2011b; Keefe et al., 2011a) (Figure 13.1). To date, translations have been made available in over 15 languages with several more translations underway. The key metric, of course, is whether the MCCB is sensitive to change during pharmacological treatment. As its use has increased substantially in ongoing add-on trials, a wealth of data regarding this issue will be available in the next few years, and very recent unpublished results are promising (Hilt et al., 2011).

Challenge of cognition clinical trial implementation

Multisite trials to assess the effects of an intervention on cognitive outcomes in schizophrenia present a large number of challenges that need to be met for cognitive data to be collected reliably and efficiently (Keefe and Kraus, 2009). Many clinical investigators do not have substantial experience with cognitive assessment, although this is clearly changing over time. Thus, sites and testers must be trained and certified on the test battery and related procedures to assure test fidelity and consistency across sites. As described in the MCCB manual and as mandated by the American Psychological Association's *Standards for Educational and Psychological Testing*, psychological tests must be administered or supervised by a psychologist (APA, 1999), who can perform these duties at a central site. To maintain high quality cognitive data throughout the course of a trial and reduce "rater drift," it is important that review processes are established, followed, and refreshed regularly. Because personnel who conduct testing at a site may depart the site, plans must be in place for adding replacement testers. Test selection should address the scientific hypotheses of the investigators, yet the tests chosen must be efficient to implement without leading to excessive missing data, which can have strong deleterious effects on statistical power (Cohen, 1977). Finally, the data analytical plan should focus on a single or small number of outcome measures so that statistical power is not compromised. The manner of approach for all of these issues will depend upon the phase of development of the compound or behavioral intervention.

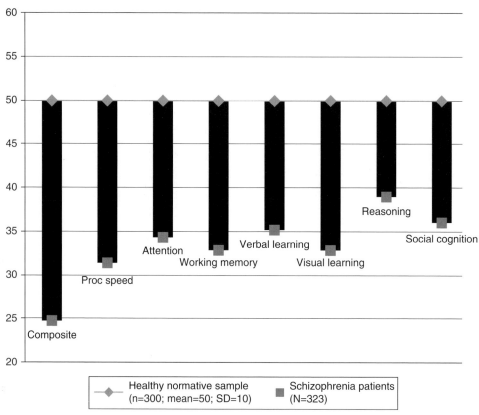

Figure 13.1. Severity and profile of cognitive impairment in schizophrenia using the MATRICS Consensus Cognitive Battery. (Reprinted with permission from Keefe et al., 2011b.)

Early-phase trials

While the MCCB has been established as the gold standard for schizophrenia registration trials, it is possible that earlier-phase work may benefit from the use of measures that assess cognition in a manner that is closer to the actual neurobiological circuits that mediate cognitive function or the pharmacological mechanism of the compound under examination. To meet the need for more precise assessment instruments for measuring changes in specific cognitive functions in treatment studies, cognitive neuroscience methods with known linkages to specific brain systems and their biochemistry provide a logical alternative assessment strategy for the cognitive impairments to be targeted in schizophrenia treatment trials. These methods can potentially distinguish specific cognitive deficits from generalized deficits. For instance, while list-learning tests may assess memory in a manner that is clinically relevant and correlated with important functional skills, the development of a treatment for memory impairment may need a more sensitive task that better reflects the biological processes involved in the acquisition and storage of representations.

A large variety of such tests are available in the cognitive neuroscience literature, many of which have been utilized in schizophrenia research (Carter and Barch, 2007; Carter et al.,

Table 13.2. Criteria for selecting which cognitive constructs and mechanisms should be used for cognition treatment studies in schizophrenia

(a)	Construct validity and link to cognitive mechanisms
(b)	Link to neural circuit
(c)	Link to neural systems through pharmacology
(d)	Availability of animal model
(e)	Amenable for use in human neuroimaging
(f)	Evidence of impairment in schizophrenia
(g)	Linked to functional outcome in schizophrenia
(h)	Good psychometric characteristics
(i)	Multisite implementation potential

2008). In order to expedite the use of these tests for early-phase drug development, the National Institute of Mental Health sponsored a series of meetings and funding sources called the Cognitive Neuroscience Treatment Research to Improve Cognition in Schizophrenia (CTNRICS). More than 140 academic and industry experts in basic cognitive neuroscience, cognitive research in schizophrenia, and treatment of schizophrenia were surveyed to determine the most important criteria for selecting which cognitive constructs and mechanisms should be used for cognition treatment studies in schizophrenia. The most highly rated criteria are listed in Table 13.2. A subset of the tests that met these criteria has been further developed for early-phase trials including the following tests assessing four cognitive constructs:

- Goal maintenance: the Dot Probe Expectancy Task (DPX), a variation on the Expectancy AX-Continuous Performance Test (CPT)
- Relational encoding and retrieval: the Relational and Item Specific Encoding Task (RISE)
- Gain control: the Contrast–Contrast Effect Task (CCE)
- Visual integration: the Jitter Orientation Visual Integration Task (JOVI)

These tests are available for download by researchers and clinical trialists at http://cntrics. ucdavis.edu/.

One of the critical issues associated with sophisticated cognitive neuroscience tests is whether these tests will manifest the substantial and consistent correlations seen between standard neuropsychological tests and indices of everyday functioning. These standard tests may be so strongly correlated with everyday functioning that they are global and nonspecific. Individuals with highly localized lesions in focal brain regions often manifest levels of everyday disability that are less than those seen in schizophrenia. Sophisticated and complex cognitive neuroscience tests may prove to be highly sensitive to focal brain functioning and only modestly sensitive to disability. If this is found, then their use for early-stage research would have to be carefully considered. As one of the primary goals of developing treatments for cognitive impairment in schizophrenia is to reduce disability, if task performance is uncorrelated with disability, then it seems implausible to think that improving performance would reduce disability.

Issues of implementation for trials using cognitive neuroscience tests

As described earlier, most of the previous work on the effects of pharmacological interventions on cognition in patients with schizophrenia has involved standard neuropsychological tests that have a long history of use in neuropsychiatric populations including schizophrenia. These tests have been chosen as outcome measures in clinical trials partly due to the ease with which they can be implemented in a standardized manner. Tests that have not been used extensively, even if expertly conceptualized, may not have the psychometric characteristics and utility necessary for use in clinical trials. The possibility of multisite trials involving cognitive neuroscience tasks, which may require more attention to the details of the methods, more complex instrumentation, and greater expertise with complex assessment methodology, present a series of challenges for our field (Keefe and Harvey, 2008). These tasks are almost always developed in a single laboratory, although different versions may be developed at multiple labs simultaneously. Usually, considerably more work has been done with healthy subjects performing these procedures. In almost all cases, cognitive neuroscience procedures involve computerized stimulus presentation and subject response data collected with electronic data capture. However, it is very important to note, and is often misunderstood, that many computerized presentations of standard tasks do not qualify as cognitive neuroscience tasks. These tests, some of which are described later, often measure the exact same constructs as does pen-and-paper testing.

As most cognitive neuroscience tasks are developed in individual laboratories, their methods allow great attention to detail and essentially no need for clear communication of assessment procedures to other investigators, who may have only modest levels of assessment (or even research) experience. Multisite clinical trials differ from these single-site investigations in a variety of ways. First, the collection of data from different testers, sites, and patient populations, and the diffusion of responsibility associated with multisite clinical trials, can reduce data quality and produce heterogeneity of results, including increased variance in scores across sites. Data quality from sites with little experience of administering cognitive tests may be particularly jeopardized. While some of these site effects (e.g., variation in characteristics of patient samples) may be controlled statistically, the systematic error that is due to administration errors across different sites cannot be controlled statistically and needs to be minimized. Control over the systematic error arising from inaccurate administration of neuropsychological tests needs to be addressed early on in the research design process.

Co-primary measures of functional capacity

This topic is discussed in great detail in Chapter 14 of this book. However, it is important to understand the measurement of functioning in the specific context of schizophrenia clinical trials that aim to satisfy regulatory expectations. The FDA historically has required a co-primary measure in cognitive enhancement studies in dementia. This requirement was designed to ensure that changes in cognition on a performance-based test led to a clinically meaningful change in everyday functioning. Similarly, a co-primary measure has been required for schizophrenia cognitive enhancement trials. The existence of this FDA requirement led to a comprehensive collaborative study, the Validation of Intermediate Measures (VIM) study (Green et al., 2011), funded by grants from the pharmaceutical industry to the Foundation for the National Institute of Mental Health (F-NIMH), comparing a variety of performance-based and interview-based outcome measures. The VIM results indicated that performance-based measures of functional capacity were superior to interview-based assessments of cognitive functioning in terms of their convergence with the MCCB, while the two sets of measures were similar in relation to interview-based assessments of functional outcomes. One of the challenges of utilizing interview-based assessments is that informants are generally needed to enhance reliability and validity (Keefe et al., 2006a). On the other hand, few existing performance-based measures were developed specifically for schizophrenia clinical trials, and may have some psychometric weaknesses such as ceiling effects (Keefe et al., 2011b) and increased practice effects.

Interview-based measures

Because these tools pose questions about common cognitive experiences, they may be considered more face valid than standard cognitive test batteries. Step-wise regression analysis indicates that both of the interview-based assessments described as follows account for significant variance in real-world functioning beyond that explained by standard cognitive test batteries and measures of functional capacity, and thus may tap into aspects of cognition not fully overlapping those assessed by standard cognitive test batteries (Keefe et al., 2006a; Ventura et al., 2010).

The Schizophrenia Cognition Rating Scale (SCoRS) is a 20-item interview-based assessment covering all seven cognitive domains tested in the MATRICS battery, and takes approximately 12 minutes to complete. It is administered separately to the patient and to an informant (family, friend, social worker, etc.). The interviewer is asked to rate the patient's level of difficulty performing various cognitive functions on a four-point scale, with four indicating that the patient is having extreme difficulty and one indicating no difficulty. Upon completion of the 20 items, the interviewer is asked to give a global rating of the patient's cognitive functioning on a scale of one to 10. After the interview is administered to both the patient and the informant, the interviewer ranks the patient on all 20 items and gives a global score, based on the responses of both the patient and informant as well as the interviewer's observations of the patient. The SCoRS is available in several languages. Empirical evaluations of the SCoRS have demonstrated high interrater reliability and moderate and significant correlations with measures of performance-based cognition, performance-based assessment of function, and real-world assessment of function. Because patient ratings have been found to account for little variance in cognitive performance, functional capacity, or real-world functioning beyond that accounted for by informant ratings (Keefe et al., 2006a), it is possible that informant ratings alone could be collected in cases when an informant has sufficient contact with the patient.

The Cognitive Assessment Interview (CAI) contains 10 items selected from a longer interview-based assessment, the CGI-CogS, by means of classical test theory and item response theory (Ventura et al., 2010). Like the SCoRS, the CAI items cover all seven MATRICS domains and are administered to patients and informants and subsequently rated by the interviewer. When an informant is not available, the CAI may be preferred over the SCoRS because the patient-only assessment demonstrates better test–retest reliability and relation to performance-based measures of cognition (Green et al., 2008). Although the CAI has fewer items, the probe questions are extensive and may require more time than those of the SCoRS (Green et al., 2011).

Additional cognitive outcome measures

In addition to the MCCB and specific cognitive neuroscience measures described previously, there are a variety of additional methods that can be used to assess cognition in schizophrenia clinical trials. Some of the available methods are described as follows.

The instruments typically used to measure cognitive function in schizophrenia fall into two main categories: (1) performance-based assessment batteries composed of standard (mostly paper-and-pencil based) neuropsychological tests; and (2) computerized performance-based test batteries. The instruments vary widely in their required testing time. A thorough neuropsychological assessment can require several hours of assessment time and enables a full evaluation of cognitive strengths and weaknesses across a broad range of neuropsychological domains. Such an assessment is usually completed or supervised by a licensed psychologist. The batteries described here are relatively brief. They capture much of the variance in overall cognition as measured by the composite score of more comprehensive batteries. The list of instruments described is not exhaustive but represents the most commonly used tools for measuring cognition in schizophrenia.

Paper-and-pencil batteries

Standard neuropsychological test batteries offer several advantages. The psychometric properties of the tests are generally well established and normative data are available in many cases. The interpersonal interaction that is fundamental to the administration of these batteries allows greater flexibility in testing people with schizophrenia, and may feel less intimidating to some patients than the computer-based batteries. An engaged tester is more likely to be able to determine reasons for odd or outlying scores. The pencil-and-paper testing process generally results in a higher completion rate than computerized tests in patients with schizophrenia (Harvey et al., 2011; Silverstein et al., 2010). The weaknesses of traditional neuropsychological tests are that they tend to require more training, refresher courses, and data review than do automated computerized batteries.

The Repeatable Battery for the Assessment of Neuropsychological Status (RBANS) is a brief (45-minute) assessment originally designed to test cognitive performance in elderly patients. It has shown utility in providing reliable assessment of cognitive performance in schizophrenia patient populations (Weber, 2003; Wilk et al., 2002). The performance of schizophrenia patients on the RBANS has been shown to be highly correlated with performance on the much longer Wechsler Adult Intelligence Scale (WAIS)-III and Wechsler Memory Test (WMS)-III batteries (Gold et al., 1999; Hobart et al., 1999). Because it was designed to be administered repeatedly, the RBANS does not suffer from large practice effects. However, because the battery was developed to test for dementia, it is composed largely of tests of memory, language, and visual perception, and may suffer from ceiling effects on some subtests when used in a schizophrenia patient population. Additionally, the battery lacks measures of motor and executive and working memory performance, cognitive domains thought to be important in the cognitive impairment observed in schizophrenia. Although it has been utilized in a few small clinical trials (Olincy et al., 2006), the RBANS is most appealing as a tool for assessment of cognition in routine clinical practice due to its relative brevity.

The Brief Assessment of Cognition in Schizophrenia (BACS) battery retains the positive attributes of the RBANS (brevity of administration and scoring, repeatability, and portability) while more completely assessing the extent of cognitive impairment over multiple domains thought to be effected by schizophrenia (executive functions, verbal fluency, attention, verbal memory, working memory, and motor speed). The BACS is available in over 30 languages, has alternate forms to minimize practice effects, requires approximately 30 minutes to complete, and is devised for easy administration and scoring. A spreadsheet is available for generation of composite scores by comparison to a normative sample of 400 healthy controls. Its sensitivity, reliability, validity, and comparability of forms have been established empirically (Keefe et al., 2004a). The BACS also has clear functional relevance, as the composite score is strongly related to functional measures such as independent living skills (r=0.45) and performance-based assessment of functioning (r=0.56) (Keefe et al., 2006b). The BACS has been used as a cognitive measure in several clinical trials (Hill et al., 2008), usually as a secondary outcome when time concerns precluded using the MCCB, and has been found to be sensitive to treatment effects (Geffen et al., 2012).

Two very short batteries are the Brief Cognitive Assessment (BCA) and the Brief Cognitive Assessment Tool for Schizophrenia (B-CATS). These batteries are compositions of existing tests that were designed to assess cognition in schizophrenia patients in 15 minutes. They have good test–retest reliability, strong correlations with larger batteries (Hurford et al., 2011; Velligan et al., 2004), and good correlations with measures of functional ability. The extreme brevity of the BCA and the B-CATS allow their use in circumstances when longer assessment is not possible due to patient tolerability or resource challenges.

Promise and challenge of computerized testing

The advantages of computerized test batteries are that they allow standardized stimulus presentation and scoring, response measures of response latencies, and immediate direct data transfer to study databases. These methods minimize rater error and reduce the costs required for human quality assurance. However, computerized testing does not eliminate the need for training. While tester administration errors are minimized, computerized methods can hide invalid assessment techniques, particularly with poorly trained testers. Computerized testing may not be valid for patients with severe impairment, low education, or less than average computer experience (Iverson et al., 2009), especially in cases where the patient–test interface requires flexibility or interruptions are possible.

The drawbacks of computerized tests can lead to a higher rate of invalid or missing data in the assessment of people with schizophrenia compared to standardized test procedures (Harvey et al., 2011; Keefe et al., 2007). As an example, in the CATIE study, the three tests with the most missing data were all computerized. In fact, by the third assessment of the patients, 407 of the 1332 (31%) cases were missing at least one data point on a computerized test, as compared to 40 out of 1332 cases (3%) with a missing assessment on the Hopkins Verbal Learning Test (HVLT). In a comparison of the various reasons that computerized and noncomputerized tests were missing at the baseline assessment of the CATIE schizophrenia trial, the most likely reasons for cognitive test data to be missing were the patient's inability to understand the task demands, computer malfunction, and patient's refusal, all of which were far greater in the computerized tests. These data are consistent with that of other studies assessing cognition in first-episode patients in industry trials. In a study of first-episode patients with schizophrenia randomized to treatment with risperidone or haloperidol, 16% of the patients were missing their CPT assessment at the baseline and another 8% were missing their three-month follow-up. In contrast, the rates of missing data for the multi-trial list learning test in that study were 4% at baseline and an additional 1% at the three-month follow-up (Harvey et al., 2005). Similar rates of attrition were reported in another first-episode study (Keefe et al., 2004b) composed solely of academic sites, where 12% of cases were missing the CPT and 4% were missing their list learning performance data.

It may be instructive to note that these testing challenges are not limited to patients with schizophrenia. Very similar rates of missing data were found in a study of the treatment of traumatic brain injury with cholinesterase inhibitors (Silver et al., 2006). In that study, every case record form for every patient was monitored for accuracy within 24 hours of assessment, and the rate of missing data on a paper-and-pencil VLT was 0%. However, data were missing from the computerized Cambridge Neuropsychological Test Automated Battery (CANTAB) assessment on up to 14% of cases across the different dependent variables.

Most recently, data utilizing a computerized test battery in a largely positive clinical trial examining the effects of a broad spectrum antipsychotic agent on symptoms and cognition found positive cognitive effects, but 40% of subjects were not able to produce valid data (Harvey et al., 2011).

These data are not presented to suggest that computerized assessments are unsuitable for use in clinical trials in schizophrenia. In fact, changes in the identical pairs version of the CPT administration system, including more practice trials and a change in the subject response required, have been associated with the substantial improvement in completion rates from the earlier studies employing the CPT (Keefe et al., 2011b). Instead, these computerized assessments need to be evaluated for their ability to be participant friendly, as well as tester friendly in order to obtain suitable completion rates in clinical trials. Although test batteries that are completely computerized may enable patients and testers to become more easily accustomed to this method than test batteries that combine computerized and pen-and-paper tests, it would be an error to assume that completely automated data collection procedures will assure that testing will be completed on all patients.

The CANTAB schizophrenia battery is composed of eight tests covering all seven of the MATRICS domains and requiring 70 minutes of assessment time. The CANTAB is presented on a touch screen computer and the nonverbal nature of most of the tests make it an ideal battery for use in multilingual contexts. The neural bases of the CANTAB tests have been well established in animal models and human imaging, thus allowing interpretation of results to be informed by this vast literature. The test–retest reliabilities of select CANTAB tests mostly appear promising (Barnett et al., 2010).

The CogState schizophrenia battery is composed of eight tests covering all seven of the domains of cognition recommended by the MATRICS initiative. Composite scores for the CogState schizophrenia battery correlate strongly with MCCB composite scores in schizophrenia subjects ($r=0.83$), while correlations between CogState and MCCB domain scores ranged from moderate to strong (Pietrzak et al., 2009). The battery requires approximately 35 minutes to complete and is suitable for testing in most countries due to the use of culture-neutral stimuli. The battery has been used in a few recent clinical trials, with some potential sensitivity to treatment effects reported in abstracts (Harvey et al., 2011; Hosford et al., 2011) and press releases but as of this printing not yet in the peer-reviewed literature.

The Cognitive Drug Research (CDR) battery was designed for repeated testing in clinical trials and has been used to study effects of disease and treatment on cognition in a variety of conditions, including schizophrenia. The standard CDR can be completed in approximately 20 minutes and assesses the domains of power of attention, continuity of attention, working memory, episodic memory, and speed of memory. Individual tests can be removed from or added to the battery, which relies heavily on timed testing. The CDR has been translated into close to 60 languages and has more than 70 parallel forms.

References

American Psychological Association. (1999). *Standards for Educational and Psychological Testing*. Washington, DC: APA Publications.

AstraZeneca and Targacept announce results from trial of AZD3480 for cognitive dysfunction in schizophrenia. (2008). Available at: http://www.news-medical.net/news/2008/12/10/43968.aspx (Accessed: November 6, 2011).

Barnett, J. H., Robbins, T. W., Leeson, V. C., et al. (2010). Assessing cognitive function in clinical trials of schizophrenia. *Neuroscience and Biobehavioral Reviews*, **34**, 1161–1177.

Bowie, C. R., Reichenberg, A., Rieckmann, N., et al. (2004). Stability and functional correlates of memory-based classification in older schizophrenia patients. *American Journal of Geriatric Psychiatry*, **12**, 376–378.

Bonner-Jackson, A., Grossman, L. S., Harrow, M., et al. (2010). Neurocognition in schizophrenia: a 20-year multi-follow-up of the course of processing speed and stored knowledge. *Comprehensive Psychiatry*, **51**, 471–479.

Buchanan, R. W., Davis, M., Goff, D., et al. (2005). A summary of the FDA-NIMH-MATRICS workshop on clinical trial designs for neurocognitive drugs for schizophrenia. *Schizophrenia Bulletin*, **31**, 5–19.

Buchanan, R. W., Javitt, D. C., Marder, S. R., et al. (2007). The Cognitive and Negative Symptoms in Schizophrenia Trial (CONSIST): the efficacy of glutamatergic agents for negative symptoms and cognitive impairments. *American Journal of Psychiatry*, **164**, 1593–1602.

Buchanan, R. W., Conley, R. R., Dickinson, D., et al. (2008). Galantamine for the treatment of cognitive impairments in people with schizophrenia. *American Journal of Psychiatry*, **165**, 82–89.

Buchanan, R. W., Keefe, R. S. E., Umbricht, D., et al. (2011a). The FDA-NIMH-MATRICS guidelines for clinical trial design of cognitive-enhancing drugs: what do we know

5 years later? *Schizophrenia Bulletin*, **37**, 1209–1217.

Buchanan, R. W., Keefe, R. S., Lieberman, J. A., et al. (2011b). A randomized clinical trial of MK-0777 for the treatment of cognitive impairments in people with schizophrenia. *Biological Psychiatry*, **69**, 442–449.

Carter, C. S. & Barch, D. M. (2007). Cognitive neuroscience-based approaches to measuring and improving treatment effects on cognition in schizophrenia. The CNTRICS initiative. *Schizophrenia Bulletin*, **33**, 1131–1137.

Carter, C. S., Heckers, S., Nichols, T., et al. (2008). CNTRICS final task selection: social cognitive and affective neuroscience-based measures. *Schizophrenia Bulletin*, **35**, 153–162.

Cohen, J. (1977). *Statistical Power Analysis for the Behavioral Sciences*. New York, NY: Academic Press.

Davidson, M., Galderisi, S., Weiser, M., et al. (2009). Cognitive effects of antipsychotic drugs in first-episode schizophrenia and schizophreniform disorder: a randomized, open-label clinical trial (EUFEST). *American Journal of Psychiatry*, **166**, 675–682.

Eack, S. M., Greenwald, D. P., Hogarty, S. S., et al. (2009). Cognitive enhancement therapy for early-course schizophrenia: effects of a two-year randomized controlled trial. *Psychiatric Services*, **60**, 1468–1476.

Eack, S. M., Hogarty, G. E., Cho, R. Y., et al. (2010). Neuroprotective effects of cognitive enhancement therapy against gray matter loss in early schizophrenia: results from a 2-year randomized controlled trial. *Archives of General Psychiatry*, **67**, 674–682.

Friedman, J. I., Carpenter, D., Lu, J., et al. (2008). A pilot study of adjunctive atomoxetine treatment to second-generation antipsychotics for cognitive impairment in schizophrenia. *Journal of Clinical Psychopharmacology*, **28**, 59–63.

Geffen, Y., Keefe, R., Rabinowtiz, J., et al. (2012). BL-1020 a new GABA-enhanced antipsychotic: results of six-week, randomized, double-blind, controlled, efficacy and safety study. [In Press].

Goff, D. C., Lamberti, J. S., Leon, A. C., et al. (2008a). A placebo-controlled add-on trial of the Ampakine, CX516, for cognitive deficits in schizophrenia. *Neuropsychopharmacology*, 33, 465–472.

Goff, D. D., Cather, C., Gottlieb, J. D., et al. (2008b). Once-weekly D-cycloserine effects on negative symptoms and cognition in schizophrenia: an exploratory study. *Schizophrenia Research*, 106, 320–327.

Gold, J. M., Queern, C., Iannone, V. N., et al. (1999). Repeatable battery for the assessment of neuropsychological status as a screening test in schizophrenia, I: sensitivity, reliability, and validity. *American Journal of Psychiatry*, 156, 1944–1950.

Green, M. F., Nuechterlein, K. H., Gold, J. M., et al. (2004). Approaching a consensus cognitive battery for clinical trials in schizophrenia: the NIMH-MATRICS conference to select cognitive domains and test criteria. *Biological Psychiatry*, 56, 301–307.

Green, M. F., Nuechterlein, K. H., Kern, R. S, et al. (2008). Functional co-primary measures for clinical trials in schizophrenia: results from the MATRICS psychometric and standardization study. *American Journal of Psychiatry*, 165, 221–228.

Green, M. F., Schooler, N. R., Kern, R. S., et al. (2011). Evaluation of functionally meaningful measures for clinical trials of cognition enhancement in schizophrenia. *American Journal of Psychiatry*, 168, 400–407.

Harvey, P. D., Rabinowitz, J., Eerdekens, M., et al. (2005). Treatment of cognitive impairment in early psychosis: a comparison of risperidone and haloperidol in a large long-term trial. *American Journal of Psychiatry*, 162, 1888–1895.

Harvey, P. D., Green, M. F., Nuechterlein, K. H. (2010). Latest developments in the MATRICS process. *Psychiatry (Edgmont)*, 7, 49–52.

Harvey, P., Pikalov, A., Cucchiaro, J., et al. (2011). Cognitive performance in patients with acute schizophrenia treated with Lurasidone: a double-blind, placebo-controlled trial. Abstract/poster presented at the 51st Annual NCDEU Meeting, Boca Raton, FL, June 13–16.

Hill, S. K., Sweeney, J. A., Hamer, R. M., et al. (2008). Efficiency of the CATIE and BACS neuropsychological batteries in assessing cognitive effects of antipsychotic treatments in schizophrenia. *Journal of the International Neuropsychological Society*, 14, 209–221.

Hilt, D., Meltzer, H., Gawry, M., et al. (2011). EVP-6124, and Alpha-7 nicotinic partial agonist, produces positive effects on cognition, clinical function, and negative symptoms in patients with chronic schizophrenia on stable antipsychotic therapy. Abstract/poster presented at the 50th ACNP Annual Meeting, Waikoloa, HI, December 4–8.

Hobart, M. P., Goldberg, R., Bartko, J. J., et al. (1999). Repeatable battery for the assessment of neuropsychological status as a screening test in schizophrenia, II: convergent/discriminant validity and diagnostic group comparisons. *American Journal of Psychiatry*, 156, 1951–1957.

Honer, W. G., Thornton, A. E., Chen, E. Y., et al. (2006). Clozapine alone versus clozapine and risperidone with refractory schizophrenia. *New England Journal of Medicine*, 354, 472–482.

Hosford, D., Dunbar, G., Lieberman, J., et al. (2011). The alpha7 neuronal nicotinic receptor (NNR) modulator TC-5619 had beneficial effects and was generally well tolerated in a phase 2 trial in cognitive dysfunction in schizophrenia (CDS). Abstract/poster presented at the 50th ACNP Annual Meeting, Waikoloa, HI, December 4–8.

Hurford, I. M., Marder, S. R., Keefe, R. S. E., et al. (2011). A brief cognitive assessment tool for schizophrenia: construction of a tool for clinicians. *Schizophrenia Bulletin*, 37, 538–545.

Iverson, G. L., Brooks, B. L., Ashton, V. L., et al. (2009). Does familiarity with computers affect computerized neuropsychological test performance? *Journal of Clinical and Experimental Neuropsychology*, 31, 594–604.

Javitt, D. C., Buchanan, R. W., Keefe, R. S. E., et al. (2011). Effect of the neuroprotective peptide davunetide (AL-108) on cognition and functional capacity in schizophrenia. *Schizophrenia Research* [Epub ahead of print].

Kane, J. M., D'Souza, D. C., Patkar, A. A., et al. (2010). Armodafinil as adjunctive therapy in adults with cognitive deficits associated with schizophrenia: a 4-week, double-blind, placebo-controlled study. *Journal of Clinical Psychiatry*, **71**, 1475–1481.

Keefe, R. S. E., Goldberg, T. E., Harvey, P. D., et al. (2004a). The brief assessment of cognition in schizophrenia: reliability, sensitivity, and comparison with a standard neurocognitive battery. *Schizophrenia Research*, **68**, 283–297.

Keefe, R. S. E., Seidman, L. J., Christensen, B. K., et al. (2004b). Comparative effect of atypical and conventional antipsychotic drugs on neurocognition in first-episode psychosis: a randomized double-blind trial of olanzapine versus low-dose haloperidol. *American Journal of Psychiatry*, **161**, 985–995.

Keefe, R. S. E., Poe, M., Walker, T. M., et al. (2006a). The Schizophrenia Cognition Rating Scale (SCoRS): interview-based assessment and its relationship to cognition, real-world functioning and functional capacity. *American Journal of Psychiatry*, **163**, 426–432.

Keefe, R. S., Poe, M., Walker, T. M., et al. (2006b). The relationship of the brief assessment of cognition in schizophrenia (BACS) to functional capacity and real-world functional outcome. *Journal of Clinical and Experimental Neuropsychology*, **28**, 260–269.

Keefe, R. S. E., Bilder, R. M., Davis, S. M., et al. (2007). Neurocognitive effects of antipsychotic medications in patients with chronic schizophrenia in the CATIE trial. *Archives of General Psychiatry*, **64**, 633–647.

Keefe, R. S. & Harvey, P. D. (2008). Implementation considerations for multisite clinical trials with cognitive neuroscience tasks. *Schizophrenia Bulletin*, **34**, 656–663.

Keefe, R. S. E. & Kraus, M. S. (2009). Measuring memory-prediction errors and their consequences in youth at risk for schizophrenia. *Annals of the Academy of Medicine, Singapore*, **38**, 414–416.

Keefe, R. S., Buchanan, R. W., Marder, S. R., et al. (2011a). Clinical trials of potential cognitive-enhancing drugs in schizophrenia: what have we learned so far? *Schizophrenia Bulletin* [Epub ahead of print].

Keefe, R. S., Fox, K. H., Harvey, P. D., et al. (2011b). Characteristics of the MATRICS Consensus Cognitive Battery in a 29-site antipsychotic schizophrenia clinical trial. *Schizophrenia Research*, **125**, 161–168.

Kelly, D. L., Buchanan, R. W., Boggs, D. L., et al. (2009). A randomized double-blind trial of atomoxetine for cognitive impairments in 32 people with schizophrenia. *Journal of Clinical Psychiatry*, **70**, 518–525.

Kern, R. S., Nuechterlein, K. H., Green, M. F., et al. (2008). The MATRICS Consensus Cognitive Battery, part 2: co-norming and standardization. *American Journal of Psychiatry*, **165**, 214–220.

Kraemer, H. C., Mintz, J., Noda, A., et al. (2006). Caution regarding the use of pilot studies to guide power calculations for study proposals. *Archives of General Psychiatry*, **63**, 484–489.

Leon, A. C. (2008). Implications of clinical trial design on sample size requirements. *Schizophrenia Bulletin*, **34**, 664–669.

Leon, A. C., Davis, L. L., Kraemer, H. C. (2011) The role and interpretation of pilot studies in clinical research. *Journal of Psychiatric Research*, **46**, 626–629.

Levkovitz, Y., Mendlovich, S., Riwkes, S., et al. (2010). A double-blind, randomized study of minocycline for the treatment of negative and cognitive symptoms in early-phase schizophrenia. *Journal of Clinical Psychiatry*, **71**, 138–149.

Lieberman, J. A., Papadakis, K., Csernansky, J., et al. (2009). A randomized, placebo-controlled study of memantine as adjunctive treatment in patients with schizophrenia. *Neuropsychopharmacology*, **34**, 1322–1329.

Marder, S. R. (2011). Lessons from MATRICS. *Schizophrenia Bulletin*, **37**, 233–234.

Memory Pharmaceuticals Achieves Enrollment Goal for Phase 2 Study of MEM 3454 in Cognitive Impairment Associated with Schizophrenia (2008). Available at: http://www.life-sciences-germany.com/news/press-release-memory-pharmaceuticals-corporation-roche-group-2008-2001-89665.html. (Accessed: November 6, 2011).

Nuechterlein, K. H., Green, M. F., Kern, R. S., et al. (2008). The MATRICS consensus cognitive battery: Part 1. Test selection, reliability, and validity. *American Journal of Psychiatry*, **165**, 203–213.

Olincy, A., Harris, J. G., Johnson, L. L., et al. (2006). Proof-of-concept trial of an alpha7 nicotinic agonist in schizophrenia. *Archives of General Psychiatry*, **63**, 630–638.

Pietrzak, R. H., Olver, J., Norman, T., et al. (2009). A comparison of the CogState schizophrenia battery and the measurement and treatment research to improve cognition in schizophrenia (MATRICS) battery in assessing cognitive impairment in chronic schizophrenia. *Journal of Clinical and Experimental Neuropsychology*, **31**, 848–859.

Rund, B. R. (1998). A review of longitudinal studies of cognitive functions in schizophrenia patients. *Schizophrenia Bulletin*, **24**, 425–435.

Silver, J. M., Koumaras, B., Chen, M., et al. (2006). The effects of rivastigmine on cognitive function in patients with traumatic brain injury. *Neurology*, **67**, 748–755.

Silverstein, S. M., Jaeger, J., Donovan-Lepore, A. M., et al. (2010). A comparative study of the MATRICS and IntegNeuro cognitive assessment batteries. *Journal of Clinical and Experimental Neuropsychology*, **32**, 937–952.

Sponheim, S. R., Jung, R. E., Seidman, L. J., et al. (2010). Cognitive deficits in recent-onset and chronic schizophrenia. *Journal of Clinical Research*, **44**, 421–428.

Velligan, D. I., DiCocco, M., Bow-Thomas, C. C, et al. (2004). A brief cognitive assessment for use with schizophrenia patients in community clinics. *Schizophrenia Research*, **71**, 273–283.

Ventura, J., Reise, S. P., Keefe, R. S. E., et al. (2010). The Cognitive Assessment Interview (CAI): development and validation of an empirically derived, brief interview-based measure of cognition. *Schizophrenia Research*, **121**, 24–31.

Weber, B. (2003). RBANS has reasonable test–retest reliability in schizophrenia. *Evidence Based Mental Health*, **6**, 22.

Wilk, C. M., Gold, J. M., Bartko, J. J., et al. (2002). Test–retest stability of the repeatable battery for the assessment of neuropsychological status in schizophrenia. *American Journal of Psychiatry*, **159**, 838–844.

Wykes, T., Reeder, C., Landau, S., et al. (2009). Does age matter? Effects of cognitive rehabilitation across the age span. *Schizophrenia Research*, **113**, 252–258.

Zanello, A., Curtis, L., Badan, BâM., et al. (2009). Working memory impairments in first-episode psychosis and chronic schizophrenia. *Psychiatric Research*, **165**, 10–18.

Performance-based measures of functioning in schizophrenia

Colin A. Depp, Laura Vergel de Dios, Brent Mausbach, and Thomas Patterson

Introduction

Over the past decade, a substantial amount of research attention has been paid to the measurement of everyday functional outcomes in schizophrenia. Two concurrent trends have increased the emphasis on measurement of everyday functioning in schizophrenia, which had previously not received the same rigorous attention as had the quantification of cognitive deficits or psychotic symptoms. First, stakeholders from consumer, family, and mental health agency groups have raised the prominence of recovery in mental health treatment. While no consensus definition exists, the core elements of recovery typically center on functional outcomes (e.g., employment, independence) rather than on symptom alleviation (Bellack, 2006). Second, the recognition of the high prevalence and severity of cognitive impairments in schizophrenia has led to a number of international initiatives that are paving the way for clinical trials of cognitive remediation strategies described elsewhere in this volume (e.g., Measurement and Treatment Research to Improve Cognition in Schizophrenia [MATRICS], Treatment Units for Research on Neurocognition and Schizophrenia [TURNS], and Cognitive Neuroscience Treatment Research to Improve Cognition in Schizophrenia [CNTRICS]). In considering what the endpoint of such clinical trials should be, a joint U.S. Food and Drug Administration (FDA) and National Institute of Mental Health (NIMH) panel on cognitive remediation in schizophrenia led to the determination that functional outcomes should be included as a "co-primary" outcome in such studies (Buchanan et al., 2005). This determination was based on the notion that functional outcomes are more face-valid and meaningful to stakeholders than are measures of neurocognitive performance. Subsequently, the demand emerged to rigorously measure functional outcomes that are reliable, valid, and sensitive to change.

Unfortunately for the practical need, the measurement of functioning turns out to be quite challenging. By everyday functioning we mean the capacity to perform (or the actual performance of) daily tasks that are essential for maintenance of social and occupational roles (Marcotte & Grant, 2009). As a construct, functional outcome has been measured by diverse methods ranging from self-report, clinician report, proxy report (from family members or other informants), verifiable milestones such as employment and residential independence, and performance-based measures. A number of psychometric studies conducted over the past decade have indicated that, among these various methods, performance-based measures possess advantages in the assessment of functional outcomes in schizophrenia, particularly in clinical trials. In this chapter, we describe the role of performance-based measures in assessing functional outcomes in schizophrenia; we provide

Cognitive Impairment in Schizophrenia, ed. Philip D. Harvey. Published by Cambridge University Press. © Cambridge University Press 2013.

a practical overview of the most commonly used measures, and we describe recent evidence for these measures' psychometric properties and validity. We conclude with a discussion of areas in need of further development and research.

What are performance-based measures?

As a class, performance-based assessments of functioning share several characteristics. Each involves a standardized set of stimuli with which a respondent is presented, and these stimuli invoke one or a number of life skills that are evaluated relative to normative performance. Importantly, the stimuli and life skills are designed to maximize ecological validity, approximating real-life contexts for the rated behaviors. Thus, the goal is to simulate, as closely as possible, the features of a common situation that would be encountered in a real-world setting, yet in which the respondent's skill–performance can be evaluated in a standardized and objective manner in a laboratory setting. Performance-based measures are similar in some respects to direct observation of task performance, with the difference that behaviors are observed in a simulated rather than a real-world environment. Performance-based measures differ with respect to their focus on specific skills, ranging from multi-domain assessments of various independent living skills (e.g., managing medications or finances) to assessments focused on specific abilities (e.g., social functioning) (see Table 14.1 for examples in schizophrenia). Most commonly, these tests involve interaction with tangible "props" that seek to recreate an environment (e.g., bus schedules), although virtual and computerized tasks are emerging and are described later in this chapter.

There is a long history of use of performance-based measures in the assessment of disability in older adults (for review, see Moore et al., 2007). More recently, these measures have been applied to schizophrenia and other mental health problems. Moore et al. (2007) comprehensively reviewed 31 performance-based instruments designed for both patient populations (of various disorders) and healthy controls. Notably, the review concluded that while a majority of measures possessed good internal consistency as well as concurrent validity (correspondence with other measures such as self-report and neurocognitive tests), measures varied in regard to their predictive validity; that is, their ability to predict actual real-world functioning. At the time of that review, only two measures (the University of California at San Diego [UCSD] Performance-Based Skills Assessment [UPSA] and the Independent Living Scales [ILS]) had appreciable data in psychiatric populations, and since that time a number of additional measures have generated data and more validation studies have been conducted.

Conceptual role of performance-based measures in identifying the determinants of disability in schizophrenia

Performance-based tasks assess for the quality of functional skills, performed under ideal conditions, what is typically referred to as functional capacity. In other words, performance-based measures assess what one "can do," whereas other functional measurement modalities identify what an individual "actually does." Among people with schizophrenia, it is clear that while an individual may possess the capacity to perform tasks of independent living (e.g., read a bus schedule), he/she may encounter a number of barriers to engaging in those tasks in the real world. Barriers may include diminished motivation and other negative symptoms (e.g., avolition), positive symptoms (e.g., paranoia limiting willingness to use public transportation), and environmental factors (e.g., lack of financial

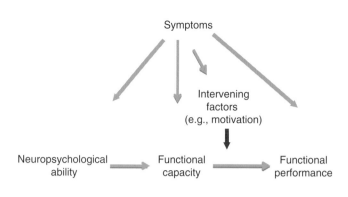

Figure 14.1. Model specifying the role of measures of functional capacity.

resources). Functional capacity, as measured by performance-based assessments, consists of the skills underlying everyday functional behaviors – skills that are necessary but sometimes not sufficient to engage successfully in functionally relevant behaviors.

Accordingly, a number of studies have used structural equation modeling to evaluate the relationships among indicators of neurocognitive ability, functional capacity as measured by performance-based measures, and clinician- and informant-rated measures (Figure 14.1). Bowie et al. (2008) found that the best-fitting model in schizophrenia, more recently replicated in a different sample (Bowie et al., 2010), is one in which performance-based measures of functioning mediate the relationship between neurocognitive ability and real-world functioning. In other words, the influence of cognitive impairment in reducing functioning is dependent, to a large extent, on the capacity to perform those functional tasks. Thus, if future interventions could improve cognitive ability in schizophrenia, these improvements should be observable on performance-based measures of functioning, which would in turn produce improvement in real-world functional performance. In addition, scores on performance-based measures appear largely unrelated to positive psychotic symptoms in schizophrenia. For this reason, performance-based measures are useful in clinical trials (such as for cognitive remediation), in which the treatment would not be expected to affect positive symptoms.

Advantages of performance-based measures over other modalities
Avoidance of self-report biases
Self-report measures of functioning that are frequently employed in evaluating persons with schizophrenia include the World Health Organization Disability Assessment Schedule (WHODAS) and SF-36. The advantages of self-report are the ease of administration and lack of any requirement for props or informants. Nevertheless, a substantial body of literature suggests that self-reported ratings of functioning among people with schizophrenia do not correspond well with clinician and informant reports. Indeed, accurate self-appraisal is difficult even for persons without psychiatric illnesses, due to various cognitive biases in global ratings of performance, such as overemphasis on recent or salient experiences (Podsakoff et al., 2003). In schizophrenia, poor insight into one's illness and behavior further reduces the accuracy of self-reports, often contributing to overestimation of one's ability to perform tasks.

A number of studies have examined the predictors of inaccuracy in self-report of functioning in schizophrenia. Bowie et al. (2007) assessed 67 patients with schizophrenia and their informants. Patients' self-reports of their functional status were related to their subjective ratings of their quality of life, but unrelated to their actual performance on functional capacity and neuropsychological tests as well as to informant reports of their functional status. Patients were categorized as "underestimated," "overestimated," or "accurate," based on the convergence (or lack thereof) between their self-reports and reports by informants. Patients who accurately rated their functional status tended to have better social skills, while overestimating patients were the most cognitively and functionally impaired.

Variation in informant validity

Because of their concerns about the validity of self-reports, researchers often turn to informant reports, either from clinicians or nonclinician family members and close associates. Examples of such instruments include the Specific Levels of Functioning Scale (SLOF) (Schneider & Struening, 1983) and the Independent Living Skills Survey (ILSS) (Wallace, 2000). For example, the ILSS-informant is rated on a zero (never) to four (always) scale with a "no opportunity" choice available for those tasks that some patients may not have the opportunity to perform in their community.

A common problem for many patients is the lack of available or knowledgeable informants, whether family, friends, or clinicians. Anecdotal evidence suggests that it is often difficult to obtain ratings from treating clinicians due to constraints on their time. In addition, informant- and clinician-rated measures vary considerably in their degree of convergence with patient self-report and performance-based measures. This was among the initial findings from the Validating Real-World Outcomes (VALERO) study, whose aim is to identify the best scales for measuring real-world functioning (Harvey et al., 2011). The investigators assessed patients with schizophrenia on neurocognitive tests (MATRICS Consensus Cognitive Battery [MCCB]) and functional capacity tests (UPSA-B, advanced finances of the Everyday Functioning Battery [EFB]), and they had informants, participants, and the interviewer complete several real-world functional outcomes rating scales (SLOF, ILSS, among others).

Sabbag et al. (2011) analyzed whether patient self-reports of real-world functioning were related to informant reports (friend/family or clinician), and whether the patient's or the informant's rating was better related to the patient's actual performance on tests of functioning and cognition. Out of six scales, patient and friend/family reports correlated on four scales, while patient and clinician reports correlated on only two scales. In terms of convergence of functional rating scales with performance measures, only one out of 12 correlations were significant for the patient and friend/relative informant. However, with the small group of clinician informants, four out of six rating scales correlated with functional performance tests, and two out of six scales correlated with performance on neuropsychological measures.

Limited responsiveness of functional milestones

The attainment of such functional milestones as marriage, employment, and independent living are the ultimate indicators of functional success in the community. In a sense, all other measures can be considered proxy indicators of these attainments. Yet there are problems with using such milestones as endpoints in clinical trials. First, the base rate of certain functional attainments is often low in schizophrenia (e.g., fewer than 20% of patients are employed in paid work), and there is an unfortunately low likelihood that, within a six-month period of a clinical trial, functional milestones will change (Buchanan et al., 2011). Second, socioeconomic status and environmental factors vary substantially among patients, and such factors as the availability of disability payments make it such that patients with similar capacity to perform activities may face different barriers to the attainment of functional milestones. Such variation is particularly evident when comparing patients with schizophrenia residing in different countries. Harvey et al. (2009) compared patients with schizophrenia in Sweden to those dwelling in the United States on a performance-based measure of functioning (UPSA) and functional milestones such as independent living. Scores and psychometric properties of the UPSA in both countries were nearly identical, yet the rate of residential independence was markedly different between countries.

Infeasibility of direct observation

One might consider the direct observation of individuals performing functional tasks (e.g., medication management) in their natural living environments as a "gold standard" for functional assessment. Such studies have recently been conducted, using video capture and coding of behaviors (Bromley et al., 2011). The obvious problems with this in-person observation, and the reasons why it is rarely employed, are that continuous observation in outpatient environments is time consuming, impractical, and limited to only a subset of contexts in which the patient engages in functional activity. Moreover, the influence of being observed on the quality of functional performance is difficult to disentangle from the data.

Limitations of performance-based measures

Due to the limitations of alternative approaches to functional outcome measurement described earlier, performance-based measures can seem attractive to those conducting observational research and clinical trials. However, performance-based measures have their own limitations. Specifically, these measures generally require physical props, and they must be administered by trained raters, as is the case with neuropsychological testing. These factors limit the utility of performance-based measures in community settings. Moreover, these instruments are also limited in their applicability to cultural groups that lack exposure to or need for the skills being tested. For example, in communities where bank account ownership is rare, a test of financial management using a checkbook would likely not be able to distinguish the influences of cultural norms from impairment arising from schizophrenia. In addition, performance-based measures require effort on the participant's part, and as is the case in neuropsychological testing, poor effort may exaggerate deficits. Thus, an overall conclusion from the growing literature on measurement of functional outcomes is that each measurement modality has specific limitations and that researchers and clinicians must be aware of these limitations in interpreting functional data.

Specific performance-based measures

In what follows, we review the characteristics of some of the more frequently employed performance-based measures of functioning in schizophrenia. We describe the format, content, and available studies on reliability and validity of these measures in patients with schizophrenia. Table 14.1 summarizes the basic characteristics of selected measures.

Table 14.1. Characteristics of selected performance-based measures

Name of measure	Domains measured	Administration time (min)	Scoring	Props required
Direct Assessment of Functional Skills (Klapow et al., 1997)	Time orientation, cooking, communication, eating, transportation, shopping, finances	25	0–106	Yes–grocery items
Advanced Finances from Everyday Functioning Battery (Heaton et al., 2004)	Finances (also contains subtests on shopping, cooking, and medication management that have not been reported in schizophrenia)	40	0–13	Yes–mock checks, checkbook register, mock medication pills and dispenser, recipe and ingredients
Independent Living Skills (Wallace et al., 2000)	Memory/orientation, money management, home and transportation, health and safety, and social adjustment	45	0–140	Yes–driver's license, credit card, key
Maryland Assessment of Social Competence (Bellack et al., 1990)	Social skills and communication	20	1–5	No
Medication Management Ability Assessment (Patterson et al., 2002)	Medication adherence	15	0–25	Yes–mock medication and pills
Micro-Module Learning Test (Silverstein, 1998)	Memory, comprehension, ability to learn using feedback	30–50	0–48 or 0–42 (depending on version)	Yes–index card with paragraphs and video tape of demonstration
Social Skills Performance Assessment (Patterson et al., 2001b)	Social skills and communication	12	1–5	No
Test of Adaptive Behavior in Schizophrenia (Velligan et al., 2007)	Medication adherence, empty bathroom, shopping, closet, work skills	30–40	0–100	Yes–map, picture of empty bathroom, medication pills/bottle, prop money, doll clothes, stack of flyers

Table 14.1. (cont.)

Name of measure	Domains measured	Administration time (min)	Scoring	Props required
UCSD Performance-based Skills Assessment (Patterson et al., 2001a)	Household, communication, finances, transportation, planning	30	0–100	Yes–phone, bus map, money, grocery items
UCSD Performance-based Skills Assessment-Brief (Mausbach et al., 2007)	Communication, finances	10–15	0–100	Yes–money, phone

Direct Assessment of Functional Status (DAFS) scale (Klapow et al., 1997)
Test components (taken from Zanetti, 1998):

Time orientation: participant must be able to read a clock correctly and state the date, day, month, and year.

Communication: participants are tested on telephone skills – dialing a number from memory, a letter, a list of other numbers, etc., and must do everything they would do when using a telephone (i.e., pick up the phone, dial, hang up). They must also correctly mail out a letter to a given address and use their own return address.

Transportation: the interviewer asks the participant to identify a driver's correct response to road signs.

Finances: participants must write a check correctly, balance a checkbook, identify coins, count money, and make correct change.

Shopping: subjects are given a list of grocery items, and after a 10-minute delay, they are required to recall the items, recognize them on a larger list, and then pick out the actual items from a "mock" store.

Grooming: participants are tested on how to brush their teeth, wash their face, brush their hair, put on a coat, and tie their shoes correctly.

Eating: participants must illustrate correctly how they would eat steak and soup and describe the correct steps involved in doing so (i.e., cut the steak, take a bite).

Administration and scoring
The possible range of scores on the DAFS is 0–106. Administration takes about 25 minutes per subject.

Reliability and validity
Interrater reliability according to its authors (Klapow et al., 1997) was 0.91. Another publication (Patterson et al., 1998) reported a 0.93 reliability. The DAFS was significantly correlated ($r=0.43$) to a patient's actual independent living situation as measured on

a scale of 1–4 (1=totally dependent; 2=very dependent; 3=moderately dependent; 4=totally independent) (Palmer et al., 2002).

Maryland Assessment of Social Competence (MASC) (Bellack et al., 1990)

This test examines an individual's ability to resolve interpersonal dilemmas through conversation. It is a role play task that involves a series of three-minute conversations with a live confederate who acts as the protagonist in the scenario.

Test components

There is first a 90-second practice role play to orient the participant to this task. A description of the task scenario is presented to the individual on an index card and they must respond correctly with what role they will be playing in the scenario to move forward. Then an audio recording that describes the role play situation is played and then the confederate begins the interaction. The confederate presents a new perspective on the situation at approximately one-minute and two-minute marks of each interaction. For example, in the scene that requires the individual to talk to their landlord about fixing a leak, the first minute consists of the confederate seeming too busy for the problem; the second minute turns the situation on the participant as the confederate asks he/she what they have done about the problem; and then the confederate begins to cooperate during the last minute.

Administration and scoring

The role-plays are videotaped and scored by a trained rater and in most cases by a second rater. The participants are scored on a five-point Likert scale in three subcategories: conversational content (CC), nonverbal content (NC), and overall effectiveness (E). This task takes approximately 20 minutes to administer.

Reliability and validity

Test–retest reliability after a four-week period was good (CC, ICC=0.68; NC, ICC=0.66; E, ICC=0.69) (Green et al., 2011). The MASC is significantly correlated to both the Direct Assessment of Functional Status (DAFS, r=0.70 total score) as well as the Quality of Well-Being score (QWB, r=0.47 total score) (Patterson et al., 2001).

Micro-Module Learning Test (MMLT)

This test was developed to serve as a predictor of skills training outcomes as well as a measure of changed capacity of skills after participating in skills training interventions. The MMLT is a dynamic assessment, meaning that a participant is not scored solely on their ability to answer a question correctly or incorrectly, but rather on their ability to learn from their mistakes if they initially answer the question incorrectly. Because of this unique design, there are seven different yet psychometrically equivalent versions of the MMLT to allow for retesting.

Test components

Comprehend verbal instruction: the tester reads the participant two paragraphs from the University of California Los Angeles (UCLA) Social and Independent Living Skills module and asks three to four questions per paragraph to assess the individual's comprehension skills. If the question is answered correctly, the assessor moves on to the next question. If the question is answered incorrectly, they read a simplified version and the participant is re-asked the same question and moves on to the next question if he/she gets it right. If that answer is still wrong, the assessor reads the simplest version of the text, highlighting the correct answers with cued inflections to make the answer obvious to the participant. Regardless of whether the participant gets the answer correct, the next question is asked.

Comprehend visual demonstration (modeling): this is the same idea as the verbal instruction task except the participant watches a video that demonstrates one of the skills that was in the paragraphs read in the first task. There are six questions asked with the same protocol as detailed earlier – the participant gets three opportunities to answer a comprehension question correctly. Each time he/she answers incorrectly, a shortened version of the video is shown and on the last try, the assessor verbally explains the correct answer.

Role play: after viewing the video, the participant is asked to physically practice the skills that were demonstrated to him/her. There are five to six correct behaviors and these must all be illustrated to be scored as complete. If the participant does not complete this task correctly the first time, the assessor gives verbal feedback that details the incorrect or missing behaviors and the participant tries again. If the participant still does not complete the task correctly, the assessor gives a lengthier, more detailed feedback highlighting what the participant must do. Finally, if the participant still performs incorrectly, the tape is replayed and they must practice one final time to get any points.

Administration and scoring

For each of the three subtasks, a score of three is given if they give the correct response without any further prompting or explanations. A score of two is given if they get the answer correct after the first simplification of instructions. A score of one is given if the participant gets it correct after even further explanation, while a score of zero results from incorrect responses throughout the entire task. Each of the seven versions of the MMLT take approximately 30–50 minutes to administer.

Reliability and validity

In a small clinical sample, test–retest correlations over three-month intervals were impressive, although only eight of the 15 patients with schizophrenia had a repeat assessment (verbal instruction, 0.58, visual comprehension 0.072, role play, 0.68, overall, 0.73) (Silverstein, 2008). The MMLT was significantly correlated with several cognitive assessments, such as verbal fluency measured by (FAS) (r=0.66), verbal memory measured by Trial 5 of the Rey Auditory Verbal Learning Test (RAVLT) (r=0.60), and the theory of mind task (r=0.77) (Silverstein et al., 1998).

University of California San Diego Performance-Based Skills Assessment (Patterson et al., 2001a)

The University of California San Diego UPSA was developed in 2001 by Patterson et al. Its original purpose was to assess functioning in middle-aged and elderly patients with schizophrenia in the context of a skills–training intervention study. The test is divided into five subtests that assess different skills necessary for community functioning. It is important to note that some publications reporting on UPSA scores used a revised version (UPSA-2) that has minor changes to a few subtests. For example, in the UPSA-2, locations are altered to fit the region where the test is being administered, and the finances subtest does not require the writing of a check.

Test components

Household chores: participants are given a recipe for rice pudding and presented with a mock pantry containing some but not all of the ingredients as well as a number of distractor items. Participants are then asked to make a shopping list of the missing recipe ingredients.

Communication: participants are given a prop telephone and asked what number they would dial in the case of an emergency and what number to call for directory assistance. They then dial a phone number from memory and follow instructions on a mock medical appointment reminder letter to leave a voice mail to reschedule their appointment. Last, participants must recall the instructions listed in the letter for preparing for the medical appointment (bring your medical insurance card; no food or water for 12 hours before the appointment).

Finance: participants are presented with an assortment of coins and bills and are prompted to present the interviewer with specific amounts of money as well as the correct amount of change due after a purchase. Then they must correctly fill out a check to pay off a mock utility bill.

Transportation: subjects are given a bus schedule (preferably localized) and told where they need to go; they must then tell the rater the cost of the trip, the route they would take, the telephone number they would call for information, and where they would get off the bus for any transfers.

Planning recreational activities: subjects are given two recreational scenarios (also prefer-ably localized) and asked questions concerning them. In the first scenario, subjects are told to imagine that they will visit a certain beach on a sunny day. They are then asked to describe their plans, including how they would get there (mode of transportation), things that they would do there, and five items they would take with them for an all-day outing. The second scenario describes a trip to the zoo, including information about hours, location, attractions, and the weather forecast (cool with rain likely). Then participants must correctly report the zoo's hours of operation, what current attractions are available, and five items they would need to bring or wear to spend a full day there.

Administration and scoring

Administration takes approximately 30 minutes. The developers intended that the measure could be administered and scored by individuals with minimal training. Scores on the five subscales are combined to produce a total that has a range of 0–100.

Reliability and validity

Good validity ($r=0.48$) has been reported between UPSA performance and the real-world outcome of community independence (Twamley et al., 2002). Reliability has also been found to be high; in a study with 133 outpatients with schizophrenia (Leifker et al., 2010), reliability between UPSA at baseline and 18 months was 0.75, and between baseline and 36 months was 0.73. In a different sample (also reported by Leifker et al., 2010), repeated administration of the UPSA to 116 outpatients with schizophrenia resulted in correlations of 0.77 between baseline and six months, 0.80 between baseline and 12 months, and 0.63 between baseline and 18 months.

In a 2011 review (Green et al., 2011), evaluation of performance-based measures concluded that the UPSA correlated highly ($r=0.67$) with composite neurocognitive performance on the MCCB.

Regarding correlation of UPSA scores with reports by informants and patients, Bowie et al. (2007) found a significant correlation between UPSA scores and case manager ratings on patient activity ($r=0.42$), but no significant correlation with patient self-report ($r=0.15$).

University of California San Diego Performance-Based Skills Assessment Brief (Mausbach et al., 2007)

Test components

This brief version of the UPSA includes two of the original UPSA's subscales, namely, Communication and Finance (described previously).

Administration and scoring

The administration protocol and scoring are the same as for the original UPSA, but the UPSA-B takes approximately only 10 to 15 minutes to complete.

Reliability and validity

As reported by its developers (Mausbach et al., 2007), the UPSA-B is highly correlated ($r=0.91$) with the full UPSA. Leifker et al. (2010) reported that reliability between baseline and the 18-month follow-up was 0.75, and between baseline and 36 months was 0.73 (both identical to the full UPSA correlations). A review by Green et al. (2011) of performance-based measures concluded that the UPSA-B correlated highly ($r=0.53$) with neurocognitive performance on the MCCB but poorly with the self-reported Quality of Life Survey (QLS) ($r=0.15$).

Social Skills Performance Assessment (SSPA) (Patterson et al., 2001a)

Test components

The SSPA is a role play measure adapted from the earlier role play task of the Social Problem Solving Battery (Bellack et al., 1990). It incorporates two of the four original scenarios. Prior to the test scenarios, the subject is given one practice scene to acclimate to role-playing. Before each scene, the subject reads the scenario prompt out loud, and the interviewer makes sure the subject knows which part he or she is playing before they begin.

Scene 1: The subject plays the part of a resident in an apartment complex, and the interviewer acts as a new neighbor. The subject is instructed to welcome the new neighbor and engage in friendly conversation. To score well, the participant should approach the new neighbor with minimal prompting and initiate and sustain an appropriate conversation.

Scene 2: The subject plays the part of a tenant calling his/her landlord (played by the interviewer) about a water leak about which the tenant has already complained. To score well, the participant should be assertive and negotiate with the landlord to get the leak attended to immediately.

Administration and scoring

The SSPA can be administered by a trained paraprofessional and takes approximately 12 minutes to complete. No props are required. All of the scenes are audio-recorded, and a trained rater listens to and scores the two scenes on a scale of 1–5 along several dimensions, including interest/disinterest, fluency, clarity, focus, affect, grooming, overall conversation, and social appropriateness.

Reliability and validity

As tested by its developers (Patterson et al., 2001a), the SSPA demonstrated high (r=0.91) interrater reliability and a one-week test–retest reliability of 0.92. However, the test–retest reliability of the SSPA between baseline and longer follow-up visits (6–36 mo) among schizophrenia patients at two different sites was somewhat lower (r=0.49–0.79) (Leifker et al., 2010). A moderate correlation (0.47) was found between total SSPA score and a self-report measure of quality of life/well being (QWB) (Patterson et al., 2001a).

The SSPA was also found to be significantly (r=0.51) correlated with case manager ratings of patient interpersonal life, but it was not significantly (r=0.36) correlated with patient self-ratings on the same scale (Bowie et al., 2007).

In a clinical study examining the short-term effects of atypical antipsychotics, Harvey et al. (2006) concluded that the SSPA and neuropsychological performance were positively affected by treatment with atypical antipsychotics.

Medication Management Ability Assessment (MMAA) (Patterson et al., 2002)

The MMAA may be regarded as a modification of the Medication Management Test (MMT) (Albert et al., 1999), which was developed to assess patients with HIV.

Test components

Subjects are presented with four mock medication bottles while the interviewer describes an imaginary medication regimen (involving four different medications). Each bottle is labeled with its administration instructions (number of pills per dose, number of doses per day, and whether to take with food or on an empty stomach). Then the bottles are removed for one hour while other tests are conducted. Finally, patients are shown the bottles again and asked to narrate the course of their imaginary day, presenting the interviewer with the correct doses of each medication at the prescribed times.

Administration and scoring

The MMAA yields scores of 0–25 for the handling of each medication and 0–21 for the correct number of pills. Administration takes approximately 15 minutes (not including the initial one-hour delay). Props required include the labeled pill bottles with mock pills.

Reliability and validity

The developers of the MMAA reported excellent test–retest reliability (r=0.96) after one week (Patterson et al., 2002). Jeste et al. concluded that scores on a cognitive ability measure (Dementia Rating Scale [DRS]) were highly correlated (r=0.50) with performance on the MMAA (Jeste et al., 2003).

Everyday Functioning Battery (EFB) (Heaton et al., 2004)

Test components

This battery, which was developed to assess patients with HIV, has six subtests. To our knowledge, all of the studies that employed this measure to examine patients with schizophrenia reported data only from the Advanced Finances subtest. A description of the full battery follows.

Advanced Finances: this subtest requires the participant to pay three mock bills using mock blank checks, deposit one mock check, and keep a running total in a fictitious checkbook register. A challenging feature of this test is its requirement that participants pay off all of their bills except one (their credit card bill), and to pay an amount on that bill that will leave $100 in their checkbook register. This task is thus more demanding than the UPSA finances subtest.

Shopping: this subtest was taken directly from the DAFS (see earlier description).

Medication management: this module is an adaptation of the Medication Management Test (MMT) (revised). It requires participants to sort and organize mock pills into a daily pill dispenser, following a regimen described by the tester. They are also required to answer questions regarding each medication.

Cooking: participants are required to prepare two dishes (pasta and bread), sequencing their activities in such a way that both dishes finish cooking at approximately the same time.

Administration and scoring

The total possible score comprises 95 points (shopping, 20; cooking, 30; finances combined, 35; medication, 10), and the instrument takes approximately 40 minutes to administer. In studies utilizing only the advanced finances subtest, 13 is the maximum score.

Reliability and validity

The majority of data from the EFD stems from patients with HIV infection. There are two studies that have employed the Advanced Finances subtest in schizophrenia, one a sample of persons of Ashkenazi descent (Bowie et al., 2010) and the VALERO study (Harvey et al., 2011). To our knowledge, there have been no studies examining the incremental utility of the more complex Advanced Finances task relative to that employed in the UPSA.

Test of Adaptive Behavior in Schizophrenia (TABS) (Velligan et al., 2007)

The TABS is a performance-based test of two important factors that relate to functional ability: initiative and the ability to identify problems independently.

Test components

The TABS consists of the following five subtests: Medication management: involves taking medication as directed and being able to recognize that the current supply will not last the entire week. Subjects then must generate a solution.

Stocking an empty bathroom: identifying what products need to be put into the bathroom for everyday use.

Shopping skills: reading a map to get to a store, identifying the products needed by looking at pictures of grocery aisles, and identifying when an incorrect amount of change has been given.

Clothes closet: identifying clothing appropriate to specific situations.

Work and productivity: assembling a packet of colored flyers using an example and fixing orientation errors.

In addition to these five subtests, an examiner-rated social skills test is conducted to assess the subject's eye contact, speech, and other indicators.

Administration and scoring

For each domain, participants receive a score of 0–100. Then the mean of all domains is used as a total TABS score, with higher scores representing better functioning. Administration takes approximately 30–40 minutes. Each subtest requires different props.

Reliability and validity

As reported by its creators, test–retest reliability was 0.80 after a three-month follow-up. They also report that the TABS had a range of correlations (0.31–0.67) with neuropsychological tests of attention, memory, speed, initiation, and executive functioning. Both the full and shortened version of the TABS had high correlations with neurocognitive ability as measured by the MCCB ($r=0.61$ and 0.53, respectively) (Green et al., 2011).

Independent Living Scales (ILS) (Loeb, 1996)

This measure was developed to measure the capacity of patients with dementia for independent living in the community. Since then, it has been used with patients with schizophrenia to estimate their competence in performing daily tasks related to community living as well as personal care.

Test components

This measure is composed of five subscales:

Memory/orientation: requires that the patient be oriented to time and place, remember a shopping list, and recognize a missing object.

Money management: the patient calculates finances while keeping a budget in mind.

Managing home and transportation: the patient is tested on telephone abilities, public transportation knowledge, and home management skills.

Health and safety: tests the patient on awareness of medical problems, hazards around the house, and medical emergencies.

Social adjustment: looks at patients' concerns and attitudes about their personal relationships.

Administration and scoring

The ILS takes approximately 45 minutes to administer. Scores from the five subscales are summed for a total score ranging from 0–140.

Reliability and validity

The ILS has excellent test–retest reliability (0.90) and interrater reliability (0.98), and it strongly correlates with the Wechsler Adult Intelligence Scale – Revised (r=0.65) (Revheim & Medalia, 2004). Another study presents impressive correlations between ILS subtest scores (all but Social Adjustment) and neurocognitive scores on the DRS (ranging from r=0.61–0.72) (Baird et al., 2001).

Use of performance-based measures in treatment studies

Green et al. (2011) reported results from the MATRICS for Co-Primary and Translation (CT) study on the reliability, validity, and practicality of performance-based and interview-based measures of functional capacity and how they relate to cognitive performance and real-world functioning among patients with schizophrenia. The performance-based measures that they examined included the ILS, TABS, UPSA, and short forms of all of these measures. The interview-based measures included the Cognitive Assessment Interview (CAI) and the Clinical Global Impression Scale for Cognition (CGI–Cognition). Additional measures examined included the MCCB global composite score, the Heinrichs–Carpenter quality of life scale (QLS) summary score, and the positive and negative syndrome scale (PANSS). All performance-based and interview-based measures (both full and short versions) had high test–retest reliability (r>=68), and all three performance-based measures and their short versions were moderately to highly correlated (0.51–0.67) with cognitive functioning as measured by the MCCB. The interview-based measures were less related to cognitive functioning, with the CAI yielding 0.23 and the CGI 0.38. All measures were poorly related (r=0.15–0.30) to community functioning as measured by the QLS self-report summary score. None of the measures resulted in significant ceiling effects.

Future directions

Moving forward, it is clear that performance-based measures have an important role in both observational and treatment studies for estimating functional deficits in schizophrenia. In comparison to alternative methods, performance-based measures appear to possess greater reliability and validity as well as sensitivity to change over time. In addition, because performance is more tightly linked with cognitive impairment than with fluctuations in psychiatric symptoms, performance-based measures are particularly useful as secondary outcomes in studies of cognitive remediation for schizophrenia. However, future research employing these instruments will need to address a number of gaps. In particular, performance-based measures are not routinely employed in real-world settings. In addition, little evidence exists about the utility of these measures in other severe mental illnesses, subgroups of patients with schizophrenia (e.g., prodromal patients), and culturally diverse groups.

Increasing ease of administration

Compared to questionnaires and surveys that require only paper-and-pencil forms, performance-based measures are disadvantaged because they commonly require props to create simulated environments. One avenue to increasing ease of administration is to develop short forms of these instruments. An example of this approach is the

UPSA-Brief, which employs only two subtests of the UPSA's original five. Sensitivity and specificity of the UPSA-Brief is comparable to those of the original instrument, and the total administration time is reduced from 30 to 10 minutes. There is a short form of the TABS as well.

In addition, the need for examiners could potentially be eliminated through the use of computerized administration and virtual-reality simulation of functionally relevant environments (Freeman, 2008). Computerized neurocognitive testing is well established, but performance-based functional tests have the special requirement of ecological validity. Moreover, different subgroups (e.g., older patients) may have less familiarity with computers, which may introduce biases into the estimation of performance. However, advancement in the computerized administration of performance-based measures may increase their adoption in clinical settings.

Increasing appropriateness for adolescents

In keeping with recent increases in research attention to prodromal schizophrenia, there is great interest in assessing adolescents who are at high risk for developing the full-blown illness. The functional tasks that are relevant to adolescents are different from those relevant to younger or older adults. For example, adolescents are less likely to need to manage finances and are unlikely to be residing independently. A recent, as yet unpublished, revision to the UPSA includes subtests adapted to teens and younger adults, such as setting up a course schedule for school. Moreover, it is likely that as technological interactions become increasingly necessary for daily life, capacity to search for information on the internet and to communicate through electronic media may be a fertile area for development of new performance-based measures.

Increasing appropriateness in cultural diversity

Performance-based measures have gained enough recognition to be in demand for use in a variety of countries. The UPSA, for example, has been translated into over 20 languages and been used in 22 countries. However, simply producing a literal translation of a measure into another language does not ensure its appropriateness to the culture and society in which that language is used. Careful adaptation to each particular culture is also necessary. Specifically, performance-based measures must reflect the normative, functionally relevant tasks within a culture. For example, cooking tasks should use recipes and ingredients that are familiar to the test subjects. Little empirical data exists on performance-based measures in developing countries. One study recently conducted a cross-culture comparison in Chinese patients with schizophrenia with the UPSA, and found that education played a more substantial role in influencing the scores relative to that in comparison studies in the United States or Sweden (McIntosh et al., 2011).

Gauging disability in other severe mental illnesses

Although schizophrenia is the most disabling of mental illnesses, other illnesses can also be accompanied by functional impairment. Bipolar disorder, in particular, has recently been shown to involve stable cognitive impairments and has long been known to be associated with reduced rates of participation in employment. Recent work has suggested that scores on performance-based instruments of functioning are substantially diminished in bipolar disorder (Depp et al., 2009, 2010). Moreover, a study employing structural equation modeling revealed that the structure of the relationships between cognitive, symptom, and functional variables is similar to that seen in schizophrenia, with performance-based measures mediating the relationship between cognitive ability and real-world performance (Bowie et al., 2010). However, in contrast to schizophrenia, the influences of symptoms, particularly depressive symptoms, on real-world outcomes seem to be greater, and thus whether performance-based measures are subject to "state" effects in bipolar disorder and other affective illnesses deserves future study.

Summary and conclusions

While much ongoing work suggests that performance-based measures play an important role in gauging the functional capacity of people with schizophrenia, it is clear that more work needs to be done. At this point, empirical study indicates that performance-based measures avoid some of the shortcomings inherent in other modalities employed in the measurement of functional outcome, and that a number of performance-based instruments now appear to be reliable, convergent with neurocognitive ability and real-world performance indicators, and sensitive to change. In order for these instruments to become a part of routine clinical practice across the spectrum of severe mental illnesses, future efforts in increasing the ease of administration as well as adapting measures to capture functional activity across the spectrum of individuals with psychosis will be necessary. Such efforts will help ensure that new treatments make meaningful changes in the daily lives of people with schizophrenia.

References

Albert, S. M., Weber, C. M., Todak, G., et al. (1999). An observed performance test of medication management ability in HIV: relation to neuropsychological status and medication adherence outcomes. *AIDS and Behavior*, **3**, 121–128.

Baird, A., Podell, K., Lovell, M., et al. (2001). Complex real-world functioning and neuropsychological test performance in older adults. *Clinical Neuropsychologist*, **15**, 369–379.

Bellack, A. S. (2006). Scientific and consumer models of recovery in schizophrenia: concordance, contrasts, and implications. *Schizophrenia Bulletin*, **32**, 432–442.

Bellack, A. S., Morrison, R. L., Wixted J. T., et al. (1990). An analysis of social competence in schizophrenia. *British Journal of Psychiatry*, **156**, 809–818.

Bowie, C. R., Depp, C., McGrath J. A., et al. (2010). Prediction of real-world functional disability in chronic mental disorders: a comparison of schizophrenia and bipolar disorder. *American Journal of Psychiatry*, **167**, 1116–1124.

Bowie, C. R., Leung, W. W., Reichenberg, A., et al. (2008). Predicting schizophrenia patients' real-world behavior with specific neuropsychological and functional capacity measures. *Biological Psychiatry*, **63**, 505–511.

Bowie, C. R., Twamley, E. W., Anderson H., et al. (2007). Self-assessment of functional status in schizophrenia. *Journal of Psychiatric Research*, **41**, 1012–1018.

Bromley, E., Mikesell, L., Mates A., et al. (2011). A video ethnography approach to assessing the ecological validity of neurocognitive and functional measures in severe mental illness: results from a feasibility study. *Schizophrenia Bulletin [Epub ahead of print]*.

Buchanan, R. W., Davis, M., Goff, D., et al. (2005). A summary of the FDA-NIMH-MATRICS workshop on clinical trial design for neurocognitive drugs for schizophrenia. *Schizophrenia Bulletin*, **31**, 5–19.

Buchanan, R. W., Keefe, R. S., Umbricht, D., et al. (2011). The FDA-NIMH-MATRICS guidelines for clinical trial design of cognitive-enhancing drugs: what do we know 5 years later? *Schizophrenia Bulletin,* 37, 1209–1217.

Depp, C. A., Mausbach, B. T., Eyler, L. T., et al. (2009). Performance-based and subjective measures of functioning in middle-aged and older adults with bipolar disorder. *Journal of Nervous and Mental Disease,* 197, 471–475.

Depp, C. A., Mausbach, B. T., Harvey, P. D., et al. (2010). Social competence and observer-rated social functioning in bipolar disorder. *Bipolar Disorders,* 12, 843–850.

Freeman, D. (2008). Studying and treating schizophrenia using virtual reality: a new paradigm. *Schizophrenia Bulletin,* 34, 605–610.

Green, M. F., Schooler, N. R., Kern, R. S., et al. (2011). Evaluation of functionally meaningful measures for clinical trials of cognition enhancement in schizophrenia. *American Journal of Psychiatry,* 168, 400–407.

Harvey, P. D., Raykov, T., Twamley, E. Q., et al. (2011). Validating the measurement of real-world functional outcomes: Phase I results of the VALERO study. *American Journal of Psychiatry,* 168, 1195–1201.

Harvey, P. D., Patterson, T. L., Potter, L. S., et al. (2006). Improvement in social competence with short-term atypical antipsychotic treatment: a randomized, double-blind comparison of quetiapine versus risperidone for social competence, social cognition, and neuropsychological functioning. *American Journal of Psychiatry,* 163, 1918–1925.

Heaton, R. K., Marcotte, T. D., Mindt, M. R., et al. (2004). The impact of HIV-associated neuropsychological impairment on everyday functioning. *Journal of the International Neuropsychological Society,* 10, 317–331.

Jeste, S. D., Patterson, T. L., Palmer, B. W., et al. (2003). Cognitive predictors of medication adherence among middle-aged and older outpatients with schizophrenia. *Schizophrenia Research,* 63, 49–58.

Klapow, J. C., Evans, J., Patterson, T. L., et al. (1997). Direct assessment of functional status in older patients with schizophrenia.

American Journal of Psychiatry, 154, 1022–1024.

Leifker, F. R., Patterson, T. L., Bowie, C. R., et al. (2010). Psychometric properties of performance-based measurements of functional capacity: test–retest reliability, practice effects, and potential sensitivity to change. *Schizophrenia Research,* 119, 246–252.

Loeb, P. A. (1996). *Independent Living Scales (ILS) Manual.* San Antonio, TX: Psychological Corporation.

Marcotte, T. & Grant, I. (2009). *Neuropsychology of Everyday Functioning.* New York, NY: Guilford Press.

Mausbach, B. T., Harvey, P. D., Goldman, S. R., et al. (2007). Development of a brief scale of everyday functioning in persons with serious mental illness. *Schizophrenia Bulletin,* 33, 1364–1372.

McIntosh, B. J., Zhang, X. Y., Kosten T., et al. (2011). Performance-based assessment of functional skills in severe mental illness: results of a large-scale study in China. *Journal of Psychiatric Research,* 45, 1089–1094.

Moore, D. J., Palmer, B. W., Patterson, T. L., et al. (2007). A review of performance-based measures of functional living skills. *Journal of Psychiatric Research,* 41, 97–118.

Palmer, B. W., Heaton, R. K., Gladsjo, J. A., et al. (2002). Heterogeneity in functional status among older outpatients with schizophrenia: employment history, living situation, and driving. *Schizophrenia Research,* 55, 205–215.

Patterson, T. L., Goldman, S., McKibbin, C. L., et al. (2001a). UCSD Performance-Based Skills Assessment: development of a new measure of everyday functioning for severely mentally ill adults. *Schizophrenia Bulletin,* 27, 235–245.

Patterson, T. L., Klapow, J. C., Eastham, J. H., et al. (1998). Correlates of functional status in older patients with schizophrenia. *Psychiatry Research,* 80, 41–52.

Patterson, T. L., Lacro, J., McKibbin, C. L., et al. (2002). Medication management ability assessment: results from a performance-based measure in older outpatients with schizophrenia. *Journal of Clinical Psychopharmacology*, **22**, 11–19.

Patterson, T. L., Moscona, S., McKibbin, C. L., et al. (2001b). Social skills performance assessment among older patients with schizophrenia. *Schizophrenia Research*, **48**, 351–360.

Podsakoff, P. M., MacKenzie, S. B., Lee, J. Y., et al. (2003). Common method biases in behavioral research: a critical review of the literature and recommended remedies. *Journal of Applied Psychology*, **88**, 879–903.

Revheim, N. & Medalia, A. (2004). The Independent Living Scales as a measure of functional outcome for schizophrenia. *Psychiatric Services*, **55**, 1052–1054.

Sabbag, S., Twamley, E., Vella, L., et al. (2011). Assessing everyday functioning in schizophrenia: not all informants seem equally informative. *Schizophrenia Research*, **131**, 250–255.

Schneider, L. C. & Struening, E. L. (1983). SLOF: A behavioral rating scale for assessing the mentally ill. *Social Work Research and Abstracts*, **19**, 9–21.

Silverstein, S. M. & Bellack, A. S. (2008). A scientific agenda for the concept of recovery as it applies to schizophrenia. *Clinical Psychology Review*, **28**, 1108–1124.

Silverstein, S. M., Schenkel, L. S., Valone, C., et al. (1998). Cognitive deficits and psychiatric rehabilitation outcomes in schizophrenia. *Psychiatric Quarterly*, **69**, 169–191.

Twamley, E. W., Doshi, R. R., Nayak, G. V., et al. (2002). Generalized cognitive impairments, ability to perform everyday tasks, and level of independence in community living situations of older patients with psychosis. *American Journal of Psychiatry*, **159**, 2013–2020.

Velligan, D. I., Diamond, P., Glahn, D. C., et al. (2007). The reliability and validity of the Test of Adaptive Behavior in Schizophrenia (TABS). *Psychiatry Research*, **151**, 55–66.

Wallace, C. J., Liberman, R. P., Tauber, R., et al. (2000). The independent living skills survey: a comprehensive measure of the community functioning of severely and persistently mentally ill individuals. *Schizophrenia Bulletin*, **26**, 631–658.

Zanetti, O., Geroldi, C., Frisoni, G. B., et al. (1999). Contrasting results between caregiver's report and direct assessment of activities of daily living in patients affected by mild and very mild dementia: the contribution of the caregiver's personal characteristics. *Journal of the American Geriatric Society*, **47**, 196–202.

Pharmacological approaches to cognitive enhancement

Philip D. Harvey

Introduction

As noted in multiple other chapters in this book, disability is common and severe in people with schizophrenia and cognitive impairments and deficits in functional capacity are associated with these impairments. Treatment of cognitive impairment has been proposed as a pathway to reduce disability and dependency, improve everyday functioning and quality of life, and reduce the personal and societal costs of the illness. These treatments can take the form of pharmacological interventions, addressed in this chapter, and remediation and rehabilitation interventions as described by Vinogradov and colleagues (Chapter 16). These approaches share some similarities in treatment targets, with both aimed at cognitive performance and eventually at everyday disability. In the rest of this chapter, we will examine the rationale for pharmacological cognitive enhancement, standard methods for trial design, candidate pharmacological mechanisms, compound selection strategies, and the results to date.

Rationale for pharmacological interventions

Cognitive impairments arise from the central nervous system (CNS), with its complex array of neurotransmitters, cortical networks, and electrochemical activity. There are multiple neurotransmitters previously isolated that are associated with cognitive performance in human and animal models. Transmitter manipulations can be beneficial or adverse and different receptor subtypes for the same transmitter can have opposite effects on the same cognitive processes. There are several ways that the transmitter influences can be used to guide treatment development (Geyer & Tamminga, 2004). They include identification of diseases marked by cognitive impairments where neurotransmitter alterations are known to be present, identification of compounds where administration of the compound has a generalized positive benefit, and identification of compounds the administration of which causes worsening in cognitive performance, where essentially opposite effects might be beneficial.

Multiple conditions are marked by the presence of cognitive impairments and are known to be associated with functional reduction in neurotransmission activity. For instance, Alzheimer's disease is marked by a reduction in cholinergic neurotransmission, demonstrated by postmortem evidence of reduced activity and also postmortem evidence of reduction in acetylcholinergic neurons. The dementia of Parkinson's disease is marked

Cognitive Impairment in Schizophrenia, ed. Philip D. Harvey. Published by Cambridge University Press. © Cambridge University Press 2013.

by similar reductions in cholinergic activity, and prior to the onset of dementia, there is reduced dopamine activation that may be associated with the milder cognitive impairments seen in that condition.

There are several mechanisms of interest that have been pursued because there are compounds that reliably produce cognitive impairments, while related compounds can reverse those impairments. Drugs that reverse cognitive deficits caused by anticholinergic compounds such as scopolamine are often those seen to have potential for treatment of cognitive deficits in Alzheimer's dementia (Vitiello et al., 1997). Given the propensity for glutamate antagonists (ketamine; phencyclidine) to induce a schizophrenia-like syndrome, including characteristic cognitive impairments, drugs that reverse those effects are also considered as potential candidates for cognitive enhancement (Krystal et al., 2003).

Amphetamine and related compounds improve cognitive functioning, with these pharmacological entities having identifiable neurotransmitter activity. These medications, while typically used for the treatment of attention deficit disorders, are well known to enhance cognitive functioning in nonclinical populations as well. Nicotine, a cholinergic agent, enhances cognitive functioning in a narrow dose range, and provides even more benefits to individuals who are addicted and in withdrawal. Finally, other compounds that affect alertness, such as modafinil, have some cognitive enhancing benefits across a variety of populations. As a result, there are several sources of information that guide the search for pharmacological compounds that improve cognition. In the following sections, we review the information that leads to specific suggestions for cognitive enhancement in schizophrenia.

Dopamine

The primary effect of antipsychotic medications is to block dopamine D2 receptors in the corpus striatum. All effective antipsychotic medications have this property and all medications that have been tried as antipsychotic medications that lack this effect have failed. Several influential theories of cognitive impairment in schizophrenia have focused on cortical/striatal dopamine balance (Davis et al., 1991). In healthy individuals, increased activation of cortical dopamine neurons is associated with reductions in striatal activity and vice versa, reflecting a regulatory relationship between these regions. In contrast, there is apparently a dysjunction in these regulatory processes in people with schizophrenia, and blockade of striatal dopamine receptors does not lead to a corresponding increase in cortical dopamine tone.

Reduced cortical dopamine activity has been a prominent idea regarding the origin of cognitive impairments in the illness (Laruelle, 2003). Many cognitive functions are related to dopaminergic activity and compounds that increase dopamine transmission, such as amphetamine, lead to improvements in these functions (Kimberg et al., 1997). For example, attention, working memory, and related executive functions are improved with amphetamine treatment and reduced regional cortical activation is associated with impaired performance on these types of tasks. Direct stimulation of cortical dopamine receptors with dopamine D1 agonists can reverse the adverse effects of aging and chronic antipsychotic treatment on working memory performance in monkeys (Castner et al., 2000), again suggesting the dopamine relevance of many of the common cognitive impairments in people with schizophrenia.

It is possible that there is a preferential loss of dopamine-containing neurons in the prefrontal cortex in people with schizophrenia. There is evidence of reduced signaling of both the synthesis regulator, tyrosine hydroxylase, and the dopamine transporter in prefrontal regions, suggesting reduced dopamine concentrations (Akil et al., 1999). Reduced dopaminergic availability can lead to upregulation of the receptor systems, which is likely to be insufficient to compensate for the reduced dopaminergic activity. Some evidence suggesting that underactivity at D1 receptors is directly related to cognitive impairments is the finding that upregulation in dopamine D1 receptors is directly correlated with impairments in working memory (Abi-Dargham et al., 2002).

Other evidence implicating dopamine in the cognitive impairments seen in schizophrenia comes from studies of the genetic variants associated with catechol-o-methyltransferase (COMT). There are two polymorphisms associated with this gene, valene and methionine (VAL and MET), with the VAL allele associated with greater catabolic potential in the dopamine receptor region and hence reduced levels of available dopamine. VAL-VAL homozygotes have been shown to have reduced levels of cognitive functions that are relevant to schizophrenia, including working memory and executive functioning (Egan et al., 2001). Although the evidence for COMT as a susceptibility gene for schizophrenia is limited, the fact that this dopamine-relevant genetic variation is broadly associated with cognitive functioning, including in individuals with schizophrenia spectrum personality disorders, again indicates the role of dopamine in the cognitive abnormalities in schizophrenia.

Glutamate

Glutamate is an excitatory transmitter that is widely distributed in the CNS, but one of the potentially important locations for these receptors is on dendritic spines. There are at least two receptor subunits for glutamate: N-methyl D-aspartate (NMDA) and α-amino-3-hydroxy-5-methyl-4-isoxazole propionic acid (AMPA), both of which are widely distributed. The NMDA antagonists such as ketamine and phencyclidine (PCP) trigger syndromes in healthy individuals that are a close analog to schizophrenia, including positive and negative symptoms, impairments in communication, and cognitive deficits. People with schizophrenia are even more sensitive to these effects than healthy individuals (Krystal et al., 2003). Similarly, reduction in dendrite density, a common postmortem finding in schizophrenia, could also lead to a corresponding reduction in glutamatergic activity.

There are two domains where glutamatergic abnormalities might cause brain changes and cognitive impairments. One is the suggestion that glutamatergic hypoactivity, as would be induced by chronic hyperdopaminergic activity, similar to the effects of PCP and ketamine, can trigger apoptosis (Benes, 2006). These programed cell death processes would be difficult to detect at postmortem because they do not necessarily cause gliosis at the time of occurrence. At the same time, this is a difficult idea to test because postmortem tissue would have to be obtained during a period of active apoptosis and these occurrences may be sporadic in nature. A second area where glutamatergic abnormalities could be related to cortical changes is through their potential direct effect on white matter. Chronic glutamatergic hyperactivity, which could be a consequence of impaired dopamine/glutamate interactions, has been proven to be toxic to oligodendrocytes (McDonald et al., 1998). This process may be due to induction of dysregulation in calcium homeostasis and increased intracellular calcium (Verity, 1992). As oligodendrocytes are damaged, demyelination can occur, which further reduces the ability of neurons to modulate glutamate activity (Matute, 1998). Thus, alterations in cortical white matter detected in diffusion tensor imaging (DTI) studies could possibly arise from glutamatergic processes, suggesting a mechanism through which psychosis, cognitive impairment, and disorganized behavior may be directly linked to each other (Olney & Farber, 1995).

A final mechanism through which glutamatergic dysregulation could impact on cognitive functioning is through disruption of dopamine input to prefrontal sites where critical cognitive operations are performed. Impaired excitatory input to cortical dopamine receptors could lead to chronic changes in their functioning, on both functional and morphological levels. One potential consequence of this process, suggested by Lewis and Sweet (2009), is that chronic reductions in excitatory input to cortical D1 receptors could lead to compensatory, but ineffective, upregulation of these neurons. This upregulation could then cause a consequential downregulation in the synthesis of gamma-aminobutyric acid (GABA). As GABA itself regulates the level of glutamatergic functioning, such a process could contribute to further dysregulation in the balance of these transmitters.

Gamma-aminobutyric acid

Postmortem data has found reduced levels of GABA signaling in a critical interneuronal subsystem: chandelier cells. Specifically, about 33% of interneurons that contain GABA are found to express essentially undetectable levels of a critical regulator of GABA synthesis: glutamic acid decarboxylase(GAD)-67 (Volk et al., 2000). Glutamic acid decarboxylase-67 is an enzyme that regulates production of GABA and it is highly responsive to excitatory input directed toward GABA-containing interneurons. Thus reduced excitatory signaling into GABA neurons would lead to reductions in synthesis of GABA. Interestingly, levels of signaling of the primary transporter of GABA, GABA transporter 1 (GAT-1), are also undetectable in these same interneurons. As GABA regulates levels of glutamatergic activity, decreased GABA functioning has the potential to contribute to the cascade of reduced cortical input, compensatory upregulation of D1 receptors, and maintenance of multisystem dysregulation of neurotransmitters.

Acetylcholine

Acetylcholine is another transmitter potentially associated with cognitive changes in schizophrenia. Specifically, the nicotinic receptor subsystems of the cholinergic system appear to be altered in people with schizophrenia. There are several lines of evidence in this regard. Expression of the nicotinic α-7 receptor in the prefrontal cortex is altered in both people with schizophrenia and their relatives (Leonard et al., 2002). Individuals with schizophrenia are more likely to smoke than the general population (Lasser et al., 2000), starting prior to the onset of their illness, as well as smoking more heavily and extracting more nicotine from cigarettes than nonschizophrenic fellow smokers (Olincy et al., 1997). There have been postmortem reports of altered nicotinic receptor density in people with schizophrenia as well, but it is challenging to rule out the effects of smoking in that regard (Freedman et al., 1995).

There has been limited evidence of alterations in muscarinic receptor systems in schizophrenia. Postmortem studies typically have not found reductions in indices of muscarinic activation or in levels of acetylcholine (Powchik et al., 1998). However, one study reported reduced levels of cholinergic neurons in the ventral striatum in schizophrenia, in the absence of any evidence of other neurodegenerative changes (Holt et al., 1999). One possible confound throughout this research is the use of antimuscarinic medications to treat extrapyramidal side effects of antipsychotic medications. The long-term effects of these medications are unknown and whether their use in early and middle life could influence the postmortem detection of illness-related alterations in muscarinic activity is uncertain.

Points of entry for cognitive enhancement

Neurotransmission is a complex phenomenon and, despite remarkable advances in neuroscience, is still only partially understood. Developing targets for cognitive enhancement requires the decision as to whether to attempt to increase activity by stimulation of receptors (agonist), reducing activity by blocking receptors (antagonist), modifying the endogenous processes of downregulation of activity, either through blocking reuptake (transport), or reducing degradation of transmitters. While many of these actions would seem to lead to the same result, the complexities of neurotransmission suggest that the situation is more involved. For instance, stimulating serotonin receptors directly has no impact on depression, but increasing serotonin activity through blocking transport is a very effective antidepressant strategy (serotonin reuptake inhibition [SRI]). We will discuss the results of studies employing these different mechanisms in the sections below.

Cognitive enhancement methodology

The US Food and Drug Administration (FDA) issues approvals for medications for specific uses. Their primary criteria for approval of an "indication" for a drug are evidence that the drug is "safe" and "effective". While psychiatric conditions are primarily defined by their symptoms in the *Diagnostic and Statistical Manual of Mental Disorders* (DSM), other aspects of these illnesses often do not benefit from treatments approved for primary indications. Clear examples of this disconnect are psychosis and agitation in dementia and cognitive impairments in schizophrenia. The FDA has previously allowed attempts to develop a treatment indication for these features, as long as it could be provided that these other features were not improved by standard, previously approved treatments. Referred to as a concern about "pseudospecificity," this means that a treatment cannot be approved for the specific treatment of an illness feature already approved for treatment. An example would be an attempt to seek an approval for treatment for "hallucinations in schizophrenia," when the same treatment is already approved for the treatment of schizophrenia (which includes hallucinations).

Beyond these issues, the FDA in the past has required that treatments aimed at cognitive enhancement be supported by evidence of clinical benefit beyond improvements in performance-based assessments. These so-called co-primary measures in studies of dementia typically have included care-giver assessments of the detectable benefits of cognitive enhancing treatments, collected in double-blind trials. While it might be asked whether our society might benefit if similar expectations were imposed for approval of treatments such as collagen injections, botox, and breast implants, similar standards to those in Alzheimer's disease have been imposed for the approval of cognitive enhancement agents in schizophrenia. Similarly, the FDA has imposed a six-month duration requirement for the active phase of "acute" treatment trials for cognitive enhancement in schizophrenia, despite the fact that antipsychotics have been approved in six-week clinical trials and that an atypical antipsychotic medication (aripiprazole) received approval for treatment-resistant depression on the basis of two three-week double-blind trials (Kahn, 2008).

Table 15.1. National Institute of Mental Health, U. S. Food and Drug Administration, Academia, and Pharmaceutical Industry Consensus Entry Criteria for Cognitive Enhancement Interventions

Criteria for enrollment into cognitive enhancement trials

Diagnosis of schizophrenia

No major change in antipsychotic medications for at least 6 weeks prior to screening

No medications that can influence cognitive functioning:
    Anticholinergics
    Amphetamines
    L-dopa

No hospitalization for psychiatric illness for at least 8 weeks prior to screening

Moderately severe or less (<5) severity rating on selected PANSS positive scale items at both screening and baseline

No evidence of current major depression

PANSS, positive and negative syndrome scale – insight item G12.

A large-scale collaborative initiative, Measurement and Treatment Research to Improve Cognition in Schizophrenia (MATRICS), was undertaken to develop a consensus between the FDA, the pharmaceutical industry, the National Institute of Mental Health (NIMH), and academia. Funded by the NIMH, this initiative had several consensus conferences aimed at measurement of cognition and co-primary outcomes, research design, and pharmacological target selection. Several critical outcomes from this project were realized. A cognitive battery was identified by consensus, tested, normed, and validated (Kern et al., 2008). A consensus research design was proposed (Buchanan et al., 2005) and then revised after five years of experience (Buchanan et al., 2011b). In an extension of this process, a preferred co-primary assessment method and outcomes measures were identified after an extensive consensus and validation process (Green et al., 2011).

Thus, to date, there is a path toward approval for cognitive enhancing medications in schizophrenia. Table 15.1 presents the critical features of this regulatory pathway. Included are patient populations, trial design and duration, and primary and co-primary outcomes measures. There are several critical corollary features of this design. These include:

1. Functional improvements in the real world are not required for approval of a treatment.
2. Two global performance-based measures are the critical outcomes and statistical correction is not required.
3. No a priori magnitude of improvement is specified, other than significantly greater improvement than the placebo in an add-on design.
4. Treatments that improve both clinical symptoms and cognition may not be qualified for dual indications but would receive acknowledgment of these benefits elsewhere.

As noted in point three, the typical research design aimed at indications for the treatment of cognitive impairments will be an add-on "polypharmacy" approach. This design would result in interpretable results from a clinical trial, in that active treatment added to standing treatment compared to placebo treatment, on two separate outcomes measures, would only have to achieve an a priori level of statistical significance of $P<0.05$ each.

Previous mechanisms of action studied

There have been multiple previous cognitive enhancement studies. This review will focus on only those studies with adequate methodology: randomized assignment and double-blind treatment strategies. The review will not be limited by sample size, because potentially interesting but not definitive information can come from smaller trials. In areas such as the study of widely available medications such as cholinesterase inhibitors, we weight large-scale studies more than smaller ones, even with double-blind methods. We will not exclude studies that included patients with schizoaffective disorder, but will not review studies that focused on psychotic disorders broadly defined. We will not exclude studies where medications that would not be viable long-term treatments (e.g., amphetamine, tolcapone) are studied. In addition, because of consistently small treatment effects and several previous meta-analytic reviews (Harvey & Keefe, 2001; Woodward et al., 2005), we will not examine studies of atypical antipsychotic medications as cognitive enhancers. Table 15.2 gives a listing of the compounds used in previous studies and their putative mechanisms of action.

Acetylcholinesterase inhibitors

Several adequately powered studies have examined the benefits of acetylcholinesterase inhibitors on cognitive functioning. In the largest of these studies, Keefe et al. (2008) reported on a large-scale randomized comparison of donepezil compared to the placebo in clinically stable outpatients with schizophrenia. The results of the study were strikingly negative, with performance at the 12-week endpoint significantly worse on active treatment than on the placebo. Reporting on a small-sample study, Sharma et al. (2006) found that there was no global cognitive benefit from treatment with rivastigmine in a double-blind placebo-controlled study. There was a small sample size (total n=21) and there were no significant differences associated with the treatment compared to the placebo on any of the cognitive outcomes measures. In an adequately powered study, Buchanan et al. (2007a) reported that galantamine treatment of schizophrenia was also not associated with significant global benefit for active treatment compared to the placebo. This result was consistent with the report of an industry study (clinicaltrials.gov; NCT00077727) that also found no global benefit of galantamine treatment. Using a creative approach to data analysis, Buchanan et al. (2007a) performed a "heterogeneity of effect analysis" to go beyond effects based on the global composite score. Tests that improved significantly included measures of verbal memory. However, galantamine treatment appeared to interfere with practice effects on a distraction version of a continuous performance test. Thus, there was some signal of differential effects of galantamine across cognitive abilities but no global improvements.

Nicotinic agonists

Two nicotinic receptor complexes have been the target of intervention, the alpha-7 and the alpha4-beta2 subunits. Some of the compounds tested to date have primary effects on one subunit or the other and some compounds affect multiple receptor subunits. Two studies, one of which was published and one of which was described on the worldwide web, have examined different nicotinic receptor agonists. In the first study (Freedman et al., 2008), DMXB, an alpha-7 partial agonist, was compared in a twice-daily dosing regimen to a placebo, with changes in negative symptoms and cognitive impairment as the outcomes of interest. A total of 29 patients received the placebo and two different doses of DMXB in a

Table 15.2. Compounds employed and mechanisms of action in previous cognitive enhancement studies

General pharmacological domain	Specific compounds	Specific actions of the compounds
Cholinergic		
Muscarinic	Donepezil	Acetylcholinesterase inhibition
	Galantamine	Acetylcholinesterase inhibition
	Rivastigmine	Acetylcholinesterase inhibition
Nicotinic	DMX-B	alpha-7 partial agonist
	AZD3480	alpha4-beta2 agonist
Glutamatergic	Glycine	NMDA cotransmitter
	d-cyloserine	NMDA glycine site partial agonist
	CX-516	AMPA-kine (allosteric modulator)
	Lamotrigine	Glutamate release regulation
Noradrenergic	Guanfacine	Alpha2 agonist
	Atomoxetine	Transport inhibitor
γ-amino butyric acid	Flumazenil	GABAA antagonist
	MK-0777	GABAA$_{23}$ antagonist
Serotonergic	Tandospirone	5-HT1A partial agonist
	Buspirone	5-HT1A partial agonist
Dopaminergic	Tolcapone	COMT inhibitor
Stimulant	Amphetamine	Monoamine agonist and transport inhibitor
Alertness agents	Modafinil	Unknown (dopamine transport inhibitor?)
Cannabinoid	Rimonabant	CB1 inverse agonist
Neuroactive peptide	Davunitide	Promotion of dendritic outgrowth

cross-over design. The results indicated some improvements in negative symptoms, but no detectable cognitive effects. Furthermore, all participants were non-smokers and there may be intrinsic differences between people with schizophrenia who do and do not smoke, with these differences possibly reflected in their response to nicotinic stimulation. Negative results were also reported in a larger-scale double-blind placebo-controlled parallel design study conducted by Astra-Zeneca and Targacept Pharma (www.astrazeneca.com/itemid4376018). They used AZD3480, which is an alpha4-beta2 agonist, and found that there were no cognitive improvements at any of their endpoints.

Glutamatergic interventions

There have been several attempts to improve cognition using a variety of approaches involving the glutamatergic system, including NMDA and AMPA receptor subtypes, as well as the NMDA obligatory cotransmitter glycine. In a large-scale and systematic research effort, the investigators in the Cognitive and Negative Symptoms in Schizophrenia Trial (CONSIST) (Buchanan et al., 2007b) used two different agents to influence the NMDA receptor system. These two compounds were chosen on the basis of previous research that suggested the possibility that they improved either cognition or negative symptoms. One of these compounds, glycine, is a cotransmitter with glutamate at its own site on the NMDA receptor, and the other, D-cycloserine, is a partial agonist at the NMDA site. In the CONSIST study, participants were randomized to one of these two active treatments or to the placebo and examined over a 16-week double-blind placebo-controlled protocol. The outcome was quite negative, in that neither active compound led to a significant benefit for either the composite cognitive score or any one of the individual cognitive items.

Goff et al. (2008) used an AMPA-kine to attempt to enhance cognition in schizophrenia patients. In these two studies with similar methods, eight weeks of AMPA-kine treatment was examined for its impact on cognitive functioning. At the eight-week endpoint, there was no significant treatment effect on the composite cognitive score or on any of the 14 individual cognitive variables.

Another strategy has been implemented to examine medications that otherwise regulate glutamatergic activity. For instance, lamotrigine, an approved anticonvulsant medication, reduces glutamatergic release and may adjust glutamatergic tone. Lamotrigine pretreatment has been shown (Anand et al., 2000) to reduce the adverse effects of ketamine administration in healthy individuals. Several studies have reported beneficial effects of lamotrigine on symptoms in people with schizophrenia (Zoccali et al., 2007), therefore an assessment of its cognitive effects seems reasonable.

In two highly similar clinical trials reported in a single paper, Goff et al. (2007) found that double-blind placebo-controlled treatment with lamotrigine was possibly associated with cognitive improvements. In the two studies, the cognitive composite score was improved by $z=0.58$ and $z=0.47$ in the lamotrigine group, with corresponding improvements in the placebo group of $z=0.21$ and $z=0.20$. The effect of treatment compared to the placebo was statistically significant in one study but not in the other. These data suggest improvements beyond the placebo that are consistent with a small effect size. Improvements of this magnitude may not be clinically significant, but the relative importance of different degrees of cognitive improvements is not well understood at present.

In summary, the complexity of the glutamatergic system is reflected in the complexity of the results obtained in studies of this mechanism. In contrast to the muscarinic cholinergic system, there is some suggestion of modest improvement effects with treatment with agents that normalize glutamatergic functions. Clearly, further research is required for the replication of these findings and to include other elements of the glutamatergic systems, such as the metabotropic system (mGlu 2/3) or glycine transport inhibitors, as potential cognitive enhancing agents (Moghaddam, 2004).

Noradrenergic interventions

Interventions aimed at the noradrenergic system have also been attempted in schizophrenia. Studies have examined both direct agonists of the noradrenergic system and compounds that inhibit the transport and degradation of noradrenaline. In a small-sample double-blind placebo-controlled study of a noradrenaline agonist, guanfacine, previously proven to enhance cognition in animals (Arnsten et al., 1988) and in attention deficit hyperactivity disorder (ADHD) (Hunt et al., 1995), Friedman et al. (2001) found cognitive benefits that were limited to attentional functions. By contrast, McClure et al. (2007) found that guanfacine had notable cognitive benefits in patients with schizotypal Parkinson's disease who were otherwise medication free. Friedman et al. (2008) found in a small-sample schizophrenia study that there were essentially no cognitive benefits from atomoxetine, the noradrenaline transport inhibitor used to treat ADHD. As a point of interest, a similar lack of cognitive benefit was reported by Kelly et al. (2009). Despite the minimal effects of atomoxetine on cognition in the study by Friedman et al., treatment with the compound had substantial effects on cortical activation in anterior cortical brain regions known to be implicated in schizophrenia.

Amphetamine

Amphetamine has a long history in schizophrenia and has been used for the treatment of many different symptoms despite its reputation as a psychotomimetic and potentiator of relapse (Angrist et al., 1980). A study by Barch and Carter (2005) suggested that a single-dose amphetamine challenge enhances cognition across multiple domains in clinically stable people with schizophrenia receiving therapeutic doses of conventional antipsychotic medications. While these results seem promising, they need to be balanced by concerns regarding the long-term safety of these interventions for people with schizophrenia. It should be noted that there are multiple amphetamine-related compounds available that could be employed if a strategy to reduce safety concerns could be developed.

Modafinil

Modafinil is an alertness-promoting medication that has a mechanism of action that may be distinct from amphetamine, but likely still involves monoaminergic mechanisms. Multiple studies have provided information regarding modafinil that is partially supportive of cognitive enhancing properties. As reviewed by Morein-Zamir et al. (2007), there are more strong findings in areas of executive functioning and attentional processes than in enhancement of memory functions. Furthermore, heterogeneity of response is clearly evident, with less severe cognitive impairment and several different genetic polymorphisms predicting better response. Cognitive enhancement in healthy individuals is also reported with modafinil, but these improvements are much more substantial in individuals who are sleep deprived at baseline (Minzenberg & Carter, 2008). A further issue with modafinil is the sporadic case reports of exacerbation of psychosis in patients with schizophrenia taking the compound. It is not clear if these are direct medication effects or if they are associated with misuse of the medication, which could then lead to sleep deprivation and associated adverse events.

Serotonergic medications

Two studies have focused on cognitive enhancement with serotonergic agonists and studies have also examined effects of more broadly active serotonergic agents such as SRI antidepressants. In the first of those studies, Sumioshi et al. (2001) reported that double-blind treatment with tandospirone, a serotonin 1A partial agonist, was associated with improvements in a limited set of cognitive functions. These included improvements in verbal immediate memory and one aspect of performance on the Wisconsin Card Sorting

Test. The benefit of this treatment on composite measures of cognitive performance was not reported and the sample size was quite small.

A second study examined the effects of buspirone (Sumyoshi et al., 2007), also a serotonin 1A partial agonist, on cognitive function. The results of this study were even less positive than those of the tandospirone trial. In this study, the only significant difference was on the Digit Symbol Test and that effect was significant at three months but not at six months. Thus, these two studies provide limited positive evidence of the benefits of serotonin 1A agonism on cognitive function in schizophrenia, and later studies, if attempted, will need to use larger sample sizes and more thorough cognitive assessment procedures.

Gamma-aminobutyric acid-based interventions

The GABA modulating compounds have been used for years as anxiolytics and these compounds, such as lorazepam, are agonists at the $GABA_A$ benzodiazepine site. In a study (Menzies et al., 2007) that employed both cognitive assessments and functional magnetic resonance imaging (fMRI) evaluations, a small sample of schizophrenia patients were compared to a similar sized sample of healthy controls (n=11 each), while receiving lorazepam, placebo, or flumazenil, an antagonist at this same GABA site. The primary cognitive outcomes measure was the N-back Working Memory Test, a commonly used test of working memory with maintenance, manipulation, and updating requirements.

In this study, flumazenil was associated with improved N-back performance under conditions of increased processing load in people with schizophrenia and simultaneously led to a normalized pattern of cortical activity associated with load response. By contrast, lorazepam led to worsened N-back performance compared with the placebo. Healthy individuals performed more poorly than the placebo group in both active pharmacological conditions. These data, albeit in a small sample and with a single cognitive test, suggest cognitive performance improvements and changes in brain activation compared to the placebo and treatments that enhance GABA activity. Furthermore, the effect is not a generalized one, because healthy individuals were adversely affected by both pharmacological manipulations. Convergence of cortical activation changes and cognitive task performance stand in contrast to previous studies of noradrenergic and cholinergic medications where brain activation was changed but behavioral performance was unaffected. That study seems quite promising and requires replication with a larger sample size and a more comprehensive cognitive assessment battery.

In a double-blind trial (Lewis et al., 2008), 15 participants with chronic schizophrenia were randomly assigned to receive four weeks of treatment with MK-0777, an agent with selective activity at $GABA_A$ receptors containing alpha(2) or alpha(3) subunits, or a matched placebo. Cognitive outcomes were the Repeatable Battery for the Assessment of Neuropsychological Status, three tests of working memory and/or cognitive control (N-back, AX Continuous Performance Test, and Preparing to Overcome Prepotency), and EEG measures of gamma band oscillations. Compared with the placebo, MK-0777 was associated with improved performance on the N-back, AX Continuous Performance Test, and Preparing to Overcome Prepotency tasks. No effects of MK-0777 were detected with the Repeatable Battery for the Assessment of Neuropsychological Status scores, with the exception of the delayed memory index.

In a much larger study, Buchanan et al. (2011a) found no benefit of this compound on the MATRICS Consensus Cognitive Battery (MCCB), the University Performance

Skills Assessment (UPSA)-B, and the same two neuroscience measures, the N-back and AX-Continuous Performance Test (CPT). Although GABA remains an interesting target, the results are not substantial to date.

Cannabinoid receptor agents

Based on findings that cannabis leads to cognitive changes similar to that seen in schizophrenia (impairments in working and episodic memory, attentional changes), there was interest in the exploration of cannabinoid agents in the treatment of cognitive deficits in schizophrenia. One trial was completed successfully with negative results (Boggs et al., 2012). In that study, rimonabant, a CB1 inverse agonist, was found to have essentially no benefits on cognition. As this compound has been removed from the market for safety concerns based on suicidal ideation and depression, there seems to be little additional promise from this mechanism.

Non-transmitter interventions

Neuroscience discoveries have identified pharmacological compounds that have effects other than transmitter manipulation/modulation. These include compounds that have other CNS effects. These have been the result of long-term interest in development of compounds that promote neurogenesis or other brain growth processes. For example, davunetide is a neuroactive peptide that appears to promote neurite outgrowth in animal models. As postmortem findings of neurite abnormalities are quite consistent, this appears to be a potentially promising intervention. In a single study examining davunetide in people with schizophrenia, Javitt et al. (2011) found that intranasal administration of one of two doses of davunitide lead to statistically significant improvements in the UPSA compared to the placebo treatment. The other higher dose was not associated with improvements in the UPSA and neither dose improved on the MCCB compared to the placebo. However, this study had a very small sample size and several of the MCCB domains improved to an extent that would have been significant with even a modestly larger sample (n=50). The effect size for UPSA change was d=0.74, which is a large and potentially quite clinically meaningful effect, and the effect size for changes on the MCCB was d=0.4, which is moderate, close to statistically significant, and potentially clinically meaningful. As interventions such as davunitide bypass some of the shortcomings of transmitter-based interventions (as described as follows), this may be a promising compound and even more promising cognitive enhancement strategy.

Why the negative results?

As can be seen in this review, with some minor exceptions, the pharmacological cognitive enhancement studies to date have been negative. These results span multiple targets and have used compounds that are known to be effective to treat cognitive impairments in other conditions such as attention deficit disorders, people with schizotypal personality disorder, and in healthy individuals. We will review several possibilities for these results.

Cognitive impairment is not modifiable by pharmacological means

There is evidence of progressive cortical volume loss in people with schizophrenia (DeLisi et al., 2006), which includes progressive loss of gray matter and reduced growth of white matter particularly in cases with multiple exacerbations (Cahn et al., 2009). It could be argued that the progressive volumetric changes constrain the ability of pharmacological treatments to induce a benefit. However, the strongest argument against the notion that progressive brain changes preclude cognitive enhancement is that behavioral cognitive remediation has been shown recently to produce cognitive changes and lead to relevant real-world functional improvements.

Use of concurrent medications may interfere with the effects of cognitive enhancers

Patients with schizophrenia are typically treated with antipsychotic medications. The entire spectrum of effects of these medications is not wholly understood and it is possible that in some way antipsychotic medications alter the effects of add-on pharmacological cognitive enhancers. This is a substantial problem, because symptomatic relapse associated with antipsychotic medication discontinuation poses a considerable clinical problem; hence simply suggesting that potential cognitive enhancing medications be tested or employed in patients who are not receiving medications is not practical. There are several ways in which antipsychotic medications could interfere with the effects of add-on pharmacotherapy. The first is through their common mechanism of antipsychotic action: dopamine D2 receptor blockade. The high levels of reduction of activity required to lead to a clinical response following exacerbations (Lauruelle et al., 1999) might lead to reductions in plasticity of other receptor systems that interact with this receptor subtype, including cholinergic, glutamatergic, and serotonergic systems. A second possibility is through the joint activity of atypical medications at the 5-HT2A receptor system. All of these medications block this receptor subtype to a greater or lesser extent and the serotonergic system is intimately involved in the regulation of multiple other neurotransmitters. A third and even more challenging possibility is that the additional pharmacological effects of antipsychotic medications in some way contribute to these negative results. While all atypical antipsychotics share serotonin/dopamine antagonism (SDA), they vary markedly in their activity at other receptors, including muscarinic, cholinergic, serotonergic (including 2A, 1A, 7, and 6A), adrenergic, and histaminergic receptors with a mix of agonist and antagonist effects.

Dosing of add-on compounds may be critically important for their efficacy

Although medication doses for treatments that are in current clinical use for other conditions (guanfacine, cholinesterase inhibitors, atomoxetine) are established for the original illnesses, it is not clear if the same doses would be required to enhance cognition in people with schizophrenia. Many of these treatments have dose-dependent side effects (e.g., nausea, hypotension) that limit the potential for dose increases in the original target populations, and concurrent antipsychotic medications may either suppress or exacerbate some of these side effects. We also do not know if doses of pro-cholinergic medications, used in illnesses such as Alzheimer's disease with substantial loss of cholinergic neurons, would be too large in people with schizophrenia, who do not have comparable loss in cholinergic functioning. Conversely, we do not know if the use of concurrent antipsychotic medications requires increased doses of medications that promote cholinergic activity. As most neurotransmitter activity is regulated by multiple other systems, it is hard to estimate a priori what is the potential dose of medications that are introduced into an already altered biological system because of antipsychotic effects.

Delivery and pharmacokinetics may lead to problems in administration

Some drugs, such as the dopamine D1 agonist SKF 38393 that has been shown to be very effective in studies of animals using direct administration into the CNS (e.g., Arnsten et al., 1994), may not cross the blood–brain barrier when administered peripherally. The consequence is that it is not currently possibly to deliver a definitive, specific D1 agonist directly into the brain. Other potentially effective cognitive enhancers either have short half-lives (alpha-7 nicotinic agonists) or lead to receptor sensitization. As a result, some treatments that have solid basic science support (D1 and alpha-7 agonists) have proven difficult to develop into medications that would be useful for treatments. New developments, such as identification and development of additional compounds, including specific precursors or pro-drugs for D1 agonists that cross the blood–brain barrier or compounds which provide allosteric modulation of cholinergic receptors may be required.

Neurotransmitters may not be the viable target for cognitive enhancement

Neurotransmitter manipulations have the potential to influence cognition, as shown in multiple previous studies. This intervention strategy is, however, predicated on the idea that neuronal targets are intact and available. This has already proven problematic in Alzheimer's disease, where cholinergic interventions may be handicapped by the widespread loss of cholinergic neurons by the time that the intervention is delivered. Similar problems may exist in schizophrenia, where abnormalities in cortical structure, circuit connectivity, and axonal/neuronal integrity possibly could reduce the beneficial effects of receptor stimulation. Behavioral interventions may actually have their effect through altering CNS circuitry or connectivity across multiple linked transmitter systems (Akbarian et al., 1996; Lim et al., 1999). If this were found to be the case, interventions aimed at neurites, circuits, and white matter may provide a more effective intervention strategy and these interventions may not be sensitive to the effects of a single transmitter system. The case of davunetide (see earlier) is a perfect example of where an intervention that has potentially direct effects on brain structure and function provides a signal of a magnitude not seen in studies of medications with known beneficial effects.

Additionally, because genetic alterations such as COMT polymorphisms can affect cognitive performance, pharmacogenetic considerations (i.e., "personalized medicine") may be a feature of future treatment development. As variation in the COMT genotype has been shown to influence cognitive performance and response to pharmacological agents (as well as the effect of tolcapone) (Giakoumaki et al., 2008), it will be important to consider new developments in genetics when evaluating the possible benefits of new pharmacological cognitive enhancers.

Conclusions

Cognitive enhancement in schizophrenia is a critical treatment goal but has proven to be quite a challenging target. A regulatory pathway and research design as well as outcomes measures have been identified to facilitate the process of development of cognitive enhancing interventions in schizophrenia. Although potential pharmacological targets have been identified, previous results have been disappointing across multiple neurotransmitter treatment targets. Optimism should arise from the findings that cognitive remediation interventions improve both cognitive performance and functional outcomes. The possible reasons for the previous failures are complex and include potential deleterious effects of antipsychotic treatments, problems associated with dosing, and, most critically, the need to consider points of intervention other than neurotransmitters.

References

Abi-Dargham, A., Mawlawi, O., Lombardo, I., et al. (2002). Prefrontal dopamine D1 receptors and working memory in schizophrenia. *Journal of Neuroscience*, **22**, 3708–3719.

Akbarian, S., Kim, J. J., Potkin, S. G., et al. (1996). Maldistribution of interstitial neurons in the prefrontal white matter of brains of schizophrenic patients. *Archives of General Psychiatry*, **53**, 425–436.

Akil, M., Pierri, J. N., Whitehead, R. E., et al. (1999). Lamina-specific alterations in the dopamine innervation of the prefrontal cortex in schizophrenic subjects. *American Journal of Psychiatry*, **156**, 1580–1589.

Anand, A., Charney, D. S., Oren, D. A., et al. (2000). Attenuation of the neuropsychiatric effects of ketamine with lamotrigine. *Archives of General Psychiatry*, **57**, 270–276.

Angrist, B., Rotrosen, J., & Gershon, S. (1980). Differential effects of amphetamine and neuroleptics on negative vs. positive symptoms in schizophrenia. *Psychopharmacology (Berl)*, **72**, 17–19.

Arnsten, A. F. T., Cai, J. X., & Goldman-Rakic, P. S. (1988). The alpha-2 adrenergic agonist guanfacine improves memory in aged monkeys without sedative or hypotensive side effects: evidence for alpha-2 receptor subtypes. *Journal of Neuroscience*, **8**, 4287–4297.

Arnsten, A. F., Cai, J. X., Murphy, B. L., et al. (1994). Dopamine D1 receptor mechanisms in the cognitive performance of young adult and aged monkeys. *Psychopharmacology (Berl)*, **116**, 143–151.

Barch, D. M. & Carter, C. S. (2005). Amphetamine improves cognitive function in medicated individuals with schizophrenia and in healthy volunteers. *Schizophrenia Research*, **77**, 43–58.

Benes, F. M. (2006). Strategies for improving sensitivity of gene expression profiling: regulation of apoptosis in the limbic lobe of schizophrenics and bipolars. *Progress Brain Research*, **158**, 153–172.

Boggs, D. L., Kelly, D. L., McMahon, R. P., et al. (2012). Rimonabant for neurocognition in schizophrenia: a 16-week double blind randomized placebo controlled trial. *Schizophrenia Research*, **134**, 207–210.

Buchanan, R. W., Conley, R. R., Dickinson, D., et al. (2007a). Galantamine for the treatment of cognitive impairments in people with schizophrenia. *American Journal of Psychiatry*, **165**, 82–89.

Buchanan, R. W., Davis, M., Goff, D., et al. (2005). A summary of the FDA-NIMH MATRICS workshop on clinical trial design for neurocognitive drugs for schizophrenia. *Schizophrenia Bulletin*, **31**, 5–19.

Buchanan, R. W., Javitt, D. C., Marder, S. R., et al. (2007b). The cognitive and negative symptoms in schizophrenia trial (CONSIST): the efficacy of glutamatergic agents for negative symptoms and cognitive impairments. *American Journal of Psychiatry*, **164**, 1593–1602.

Buchanan, R. W., Keefe, R. S., Lieberman, J. A., et al. (2011). A randomized clinical trial of MK-0777 for the treatment of cognitive impairments in people with schizophrenia. *Biological Psychiatry*, **69**, 442–449.

Buchanan, R. W., Keefe, R. S., Umbricht, D., et al. (2011b). The FDA-NIMH-MATRICS guidelines for clinical trial design of cognitive-enhancing drugs: what do we know 5 years later? *Schizophrenia Bulletin*, **37**, 1209–1217.

Cahn, W., Rais, M., Stigter, F. P., et al. (2009). Psychosis and brain volume changes during the first five years of schizophrenia. *European Neuropsychopharmacology*, **19**, 147–151.

Castner, S. A., Williams, G. V., & Goldman-Rakic, P. S. (2000). Reversal of antipsychotic-induced working memory deficits by short-term dopamine D1 receptor stimulation. *Science*, **287**, 2020–2022.

Davis, K. L., Kahn, R. S., Ko, G., et al. (1991). Dopamine in schizophrenia: a review and reconceptualization. *American Journal of Psychiatry*, **148**, 1474–1486.

DeLisi, L. E., Szulc, K. U., Bertisch, H. C., et al. (2006). Understanding structural brain changes in schizophrenia. *Dialogues in Clinical Neuroscience*, **8**, 71–78.

Egan, M. F., Goldberg, T. E., Kolachana, B. S., et al. (2001). Effect of COMT Val108/158Met genotype on frontal lobe function and risk for schizophrenia. *Proceedings of the National Academy of Sciences of the United States of America*, **98**, 6917–6922.

Freedman, R., Hall, M., Adler, L. E., et al. (1995). Evidence in postmortem brain tissue for decreased numbers of hippocampal nicotinic receptors in schizophrenia. *Biological Psychiatry*, **38**, 22–33.

Freedman, R., Olincy, A., Buchanan, R. W., et al. (2008). Initial phase 2 trial of a nicotinic agonist in schizophrenia. *American Journal of Psychiatry*, **165**, 1040–1047.

Friedman, J. I., Adler, D. N., Temporini, H. D., et al. (2001). Guanfacine treatment of cognitive impairment in schizophrenia. *Neuropsychopharmacology*, **25**, 402–409.

Friedman, J. I., Carpenter, D., Lu, J., et al. (2008). A pilot study of adjunctive atomoxetine treatment to second-generation antipsychotics for cognitive impairment in schizophrenia. *Journal of Clinical Psychopharmacology*, **28**, 59–63.

Geyer, M. A. & Tamminga, C. A. (2004). Measurement and treatment research to improve cognition in schizophrenia: neuropharmacological aspects. *Psychopharmacology (Berl)*, **174**, 1–2.

Giakoumaki, S. G., Roussos, P., & Bitsios, P. (2008). Improvement of prepulse inhibition and executive function by the COMT inhibitor tolcapone depends on COMT Val158Met polymorphism. *Neuropsychopharmacology*, **33**, 3058–3068.

Goff, D. C., Keefe, R. S. E., Citrome, L., et al. (2007). Lamotrigine as add-on therapy in schizophrenia: results of 2 placebo-controlled trials. *Journal of Clinical Psychopharmacology*, **27**, 582–589.

Goff, D. C., Lamberti, J. S., Leon, A. C., et al. (2008). A placebo-controlled add-on trial of the ampakine, CX516, for cognitive deficits in schizophrenia. *Neuropsychopharmacology*, **33**, 465–472.

Green, M. F., Schooler, N. R., Kern, R. D., et al. (2011). Evaluation of functionally-meaningful measures for clinical trials of cognition enhancement in schizophrenia. *American Journal of Psychiatry*, **168**, 400–407.

Harvey, P. D. & Keefe, R. S. E. (2001). Interpreting studies of cognitive change in schizophrenia with novel antipsychotic treatment. *American Journal of Psychiatry*, **158**, 176–184.

Holt, D. J., Herman, M. M., Hyde, T. M., et al. (1999). Evidence for a deficit in cholinergic interneurons in the striatum in schizophrenia. *Neuroscience*, **94**, 21–31.

Hunt, R. D., Arnsten, A. F. T, Asbell, M. D. (1995). An open trial of guanfacine in the treatment of attention deficit hyperactivity disorder. *Journal of the American Academy of Child and Adolescent Psychiatry*, **34**, 50–54.

Javitt, D. C., Buchanan, R. W., Keefe, R. S., et al. (2011). Effect of the neuroprotective peptide davunetide (AL-108) on cognition and functional capacity in schizophrenia. *Schizophrenia Research*, **136**, 25–31.

Kahn, A. (2008). Current evidence for aripiprazole as augmentation therapy in major depressive disorder. *Expert Reviews of Neurotherapy*, **8**, 1435–1447.

Keefe, R. S. E., Malhotra, A. K., Meltzer, H. Y., et al. (2008). Efficacy and safety of donepezil in patients with schizophrenia or schizoaffective disorder: significant placebo/practice effects in a 12-week, randomized, double-blind, placebo-controlled trial. *Neuropsychopharmacology*, **33**, 1217–1228.

Kelly, D. L., Buchanan, R. W., Boggs, D. L., et al. (2009). A randomized double-blind trial of atomoxetine for cognitive impairments in 32 people with schizophrenia. *Journal of Clinical Psychiatry*, **70**, 518–525.

Kern, R. S., Nuechterlein, K. H., Green, M. F., et al. (2008). The MATRICS consensus cognitive battery: Part 2. Co-norming and standardization. *American Journal of Psychiatry*, **165**, 214–220.

Kimberg, D. Y., Aguirre, G. K., Lease, J., et al. (1997). Cortical effects of bromocriptine, a D-2 dopamine receptor agonist, in human subjects, revealed by fMRI. *Human Brain Mapping*, **12**, 246–257.

Krystal, J. H., D'Souza, D. C., Mathalon, D., et al. (2003). NMDA receptor antagonist effects, cortical glutamatergic function, and schizophrenia: toward a paradigm shift in medication development. *Psychopharmacology (Berl)*, **169**, 215–233.

Laruelle, M. (2003). Dopamine transmission in the schizophrenic brain. In S. R. Hirsch & D. R. Weinberger (eds.), *Schizophrenia*. Oxford: Blackwell, pp. 365–387.

Laruelle, M., Abi-Dargham, A., Gil, R., et al. (1999). Increased dopamine transmission in schizophrenia: relationship to illness phases. *Biological Psychiatry*, **46**, 56–72.

Lasser, K., Boyd, J. W., Woolhandler, S., et al. (2000). Smoking and mental illness: a population based prevalence study. *Journal of the American Medical Association*, **284**, 2606–2610.

Leonard, S., Gault, J., Hopkins, J., et al. (2002). Association of promoter variants in the alpha7 nicotinic acetylcholine receptor subunit gene with an inhibitory deficit found in schizophrenia. *Archives of General Psychiatry*, **59**, 1085–1096.

Lewis, D. A., Cho, R. Y., Carter, C. S., et al. (2008). Subunit-selective modulation of GABA type A receptor neurotransmission and cognition in schizophrenia. *American Journal of Psychiatry*, **165**, 1585–1593.

Lewis, D. A. & Sweet, R. A. (2009). Schizophrenia from a neural circuitry perspective: advancing toward rational pharmacological therapies. *Journal Clinical Investigation*, **119**, 706–716.

Lim, K. O., Hedehus, M., Moseley, M., et al. (1999). Compromised white matter tract integrity in schizophrenia inferred from diffusion tensor imaging. *Archives of General Psychiatry*, **56**, 367–374.

Matute, C. (1998). Characteristics of acute and chronic kainate excitotoxic damage to the optic nerve. *Proceeding of the National Academy of Sciences of the United States of America*, **95**, 10229–10234.

McClure, M. M., Barch, D. M., Romero, M. J., et al. (2007). The effects of guanfacine on context processing abnormalities in schizotypal personality disorder. *Biological Psychiatry*, **61**, 1157–1160.

McDonald, J. W., Levine, J. M., & Qu, Y. (1998). Multiple classes of the oligodendrocyte lineage are highly vulnerable to excitotoxicity. *Neuroreport*, **9**, 2757–2762.

Menzies, L., Ooi, C., Kamath, S., et al. (2007). Effects of gamma-aminobutyric acid-modulating drugs on working memory and brain function in patients with schizophrenia. *Archives of General Psychiatry*, **64**, 156–167.

Minzenberg, M. J & Carter, C. S. (2008). Modafinil: a review of neurochemical actions and effects on cognition. *Neuropsychopharmacology*, **33**, 1477–1502.

Moghaddam, B. (2004). Targeting metabotropic glutamate receptors for treatment of the cognitive symptoms of schizophrenia. *Psychopharmacology (Berl)*, **174**, 39–44.

Morein-Zamir, S., Turner, D. C., & Sahakian, B. J. (2007). A review of the effects of modafinil on cognition in schizophrenia. *Schizophrenia Bulletin I*, **33**, 1298–1306.

Olincy, A., Young, D. A., & Freedman, R. (1997). Increased levels of the nicotine metabolite cotinine in schizophrenic smokers compared to other smokers. *Biological Psychiatry*, **42**, 1–5.

Olney, J. W. & Farber, N. B. (1995). Glutamate receptor dysfunction and schizophrenia. *Archives of General Psychiatry*, **52**, 998–1007.

Powchik, P., Davidson, M., Haroutunian, V., et al. (1998). Post-mortem studies in schizophrenia. *Schizophrenia Bulletin*, **24**, 325–342.

Sharma, T. S., Reed, C., Aasen, I., et al. (2006). Cognitive effects of adjunctive 24-week rivastigmine treatment to antipsychotics in schizophrenia: a randomized, placebo-controlled, double-blind investigation. *Schizophrenia Research*, **85**, 73–83.

Sumiyoshi, T., Matsui, M., Nohara, S., et al. (2001). Enhancement of cognitive performance in schizophrenia by addition of tandospirone to neuroleptic treatment. *American Journal of Psychiatry*, **158**, 1722–1725.

Sumiyoshi, T., Park, S., Jayathilake, K., et al. (2007). Effect of buspirone, a serotonin 1A partial agonist, on cognitive function in schizophrenia: a randomized, double-blind, placebo-controlled study. *Schizophrenia Research*, **95**, 158–168.

Verity, M. A. (1992). Ca(2+)-dependent processes as mediators of neurotoxicity. *Neurotoxicology*, **13**, 139–147.

Vitiello, B., Martin, A., Hill, J., et al. (1997). Cognitive and behavioral effects of cholinergic, dopaminergic, and serotonergic blockade in humans. *Neuropharmacology*, **16**, 15–24.

Volk, D. W., Austin, M. C., Pierri, J. N et al. (2000). Decreased glutamic acid decarboxylase 67 messenger RNA expression in a subset of prefrontal cortical gamma-aminobutyric acid neurons in subjects with schizophrenia. *Archives of General Psychiatry*, **57**, 237–245.

Woodward, N. D., Purdon, S. E., Meltzer, H. Y., et al. (2005). A meta-analysis of cognitive change to clozapine, olanzapine, quetiapine, and risperidone in schizophrenia. *International Journal of Neuropsychopharmacology*, **8**, 457–472.

Zoccali, R., Muscatello, M. R., Bruno, A., et al. (2007). The effect of lamotrigine augmentation of clozapine in a sample of treatment-resistant schizophrenic patients: a double-blind, placebo-controlled study. *Schizophrenia Research*, **93**, 109–116.

Chapter

16

Computerized cognitive training in schizophrenia: current knowledge and future directions

Melissa Fisher, Karuna Subramaniam, Rogerio Panizzutti, and Sophia Vinogradov

Acknowledgments

The authors gratefully acknowledge Gina Poelke, Rachel So, Virginia Powell, and Coleman Garrett for help during preparation of this chapter.

Introduction

The past 15 years have seen explosive growth in research and clinical interest in cognitive remediation for schizophrenia. Meta-analytic work confirms that a wide range of non-computerized and computerized approaches results in moderate increases in global cognition measures, but many questions remain. What are the similarities and differences among the various approaches? Which ones produce the most robust and enduring effects? What are the critical neural mechanisms that support a positive response to cognitive training interventions?[1] How can we use the current knowledge to perform high-impact research that will translate into meaningful new treatments for our patients?

In this overview, we will provide some emerging answers to these questions. First, we will briefly review the conclusions that can be drawn from recent meta-analytic work on the last 20 years of cognitive training studies in schizophrenia. Next, we will focus on currently available computerized cognitive and social cognitive training programs, examine their salient features, and discuss what we know about their effects. Finally, we will present data on neurobiological mechanisms that appear to be key aspects of successful cognitive training, and present recommendations for future research.

What do we know from prior meta-analytic work?

In 2007, McGurk et al. published an important meta-analysis of 26 randomized controlled trials of cognitive training in schizophrenia dating from 1968 to 2006 and using various approaches ranging from noncomputerized attention training to computerized training of multiple cognitive functions provided with psychiatric rehabilitation (McGurk et al., 2007a). The study demonstrated a small to medium effect size for improvements in cognitive performance

---

[1] We will use the term cognitive training rather than cognitive remediation, as it is our view that the optimal approaches harness physiological neuroplasticity mechanisms that are present in healthy individuals as well as those with illness.

Cognitive Impairment in Schizophrenia, ed. Philip D. Harvey. Published by Cambridge University Press. © Cambridge University Press 2013.

(0.41), with a slightly lower effect size for psychosocial functioning (0.36); however, when adjunctive psychiatric rehabilitation was provided with cognitive training, the effects on functional outcome were significantly stronger. Additional moderator variables were examined including hours of training and type of method (i.e., drill and practice versus drill and practice plus strategy coaching). The results showed no significant heterogeneity in effect sizes on various Measurement and Treatment Research to Improve Cognition in Schizophrenia (MATRICS)-defined cognitive domains based on either the type of method or on the hours of training, with the exception of verbal learning and memory. In this one domain, a larger effect size was associated with more hours of training (0.57) compared with fewer hours (0.29) and with computerized drill-and-practice (0.48) compared with drill-and-practice plus strategy-coaching (0.23).

In 2011, Wykes et al. published a comprehensive meta-analysis of 40 studies undertaken from 1973 to June 2009, rating the trial methodology of each study using a metric developed by this group called the clinical trials assessment measure (assessing sample characteristics, allocation to treatment, comparison treatments, etc.) (Wykes et al., 2011). As in the McGurk et al. (2007a) study, many different forms of training were represented, had been studied in various combinations with other therapies or psychosocial rehabilitation, and were compared to a large assortment of active and passive "control conditions," including treatment as usual, supportive therapy, and computer skills exercises. A mean global cognition effect size of 0.45 was found, with heterogeneity of effect sizes in global cognition, speed of processing, and reasoning and problem solving; however, the meta-analysis did not find that type of training, participant characteristics, or trial quality could account for this heterogeneity in cognitive outcomes.

In an exploratory analysis, functional outcomes were significantly better in the four studies where cognitive training was combined with some other form of rehabilitation and when it included strategy-coaching relative to when drill-and-practice was delivered with rehabilitation. However, this interpretation was based on a comparison of a very small number of studies using widely different methods and designs. Similar to McGurk et al. (2007a), Wykes et al. (2011) found significantly stronger effects on functioning when cognitive training was provided together with other psychosocial rehabilitation, but less than one-third of the studies reviewed in each of these meta-analyses provided such adjunctive rehabilitation.

We posit that it is premature to draw too many definitive conclusions from the current meta-analyses, given the wide disparity in assessment measures, study designs, cognitive training methodologies, and control groups used. For example, in both meta-analyses (McGurk, et al., 2007a; Wykes et al., 2011), the primary outcome measure was designated as the "global cognitive effect," in most cases. However, some studies assessed only one or two cognitive domains with one or two measures, while others provided a comprehensive neuropsychological battery. Until the field adopts standardized assessment tools (e.g., MATRICS consensus cognitive battery), it will be difficult to make meaningful comparisons among studies or to perform highly informative meta-analyses.

Another issue is that the field has not yet adopted a uniform method of calculating effect sizes between studies. We found several discrepancies between the effect sizes reported by both McGurk et al. (2007a) and Wykes et al. (2011). In some cases, the discrepancies were quite large. This is likely the result of differences in the effect size calculations used in each study. Wykes et al. (2011) reported effect sizes listed in the published manuscripts. If these were unavailable, effect sizes were calculated with statistics that controlled for baseline differences. If these were unavailable, the post-treatment group means were used. In studies

Table 16.1. Cognitive domains showing significant heterogeneity in meta-analytic studies of cognitive training in schizophrenia

Meta-analysis	Cognitive domain	Effect size (Cohen's d)	Moderator variables identified	Moderator variables ruled out
McGurk et al., 2007a	Verbal learning and memory	0.39	More hours of training (d=0.57), drill-and-practice (d=0.48)	Participant characteristics, setting, control condition, adjunctive psychiatric rehabilitation
Wykes et al., 2011	Global cognition	0.45	None identified	Participant characteristics, methodological rigor, training approach (drill-and-practice vs. drill-and-strategy coaching), adjunctive psychiatric rehabilitation, computer use, therapy duration
	Speed of processing	0.26		
	Verbal learning and memory	0.41		
	Reasoning and problem solving	0.57		

with active and passive control groups, the statistics from the active control group were used where possible. McGurk et al. (2007a) used similar procedures; however, there were no statistical procedures that controlled for baseline and the effect sizes from both active and passive control groups were reported.

A third meta-analysis published in 2011 examined 16 randomized controlled trials of computer-assisted cognitive training in schizophrenia performed between 1991 and 2007, studying 12 different computerized programs, including some that focused on general cognitive abilities such as attention or working memory and some that focused on social cognition (Grynszpan et al., 2011). A mean general cognition effect size of 0.38 was found, while a substantially larger effect size of 0.64 was found in social cognition. Similar to the meta-analyses of McGurk et al. (2007a) and Wykes et al. (2011), the results showed no effect of potential moderator variables including age, treatment duration, weekly frequency, control condition type, and whether the training targeted specific domains or was nonspecific.

What can we conclude from the meta-analytic work to date? First, it appears that a wide range of approaches providing various forms of cognitive stimulation for variable amounts of time and treatment intensity *all* have a modest beneficial effect in schizophrenia. The overall lack of effect of moderator variables such as control condition type, the nature of training, and treatment duration, strongly suggest that thus far the approaches have been very nonspecific and have been working through a beneficial mechanism of general cognitive/affective engagement in patients. At the same time, heterogeneity of effect sizes has been identified for verbal learning and memory by McGurk et al. (2007a) (moderator variables: hours of training, drill-and-practice) and for global cognition, speed of processing, and reasoning/problem solving by Wykes et al. (2011) (moderator variables not identified) (Table 16.1). These findings indicate that some aspects of treatment delivery – as yet incompletely identified – have an influence on the degree of improvement that can be obtained in specific cognitive domains as well as in overall cognition.

What do we know about computerized cognitive training in schizophrenia?

In this section, we compare the four most frequently studied computerized programs in order to identify key components that appear to contribute to behavioral improvement in patients. We limit our review to programs that have been used in three or more studies aiming to improve cognition in schizophrenia. Neuropsychological tests are categorized into cognitive domains recommended by the MATRICS committee (Nuechterlein et al., 2004). Table 16.2 presents a summary of the key features and scientific rationale for the design of each of the programs reviewed. We then provide a brief review of studies that have targeted social cognition using computerized training.

Table 16.2. Scientific rationale and key features of commonly used computerized cognitive training programs in schizophrenia

Program	Scientific rationale	Key features
CogRehab, *Psychological Software Services*	Originally developed for traumatic brain injury. Based on the theoretical argument that diffuse traumatic lesions rarely have just one behavioral effect, and the degree to which a single behavior will be normal (or pathological) may depend on its interactions with other functional systems (Chen et al., 1997)	• hierarchical approach: training of fundamental cognitive functions followed by more complex functions • 8 modules target 4 domains: simple attention and executive skills, visuospatial skills, memory, and problem solving • 2 modules of increasing complexity within each domain • exercises follow a standard sequence and progression of difficulty. Subjects graduate to new tasks after reaching a prescribed performance level
CogPack, *Marker Software*	Information on rationale and approach were unavailable	• 64 programs for testing and training, each with several variants for visuomotor, comprehension, reaction, vigilance, memory, language, intellectual and professional skills • exercises can be edited and expanded • difficulty level and the sequence of exercises can be modified
Neuropsychological and educational approach to remediation (NEAR), Alice Medalia, Columbia University, *http://www. cognitive-remediation. org/id7.html*	Developed for mental and medical illness. Makes extensive use of educational techniques designed to promote learning by increasing motivation and task engagement	• holistic approach: incorporates ideas from educational psychology, learning theory, rehabilitation psychology, and neuropsychology to create a comprehensive approach to remediation. Encourages the promotion of an awareness of learning style, the

Table 16.2. (cont.)

Program	Scientific rationale	Key features
		promotion of self-esteem, and improves social-emotional functioning • participants select a repertoire of educational software programs that address sustained attention, processing speed, memory, and executive functions (e.g., "Where in the USA is Carmen Sandiego?") • guidance/assistance from a therapist is provided during training
Brain fitness program (BFP) auditory module, *Posit Science Inc.*	Originally developed for children with learning disabilities but subsequently has been heavily modified and adapted for adults, with an emphasis on both individuals with schizophrenia and the cognitive decline associated with aging. Applied to patients with schizophrenia based on the known impairments in auditory processing and frontally mediated verbal memory operations	• exercises are theoretically grounded in basic principles of learning-induced neuroplasticity • intensive – many thousands of learning trials are performed for each specific exercise • neuroadaptive – the dimensions of each exercise (e.g., speed, working memory load) are parametrically and continuously modified on a trial-by-trial basis for each individual user during the course of each exercise in order to maintain performance at ~80% accuracy • attentionally engaging – each trial is gated by a "ready" signal from the user to indicate and require directed attention • rewarding – correct responses are continuously rewarded by amusing auditory and visual stimuli in order to drive high levels of training compliance and to engage reward and novelty detection systems for successful learning

CogRehab (Psychological Software Services)

The Psychological Software Services CogRehab software (Bracy, 1995), originally designed for patients with traumatic brain injury, has been used in a number of studies in schizophrenia. The exercises emphasize simple attention, executive skills, visuospatial skills, memory, and problem solving. Eight modules are completed sequentially, with two modules of increasing complexity within each cognitive domain. The developers recommend 1–3 hours per day of training over the course of one year, with weekly therapy sessions during which compensatory skills are taught, patients' progress is reviewed, and program parameters such as difficulty level are adjusted.

Cognitive enhancement therapy (CET) (Hogarty & Flesher, 1999; Hogarty et al., 2004, 2006) is a small-group approach for the treatment of social cognitive and neurocognitive deficits in schizophrenia. Subjects work in pairs and complete approximately 75 hours of computerized cognitive training exercises (attention exercises from the orientation remediation module [Ben-Yishay et al., 1987] and CogRehab exercises of memory and problem solving). Four to six months after the initiation of cognitive training, subjects participate in 1.5 hours per week of social cognitive group therapy. The total treatment is delivered over a two-year period. Hogarty et al. (2004) tested the effects of CET (n=67) relative to enriched supportive therapy (EST) (n=54) in outpatients with schizophrenia on the following composite outcome measures: speed of processing, neurocognition, cognitive style, social cognition, social adjustment, and symptoms, the latter four of which were clinician ratings or patient questionnaires. After 12 months of treatment, the CET group showed significant gains in speed of processing, global cognition, and social adjustment, while after 24 months of treatment, the CET group showed significant improvement across all measures relative to the EST group, with the exception of symptoms. The EST participants also showed clinically meaningful change after two years of treatment on many of the composites, including neurocognition, which was unexpected given that their therapy did not specifically target cognition. Further, while the cognitive testing was performed by staff blind to group assignment, unblinded staff conducted the clinician ratings, and the CET and EST conditions were not matched in terms of staff contact. A follow-up study 12 months after the completion of treatment found durability of all effects with the exception of neurocognition, and a significant relationship between early improvements in speed of processing and the long-term effects of CET on social cognition and social adjustment.

Eack et al. (2009) also examined the effects of CET (n=31) relative to EST (n=27) in individuals with recent-onset schizophrenia. After one year of CET treatment, improvements on the cognitive measures (speed of processing and global cognition) were not evident, but global cognition showed moderate improvement after two years of treatment. After both one and two years of treatment, CET subjects showed significant gains on measures of social cognition, cognitive style, social adjustment, and symptoms, and a significantly greater proportion of CET subjects were engaged in competitive employment after two years of treatment. However, similar to Hogarty et al. (2004), raters were not blind to group assignment and subjects in the CET condition received significantly more hours of clinician contact. A follow-up study one year after the completion of treatment (Eack et al., 2010) showed that the gains on social and symptom measures were broadly maintained, while the effect on employment was no longer significant (i.e., a similar proportion of EST and CET subjects was employed). Cognitive assessments were not conducted at the follow-up.

Neurocognitive enhancement therapy (NET) (Bell et al., 2001, 2003; Wexler and Bell, 2005) utilized CogRehab exercises of attention, memory, language, and executive functioning, some of which were modified for use with schizophrenia. The program has some adaptive features; as soon as subjects achieve 90% accuracy at a given difficulty level, the task is made more difficult following a prearranged hierarchy. Bell et al. (2001, 2003) compared the effects of NET plus work therapy (n=47) to the effects of work therapy alone (n=55). Subjects in the NET plus work therapy condition completed 26 weeks of 3–6 hours of cognitive training, a feedback support group, and a weekly social information processing group, and showed greater gains on measures of working memory and executive functioning compared to subjects receiving work therapy only. At the six-month follow-up, the gains in working memory were durable, with effect sizes ranging from 0.45 to 0.73, depending on the level of cognitive impairment (Bell et al., 2003). Importantly, at follow-up the NET plus work therapy subjects worked significantly more hours compared to subjects who completed work therapy alone (Wexler and Bell, 2005). In a second study, the authors tested the effects of NET in combination with a vocational program (NET+VOC) (n=38) for one year relative to subjects receiving VOC only (n=34). Similar findings emerged with NET+VOC subjects showing greater gains on measures of working memory and executive functioning, markedly better vocational outcomes at the 12-month follow-up (Greig et al., 2007; Wexler and Bell, 2005), and a significantly higher rate of employment at the 24-month follow-up (Bell et al., 2008).

Kurtz et al. (2007) used CogRehab tasks of attention and memory, two tasks of attention from Loong (1988), and a speed reading task designed to increase language processing speed. The cognitive training condition (n=23) was compared to a computer skills training condition (n=19), with a target goal of 100 hours of training over one year for both conditions. Similar to the study of Bell et al. (2001), subjects in the cognitive training group showed greater gains in working memory compared to the computer skills training group. Importantly, this study used a "dismantling" design in which both groups received equivalent computer time and equivalent staff interaction so that the effects of training could be discerned from nonspecific effects associated with hours spent on a computer and staff interactions. Interestingly, both groups showed some improvements in processing speed, working memory, episodic memory (verbal and visual), and executive functioning, indicating that nonspecific engagement and stimulation has a salutary effect on neurocognition.

We note one final study (Benedict et al., 1994) that utilized CogRehab exercises of attention, but did not find significant group differences (n=33). We speculate that this may be due to the limited number of hours of training provided (15 hours compared to 50–100 hours in the studies described previously), or due to the earlier program version and differences in exercises and outcome measures used in this study. Additionally, training focused on CogRehab exercises of attention as opposed to the working memory tasks used in the earlier studies.

In summary, in studies where CogRehab training exercises of attention and working memory have been used in sufficient doses, gains in working memory have been consistently reported (Table 16.3). Furthermore, the addition of CogRehab has provided significant benefits on work outcomes in studies that added cognitive training to work therapy or vocational programs (Table 16.4).

CogPack (Marker Software)

Designed in Germany, CogPack (Marker, 1987–2007) contains multiple exercises in each of the following sub-programs: visuomotor skills, vigilance/comprehension/reaction, language material, memory, numbers/logic, knowledge/orientation/everyday skills, and special elements (e.g., executive functioning and tone and pitch discrimination). The program has some adaptive elements (e.g., if a task is solved, the program goes on to another type of task, but if unsolved, a similar task is given). Exercises provide training across a broad range of cognitive functions including attention, psychomotor speed, learning and memory, and executive functions. According to McGurk et al. (2005, 2007b), training exercises cover the

Table 16.3. The effects of computerized cognitive training on cognition in schizophrenia

Computerized cognitive training program	Authors and sample size	Experimental and control conditions	Improvements in cognition (significant group × time interactions)
CogRehab	Hogarty et al., 2004 (n=121), 2006 (n=106)	Cognitive enhancement therapy (CET) (CogRehab + attention exercises + social cognitive group exercises) vs. enriched supportive therapy	Global cognition, speed of processing at 12 and 24 months of treatment
	Eack et al., 2009 (n=58), 2010 (n=58)	CET (CogRehab + attention exercises + social cognitive group exercises) vs. enriched supportive therapy	No cognitive gains at 12 months of treatment. Global cognition at 24 months of treatment
	Bell et al., 2001 (n=65), 2003 (n=102), 2007 (n=116); Fiszdon et al., 2004 (n=94)	CogRehab + work therapy vs. work therapy	Working memory, executive functioning
	Wexler and Bell 2005 (n=54); Greig et al., 2007 (n=62); Bell et al., 2008 (n=72)	CogRehab + vocational program vs. vocational program	Working memory, executive functioning
	Kurtz et al., 2007 (n=42)	CogRehab + day treatment vs. computer skills training + day treatment	Working memory
	Benedict et al., 1994 (n=33)	CogRehab + day treatment vs. day treatment	No significant group × time interactions
CogPack	Sartory et al., 2005 (n=42)	CogPack + inpatient treatment vs. occupational therapy + inpatient treatment	Verbal learning, verbal memory, processing speed
	Wölwer et al., 2005 (n=77)	CogPack + inpatient or outpatient treatment vs. inpatient or outpatient treatment	Verbal learning, verbal memory
	McGurk et al., 2005, 2007b (n=44)	CogPack + supported employment + outpatient treatment vs. supported employment + outpatient treatment	Verbal learning, processing speed
	Lindenmayer et al., 2008 (n=85)	CogPak + inpatient treatment vs. computer games or typing skills + inpatient treatment	Verbal learning, verbal memory, processing speed

Table 16.3. (cont.)

Computerized cognitive training program	Authors and sample size	Experimental and control conditions	Improvements in cognition (significant group × time interactions)
	McGurk et al., 2009 (n=34)	CogPack + vocational rehabilitation vs. vocational rehabilitation	Verbal learning, verbal memory, processing speed
	Cavallaro et al., 2009 (n=86); Poletti et al., 2010 (n=100)	CogPack + outpatient rehabilitation treatment vs. outpatient rehabilitation treatment	Attention, executive functioning
Neuropsychological and educational approach to remediation (NEAR)	Medalia et al., 2000 (n=28)	Educational software to enhance problem solving + inpatient treatment vs. typing instruction + inpatient treatment	Verbal comprehension
	Medalia et al., 2001 (n=54)	Education software to enhance problem solving + inpatient treatment vs. Education software to enhance memory + inpatient treatment	Problem solving
	Hodge et al., 2010 (n=40)	Education software to enhance attention, processing speed, memory, and executive functioning + inpatient or outpatient treatment vs. waiting list (inpatient or outpatient treatment)	No significant group × time interactions
PositScience Brain Fitness Program (BFP) Auditory Training Module	Fisher et al., 2009 (n=55); 2010 (n=32)	BFP auditory module + outpatient status vs. computer games + outpatient status	Verbal working memory, verbal learning, verbal memory, global cognition
	Popov et al., 2011 (n=39)	BFP auditory module + inpatient treatment vs. CogPack + inpatient treatment	Verbal working memory, verbal learning
	Keefe et al., in press (n=53)	BFP auditory training + weekly group adapted from neuropsychological and educational approach to remediation (NEAR) + outpatient status vs. computer games + weekly healthy lifestyles groups + outpatient status	Verbal learning, global cognition, auditory frequency discrimination

Table 16.4. The effects of computerized cognitive training on symptoms and functioning and durability of cognitive gains in schizophrenia

Computerized cognitive training program	Authors and sample size	Effect of training on symptoms and functioning and durability of cognitive gains
CogRehab	Hogarty et al., 2004 (n=121), 2006 (n=106)	Improvement on clinician ratings of social adjustment after 12 months Improvement on clinician ratings of cognitive style, social cognition, and social adjustment after 24 months Durability of gains in speed of processing, cognitive style, social cognition, and social adjustment at 12-month follow-up
	Eack et al., 2009 (n=58), 2010 (n=58)	Improvement on clinician ratings of cognitive style, social cognition, social adjustment, and symptoms after 12 and 24 months of treatment Greater proportion of CET subjects were employed after 24 months of treatment. Effect on employment was no longer significant at 12-month follow-up
	Bell et al., 2001 (n=65), 2003 (n=102), 2007 (n=116); Fiszdon et al., 2004 (n=94) Wexler and Bell, 2005 (n=54); Greig et al., 2007 (n=62); Bell et al., 2008 (n=72)	Greater number of hours worked at 6-month follow-up Durability of cognitive gains at 6- and 12-month follow-up Greater number of hours worked at 12-month follow-up; higher quarterly employment rates and higher cumulative rates of competitive employment over 3 quarters Improvement on the PANSS Cognitive Component, Vocational Cognitive Rating Scale and Work Behavior Inventory at 12-month follow-up
	Kurtz et al., 2007 (n=42) Benedict et al., 1994 (n=33)	None reported None reported
CogPack	Sartory et al., 2005 (n=42) Wölwer et al., 2005 (n=77) McGurk et al., 2005, 2007a (n=44)	None reported None reported Greater number of hours worked, wages earned, and more jobs worked at 1-year and 2–3-year follow-ups Improvement in PANSS Depression and Autistic Preoccupation at post-training.
	Lindenmayer et al., 2008 (n=85)	Greater number of weeks worked at 12-month follow-up

Table 16.4. (cont.)

Computerized cognitive training program	Authors and sample size	Effect of training on symptoms and functioning and durability of cognitive gains
	McGurk et al., 2009 (n=34)	Greater number of weeks worked at 12-month follow-up; greater number of internship hours and internship wages at 12-month follow-up
	Cavallaro et al., 2009 (n=86); Poletti et al., 2010 (n=100)	Improved quality of life scores at post-training; durability of effects on cognition and quality of life at 6- and 12-month follow-up
Neuropsychological and Educational Approach to Remediation (NEAR)	Medalia et al., 2000 (n=28)	Decrease on the Positive Symptom Distress Index and Global Pathology ratings completed by nurses at post-training
	Medalia et al., 2001 (n=54)	Durability of gains in problem solving at 4-week follow-up
	Hodge et al., 2010 (n=40)	No significant group x time interactions at post-training or 4-month follow-up Improvement in Social and Occupational Functioning (SOFAS) in both subject groups at post-training and 4-month follow-up
PositScience Brain Fitness Program (BFP)	Fisher et al., 2009 (n=55); 2010 (n=32)	No significant group x time interactions at posttraining or 6-month follow-up Improvements in cognition were significantly associated with improvements in functional outcome (QLS) at 6-month follow-up in cognitive training subjects
	Popov et al., 2011 (n=39)	No significant group x time interactions at post-training
	Keefe et al., in press (n=53)	No significant group x time interactions at post-training

full range of cognitive domains within the first six sessions, with subsequent sessions focusing on repeated practice of exercises across the domains.

Sartory et al. (2005) tested the effects of CogPack exercises, which targeted attention, verbal ability, spatial ability, numerical ability, memory, and fast reaction time. Inpatients with schizophrenia (n=21) completed 15, 45-minute daily sessions over a three-week period and showed significant gains on measures of immediate and delayed verbal memory as well as processing speed relative to 21 inpatients on a waiting list. Wölwer et al. (2005)

used CogPack tasks of attention, memory, and executive functioning, in combination with desk work and training of compensatory strategies (verbalization and self-instruction) among inpatients and outpatients (n=24) and also found gains on measures of verbal learning and memory compared to a "treatment as usual" schizophrenia group (n=25).

Lindenmayer et al. (2008) provided 45 inpatients with 24 hours of CogPack exercises (attention and concentration, psychomotor speed, learning and memory, and executive functions) in conjunction with a work program in a psychiatric center. Relative to a computer games control group (n=40), subjects who completed the cognitive training showed gains on measures of verbal learning, processing speed, and global cognition. Furthermore, over a 12-month follow-up period, subjects who completed the cognitive training worked more total weeks relative to subjects in the control group.

CogPack has shown positive effects on both cognition and quality of life in 50 out-patients in a rehabilitation program who completed 36 hours of exercises in verbal memory, verbal fluency, psychomotor speed and coordination, executive functioning, working memory, attention, culture, language, and simple calculation skills. Relative to subjects who completed computer-assisted non-domain-specific activities (n=36) (Cavallaro et al., 2009), subjects who completed CogPack showed gains on measures of attention, reasoning and problem solving, and the quality of life scale, as well as durability of gains at six- and 12-month follow-up (Poletti et al., 2010).

McGurk et al. (2005, 2007b) tested the effects of three months of a multimodal treatment of CogPack exercises (attention, psychomotor speed, learning and memory, and executive functions), therapist-guided compensatory strategies ("Thinking Skills for Work"), and supported employment among 23 schizophrenia outpatients versus those with participation in supported employment only (n=21). Similar to reports by Sartory et al. (2005) and Wölwer et al. (2005), subjects who completed the cognitive training showed gains on measures of verbal learning and processing speed. Importantly, over a 2–3 year period post-treatment, subjects who received cognitive training were more likely to work, held more jobs, worked more weeks and total hours, and earned more wages compared to subjects receiving supported employment alone. In a second study, the authors combined the training with vocational rehabilitation (n=18) and found similar cognitive effects and better work outcomes over a two-year follow-up period relative to vocational rehabilitation alone (n=16) (McGurk et al., 2009).

As shown in Table 16.3, CogPack has consistent positive effects on verbal learning and memory and processing speed in schizophrenia, and substantially improves vocational outcomes when combined with supported employment or vocational training programs (Table 16.4). Additional research is required to replicate the findings of improved quality of life.

Neuropsychological and educational approach to remediation

The neuropsychological and educational approach to remediation (NEAR) program (various educational software manufacturers) utilizes educational software from various manufacturers (e.g., *Where in the USA is Carmen Sandiego?*, Broderbund Software; *Memory Package*, Sunburst Software) and motivational teaching strategies from a therapist, who guides the process, monitors progress, provides instruction and feedback, and promotes a positive learning experience. In an early version of NEAR (Medalia et al., 2000), 14 inpatients completed six hours of problem-solving educational software exercises and were compared to 14 inpatients who completed a typing program. Subjects who completed the problem-solving training showed significant gains in verbal comprehension relative to the control group and some improvement in symptoms, but no significant gains on a problem-solving task. In a second study, 18 inpatients who completed ten 25-minute sessions of the problem-solving training showed significant gains on a measure of problem-solving relative to 18 subjects who completed ten 25-minute sessions of memory training, and to 18 control subjects who received standard hospital care (Medalia et al., 2001). These gains showed durability at the four-week follow-up (Medalia et al., 2002).

More recently, the NEAR program was tested in a multisite study of inpatients and outpatients (n=40) (Hodge et al., 2010). With the facilitation of a therapist, participants selected a repertoire of educational software programs designed to enhance attention, processing speed, memory, and executive functions. Within-group analyses indicated significant gains on measures of attention, speed of processing, verbal learning, verbal memory, visual memory, and social and occupational functioning among the training subject group, and durability of these effects at the four-month follow-up. However, the results were not significantly different from the change in cognition measured in a waiting list group.

Brain fitness program: auditory training (BFP, PositScience, Inc.)

The BFP is an auditory/verbal learning training program that is designed to restore and enhance auditory perceptual and working memory processes, with the goal of increasing the accuracy and temporal resolution of auditory inputs feeding working memory and long-term verbal memory processes. The BFP was originally designed to address the verbal memory impairments associated with aging, but has been applied to patients with schizophrenia based on the known impairments in auditory processing and frontally mediated verbal memory operations in the illness (Foucher et al., 2005; Friston and Frith, 1995; Javitt, et al., 2000; Kasai et al., 2002; Kawakubo et al., 2006; Light and Braff, 2005; Ragland et al., 2004; Ragland et al., 2007; Wible et al., 2001). Although many of the exercises have a heavy emphasis on perceptual processing, they also explicitly require sustained attention and working memory and repeatedly engage cognitive control and response-selection mechanisms.

The exercises have the following features: (1) intensive – many thousands of learning trials are performed for each specific exercise; (2) neuroadaptive – the dimensions of each exercise (e.g., speed, working memory load) are parametrically and continuously modified on a trial-by-trial basis for each individual user during the course of each exercise in order to maintain performance at ~80% accuracy; (3) attentionally engaging – each trial is gated by a "ready" signal from the user to indicate and require directed attention; (4) rewarding – correct responses are continuously rewarded by amusing auditory and visual stimuli in order to drive high levels of training compliance and to engage reward and novelty detection systems for successful learning.

Our group has previously reported the effects of the BFP delivered as a stand-alone treatment (Fisher et al., 2009). Twenty-nine schizophrenia outpatients completed 50 hours of the training over a 10-week period and were compared to an active computer games control condition (n=26) designed to control for the effects of computer exposure, contact with research personnel, and monetary payments. Relative to the control group, using a per protocol analysis, the auditory training showed positive effects on measures of verbal working memory, verbal learning and memory, and global cognition. Effect sizes in verbal learning and memory and in global cognition were large (Cohen's d=0.86–0.89). At a six-month no-contact follow-up, improved cognition was significantly associated with improved functional outcome.

Popov et al. (2011) tested the effects of the BFP compared to CogPack among inpatients in Germany. Patients in the BFP condition (n=20) completed 20 one-hour sessions over four weeks, while patients in the CogPack condition (n=19) followed the standard protocol recommended by the developers of 60–90 minute sessions, three times per week, for four weeks. Both subject groups showed improvement in verbal learning and verbal memory; however, the BFP group showed significantly greater gains in verbal working memory and verbal learning. Patients who completed BFP also showed normalization of auditory sensory gating deficits not seen in the CogPack group (described in the next section).

In a multisite feasibility study (Keefe et al., in press), 25 outpatients were randomized to BFP plus weekly "bridging groups" (adapted from NEAR), or to a computer games control condition plus weekly healthy lifestyles groups (n=22). Subjects completed 3–5 one-hour sessions per week for 40 sessions or 12 weeks, whichever came first. After 20 sessions, in an intent-to-treat analysis, the BFP group showed significant gains in verbal learning (d=0.69), auditory frequency discrimination (d=0.84), and global cognition (d=0.28) relative to the control group. However, at the endpoint of the study, the effects on verbal learning and global cognition did not reach significance. The authors suggest this is likely due to the study completion deadline – that nine out of the 25 auditory training subjects did not complete the entire 40 sessions within the 12-week period, which may have reduced the efficacy of the training.

Comparative effects of computerized cognitive training in schizophrenia

The computerized programs reviewed previously show some consistency in terms of their benefits on specific cognitive domains. CogRehab improved working memory in three out of six studies, executive functioning in two out of six studies (Table 16.3), and significantly improved work outcomes when combined with vocational rehabilitation (Table 16.4). CogPack showed consistent improvements in measures of verbal learning, verbal memory, and processing speed, and also improved work outcomes when combined with vocational rehabilitation. The NEAR program showed variable effects on cognition, symptoms, and functioning, likely due to the individualized nature of the program (e.g., subjects select among a repertoire of educational software and training exercises). Finally, the BFP shows consistent improvement on measures of verbal working memory, verbal learning, and global cognition in three double-blind studies with a computer games control condition, and greater improvement than CogPack in one study.

We note some similarities between the cognitive effects of CogPack and BFP. Both show enhancement of verbal learning and memory. The BFP provides intensive training of auditory and verbal processes, while CogPack provides training across a range of cognitive domains. While the BFP showed stronger effects on verbal memory when the two programs were compared head-to-head (Popov et al., 2011), one similarity they share is the use of tone and pitch discrimination exercises, which may account for the fact that they both seem to be particularly beneficial on verbal cognitive processes.

Finally, it is likely the discrepancies between studies that have used CogRehab are the result of differences in the exercises and assessment measures used, and in treatment intensity. For example, in studies where significant gains in working memory were found, subjects completed 3–6 hours of cognitive training per week over a five-month period (Bell et al., 2001, 2003) versus other studies that have used one hour per week of training over a 1–2 year period (e.g., Hogarty et al., 2004; Eack et al., 2009).

What do we know about computerized social cognitive training in schizophrenia?

Impaired social cognition is a core feature of schizophrenia and an important treatment target that is strongly associated with functional outcomes such as social and community functioning, and independent living skills (Green et al., 2008; Penn et al., 2008). While only a small number of randomized controlled trials have tested the effects of computerized social cognition training in schizophrenia, the results are promising. Further, in the meta-analysis by Grynszpan et al. (2011), computerized programs that focused on social cognition generated stronger effects than those that focused on general cognitive abilities. Given the small number of computerized social cognitive training studies performed to date, we review as follows both randomized controlled trials and pre-/post-designs of: (1) computerized social cognition training programs that have targeted specific basic social cognitive abilities, and (2) programs where computerized social cognition training was provided together with social cognitive group treatments.

Targeted computerized social cognition training programs

Developed by Eckman and colleagues, the microexpressions training tool (METT) and subtle expressions training tool (SETT) (Eckman, 2003) provide computerized training in the identification of emotional expressions. The METT focuses on commonly confused emotional expressions (anger/disgust, contempt/happy, fear/surprise, fear/sadness). During a training video, the important distinctions between the expressions are contrasted and explained; for example, "concentrate on watching how the mouth is more rounded in surprise while, in fear there is more tension and the lips are stretched horizontally." Participants practice labeling different micro-expressions before and after the video. Feedback is provided by the program, and if the participant incorrectly labels the micro-expression, it can be viewed again. The SETT teaches recognition of very small micro-signs of emotion sometimes registering in only part of the face, or when the expression is shown across the entire face it is very small. Exercises begin with easy, instructive trials, and become increasingly difficult. Participants' attention is directed to different aspects of an emotional expression (e.g., eyes, mouth) with clear instructions about the distinguishing perceptual characteristics of that emotion (e.g., "furrowed brow is characteristic of anger"). Participants then practice identifying intense and subtle displays of that expression.

Russell et al. (2006) tested the effects of a single session of METT training in 20 schizophrenia outpatients relative to 20 healthy control subjects. Both groups improved on the METT assessment as well as an emotion matching task, and after training there was no significant difference between the performance of schizophrenia and healthy subjects on either measure. In a second study, 40 outpatients with schizophrenia were allocated to one session of the METT condition (n=26) or to a repeated exposure condition (n=14), which was identical to the METT condition except that during the video training the sound was muted and no feedback was provided during practice (Russell et al., 2008). The METT group showed significant improvement on emotion recognition accuracy relative to the repeated exposure group and this effect was maintained at a one-week follow-up. Eye movement was also tracked and showed a significant association to emotion recognition accuracy prior to training. After training, the METT group directed more eye movements within feature areas of faces; however, at follow-up the difference between the METT and repeated exposure groups was at trend level only.

Our group developed a computerized program for training in facial emotion identification, social discrimination, simple social perception, and theory of mind tasks using components drawn from the METT and SETT, plus the mind-reading program (Baron-Cohen et al., 2003). The training consisted of emotion lessons (40%), emotion quizzes (40%), and emotion games (20%). During emotion lessons, subjects viewed still pictures and videos of individuals expressing a variety of emotions. Subjects were provided with descriptions of emotions, audio of voices displaying the emotions, and sentences putting the emotion into context. During emotion quizzes, subjects were asked to match videos and sound clips of people interacting or expressing emotion with text describing/defining the situations, the emotions of the people in them, or the subtext of the situation. During emotion games, subjects viewed video clips of people in busy, real-world situations, and were asked to guess what people were thinking or feeling. Subjects engaged in the social cognition training for 15 minutes per day, after they had performed one hour of the BFP. We previously found that the computerized BFP training alone provided substantial gains in neurocognition, but did not enhance social cognition (Fisher et al., 2009). However, with the addition of social cognition training we found significant improvement on several MATRICS-recommended measures of social cognition from the Mayer–Salovey–Caruso emotional intelligence test (MSCEIT) and on a self-referential source memory task in 19 outpatients with schizophrenia (Sacks et al., in press).

Training of affect recognition (TAR) is a manualized 12-session program of computer tasks and desk work focused on the remediation of facial affect recognition (Frommann et al., 2003). The program incorporates restitution and compensatory strategies, principles of errorless learning, positive reinforcement, feature abstraction, and verbalization and self-instruction. Patients work in groups of two with coaching from a therapist. The tasks become progressively more difficult and can be repeated or discontinued depending on the individual performance. In a pre-/post-design (n=16), the authors found significant improvement in affect recognition after twelve 45-minute sessions (Frommann et al., 2003). Wölwer et al. (2005) compared the effects of TAR (n=28) to the effects of CogPack (n=24) and treatment-as-usual (n=25), and found significant improvement in affect recognition among TAR subjects only and in performance in TAR subjects at posttraining that was comparable to that of healthy controls. In a second randomized controlled trial of TAR (n=20) versus Cogpack (n=18), an intent-to-treat analysis showed not only improved affect recognition but also significant improvement in prosodic affect recognition, theory of mind, social competence, and improved social functioning at trend level among TAR subjects relative to subjects in the cognitive training condition (Wölwer and Frommann, 2011). Effect sizes ranged from medium to large; however, using a per-protocol analysis, the effects on theory of mind and social competence were no longer significant.

Finally, Emotion Trainer (*Leeds Innovations*) is a commercially available computerized program designed for autistic children to teach recognition and prediction of emotional responses (e.g., recognizing core facial expressions, anticipating the emotional response from events and situations). Using a pre-/post-design, Silver et al. (2004) tested the effects of three sessions of the training spaced 2–3 days apart in 20 male inpatients with schizophrenia, and found significant improvement on two emotion identification tasks but no improvement on a differentiation of facial emotions task or a working memory task.

Computerized social cognition training provided with social cognitive group treatment

Social cognitive interaction training (SCIT) is a manualized 18–24 session intervention developed to target emotion perception, attributional style, and theory of mind. The format is primarily group-based, although a portion of the emotion perception training is computer-assisted. A pilot study of the program in seven inpatients with psychotic spectrum disorders showed significant improvement in theory of mind, trend level reductions in symptoms and hostile and aggressive biases, with moderate effect sizes (Penn et al., 2005). However, there was no significant improvement in emotion perception. To strengthen the emotion perception training, the authors added an additional session of emotion mimicry training. A second group of inpatients were treated with the revised program (n=18) once a week (one hour per session) over 18 weeks and were compared to patients receiving a coping skills training (n=10) (Combs et al., 2007). The SCIT group showed significant improvement on measures of social and emotion perception, theory of mind, attributional style, cognitive flexibility, and social function relative to the coping skills group, with moderate to large effect sizes. A third study tested the effects in an outpatient sample of SCIT plus treatment-as-usual (n=20) versus treatment-as-usual alone (n=11) (Roberts and Penn, 2009). Consistent with the study of inpatients (Combs et al., 2007), the SCIT program resulted in improved emotion perception and social skills; however, the effects on theory of mind and attributional bias were not significant, perhaps due to ceiling or floor effects.

Social cognitive skills training, a 12-session group treatment developed by Horan et al. (2009), targets four domains, including facial affect perception, social perception, attributional style, and theory of mind. The program combines some elements from TAR and SCIT (Combs et al., 2007; Frommann et al., 2003; Penn et al., 2005; Roberts and Penn, 2009; Wölwer et al., 2005; Wölwer and Frommann, 2011) and incorporates skill building strategies such as: (1) breaking down complex social cognitive processes into their component skills; (2) teaching/ training basic skills and gradually increasing complexity of skill acquisition; (3) automating these skills through repetition and practice. Outpatients with schizophrenia or schizoaffective disorder were randomly assigned to the social cognition group (n=15) or a time-matched control condition (illness self-management and relapse prevention, n=16). Out of four social cognitive outcomes, the social cognition group showed significant improvement in facial affect perception relative to the control group, with a large effect size; however, there were no significant group differences on the measures of social perception, attributional style, or theory of mind. Similar to the reports of Wölwer et al. (2005) and Sacks et al. (in press), this improvement was independent of changes in neurocognition, which suggests that social cognitive deficits in schizophrenia need to be targeted directly (i.e., training general neurocognition alone is likely insufficient to drive changes in social cognition).

Summary of computerized social cognition training in schizophrenia

The studies reviewed previously demonstrate that some aspects of social cognitive impairment in schizophrenia are highly amenable to computerized social cognitive training (Table 16.5). In particular, facial emotion perception deficits in schizophrenia

Table 16.5. The effects of computerized social cognitive training on social cognition in schizophrenia

Social cognition training program	Authors and sample size	Experimental and control conditions	Improvements in social cognition
MicroExpressions Training Tool (METT)	Russell et al., 2006 (n=40)	METT schizophrenia and healthy subjects No control group	Emotion perception
	Russell et al., 2008 (n=40)	METT vs. repeated exposure	Emotion perception, increase in eye movements directed toward feature areas of faces
METT + Subtle Expressions Training Tool (SETT) + MindReading	Sacks et al., in press (n=19)	METT + SETT + MindReading No control group	Emotion perception, social perception, and self-referential source memory
Training of Affect Recognition (TAR)	Frommann et al., 2003 (n=16)	TAR No control group	Emotion perception
	Wölwer et al., 2005 (n=77)	TAR vs. CogPack vs. treatment-as-usual	Emotion perception
	Wölwer and Frommann, 2011 (n=38)	TAR vs. CogPack	Emotion perception, prosodic affect recognition, theory of mind, and social competence
Emotion Trainer	Silver et al., 2004 (n=20)	Emotion Trainer No control group	Emotion perception
Social Cognition and Interaction Training (SCIT)	Penn et al., 2005 (n=7)	SCIT No control group	Theory of mind
	Combs et al., 2007 (n=28)	SCIT vs. coping skills group	Emotion perception, emotion discrimination, social perception, theory of mind, attributional style, and social functioning
	Roberts and Penn, 2009 (n=31)	SCIT+treatment-as-usual vs. treatment-as-usual alone	Emotion perception and social skill
Social Cognitive Skills Training (SCST)	Horan et al., 2009 (n=31)	SCST vs. illness self-management and relapse prevention skills	Emotion perception

appear very responsive to computerized training (even after only 1–3 sessions), with moderate to large effect sizes reported across most studies. As Horan et al. (2009) note, facial affect perception is the most extensively studied aspect of social cognition in schizophrenia and can be trained with highly structured programs, while other aspects of social cognition such as theory of mind are difficult to translate into structured training exercises. We suspect that the highly structured, targeted training of emotion recognition accounts for the larger effects of computerized training on social cognition relative to general cognition (Grynszpan et al., 2011).

Table 16.6. The effects of computerized cognitive training on neural activation and structure in schizophrenia

Neuroimaging findings	Authors, type and duration of training and sample size	Principal cognitive effects of training
Magnetoencephalography (MEG)	Adcock et al. (2009); training = 50 hours of Positscience, Inc. (50 hours of brain fitness program) in 29 patients; control condition patient group = 50 hours of computer games (n=26)	Normalization of hemispheric asymmetries during early auditory processes Normalization of hemispheric asymmetry was positively associated with gains in both task accuracy and verbal learning after training
	Popov et al. (2011); training = 20 hours of auditory-focused cognitive exercises (CE) training (n=20); control condition patient group = 20 hours of CogPack (n=19)	Increased attenuation of the M50 response (the MEG analog of the EEG P50 response) to the second syllable, relative to the pretraining attenuation response
	Weiss et al. (2011); training = 2.5 hours of practice on a tone discrimination task (n=7); no control condition patient group	Accuracy improved after practice, and correlated with increased mutual information between sensors in temporoparietal regions in the beta band
Functional magnetic resonance imaging (fMRI)	Wexler et al. (2000); training = two auditory verbal memory tasks for approximately 25 hours total (n=8); no control condition patient group	Significant association between behavioral improvement and increased activation of left inferior frontal gyrus
	Haut et al. (2010); training = 25 hours of CogPack plus word N-back working memory task (n=9); control condition patient group = 25 hours of social skills training (n=9)	Significant activity-behavioral associations between improved working memory performance and increased activation within left frontopolar cortex and left dorsolateral prefrontal cortex for the trained word N-back and untrained picture N-back tasks
	Bor et al. (2011); training = 28 hours of cognitive training using Rehacom software (n=8); control condition group received no additional treatment (n=9)	Significant increase in activation in left inferior frontal gyrus, cingulate gyrus, and inferior parietal lobe on an untrained N-back working memory task Increased activation in left inferior/middle frontal gyrus was associated with improvements in attention and reasoning abilities

Table 16.6. (cont.)

Neuroimaging findings	Authors, type and duration of training and sample size	Principal cognitive effects of training
	Subramaniam et al. (2012); training = 80 hours of Positscience training, Inc. (50 hours of BFP plus 30 hours of visual processing training combined with social cognition training (n=15); control condition patient group = 80 hours of computer games (n=14)	Significant improvement in reality monitoring and significant increase in medial prefrontal cortex compared to pretraining assessments Significant association between better reality monitoring performance and increased activation of medial prefrontal cortex Increased medial prefrontal cortical activation after training predicted better social functioning 6 months later
Voxel-based morphometry (VBM)	Eack et al. (2010); training = 60 hours of CogRehab with 67.5 social cognitive group training for 2 years (n=30); control condition patient group = 2 years of enriched supportive therapy (n=23)	Greater preservation of gray matter volume in left hippocampus, parahippocampal gyrus, fusiform gyrus, and amygdala. Less gray matter decline in left parahippocampal gyrus and fusiform gyrus related to greater 2-year improvement in social cognition and neurocognition, and greater gray matter increases in left amygdala were related to greater 2-year improvement in social cognition

Positive effects of social cognition training have also been shown in other social cognitive domains, but not as consistently. For example, in studies where targeted social cognitive exercises were provided in sufficient doses (e.g., 10 or more sessions), improvements were evident in multiple social cognitive domains: emotion identification, prosodic affect recognition, theory of mind, and social competence in Wölwer and Frommann (2011), and perceiving emotions, emotion management, and self-referential source memory in Sacks et al. (in press). Similarly, in studies combining computerized social cognition training with social skills group interventions, multiple social cognitive domains showed improvement (i.e., social and emotion perception, theory of mind, attributional style, and social function) particularly among inpatients (Combs et al., 2007), while fewer gains were evident among outpatients (Horan et al., 2009; Roberts and Penn, 2009).

While encouraging, results from these studies should be interpreted with caution, and several limitations are noted. First, additional randomized controlled trials with larger sample sizes are needed to adequately determine the effects of computerized social cognition training programs. Second, as with programs that target cognitive impairment, standardized social cognition measures are required in order to compare the effects between programs. Third, it is difficult to discern which components of social cognition training drive improvement, particularly in programs that also provide group-based treatment and interactions.

What do we know about the neurobiological effects of computerized cognitive training in schizophrenia?

In this section we examine what is currently known about the neurobiological effects of computerized cognitive training in schizophrenia. These findings point the way for research that will determine the critical physiological mechanisms that support successful training and that will allow for the development of optimally efficient intervention strategies.

Magnetoencephalography: improvements in neural operations during early auditory processes

Magnetoencephalography (MEG) records magnetic fields (measured by sensors outside the head) that are produced by electrical activity within the cortex. Because MEG provides a direct measure of electrical activity within the brain, with a very high temporal resolution (milliseconds), it is an excellent technique of assessing early neural operations as individuals encode and process information arising from environmental stimuli. Using MEG, we have shown that patients with schizophrenia demonstrate hemispheric asymmetric abnormalities in early neural response dynamics in the auditory cortex during discrimination of syllable pairs. After 50 hours (10 weeks) of BFP auditory training, schizophrenia subjects showed a trend toward normalization of the asymmetry, which was positively associated with gains in both task accuracy and verbal learning after training (Adcock et al., 2009).

In another MEG study, Miller and collaborators used measures of auditory sensory gating, one of the most robust findings of early auditory processing abnormalities in schizophrenia, to explore the effects of BFP auditory training and CogPack training (Popov et al., 2011). Auditory sensory gating refers to the ability of the brain to suppress the response to the second of two paired stimuli, and may reflect aspects of sensory filtering. Four weeks (approximately 20 hours) of BFP normalized sensory gating in patients with schizophrenia, while this effect was not evident in subjects who completed CogPack. These results indicate that exercises that specifically target perceptual discrimination ability in the auditory system – as opposed to providing more generalized cognitive training – can normalize early auditory gating impairments in schizophrenia.

Weiss et al. (2011) also investigated the effects of this form of cognitive training on early perceptual operations. Two MEG recordings were acquired during performance of Exercise 1 from the BFP (high or low?), a FM sweep discrimination task used to improve the acuity of auditory processing, recorded before and after 2.5 hours of task practice. Practice increased power and mutual information, an index of communication between brain areas, in temporoparietal regions. Participants showed improved accuracy after practice, and these improvements correlated with the increase in power and mutual information.

Taken together, the ensemble of emerging MEG data suggests that carefully designed computerized training of auditory processes can increase the fidelity, precision, and signal to noise ratio of auditory representations in the brain.

Functional magnetic resonance imaging: improvements in neural activation patterns during higher-order processes

Functional magnetic resonance imaging (fMRI) provides an indirect measure of neural activity through detection of changes in blood flow. Because fMRI provides much better spatial resolution (sub-millimeter thresholds) compared to MEG recordings, it is optimal for detection of neural activation in higher-order regions of the brain during more complex cognitive operations. In this section we review fMRI studies that have investigated the effects of computerized cognitive training in schizophrenia during two higher-order cognitive tasks: verbal working memory and reality-monitoring. Verbal working memory represents the short-term encoding, storing, rehearsing, and integrating of task-relevant verbal information. Reality-monitoring is a type of source memory that involves distinguishing internally generated (i.e., self-generated) information from external reality (i.e., externally presented information).

Verbal working memory

In 2000, Wexler et al. showed that training-induced improvements in verbal working memory were associated with increased activation of the left inferior frontal cortex. Of the eight patients in this uncontrolled study, three made substantial gains in verbal working memory performance after approximately 25 hours of training on the task, and these subjects also showed increased task-related fMRI activation in the left inferior frontal cortex. A significant association between performance improvement and activation increase of the left inferior frontal cortex was observed across all eight patients (Wexler et al., 2000), indicating that task-related performance gains are related to increased recruitment of relevant cortical regions.

More recently, nine patients who completed 25 hours of CogPack exercises of attention and working memory plus training on a word N-back working memory task showed increased brain activation in several regions supporting working memory processes during both a word and a picture N-back task – including the dorsolateral prefrontal cortex, frontopolar cortex, and anterior cingulate gyrus – as compared to nine patients who received behavioral social skills training (Haut et al., 2010). More importantly, there were significant activity-behavioral associations between improved working memory performance and increased activation within the regions of activity overlap for the word and picture N-back tasks (i.e., left frontopolar cortex and left dorsolateral prefrontal cortex). These findings of behavioral improvement and increased neural activation in relevant cortical regions during an untrained picture N-back task in the active training patients versus the control group suggest generalization of neurobehavioral improvements in verbal working memory to visual working memory.

Additionally, in 2011, Bor et al. compared eight patients receiving 28 hours of cognitive training, facilitated by a psychologist, of Rehacom software exercises that targeted attention, working memory, logical thinking, and executive functions versus eight patients who did not receive training (single-blind randomized trial design). The between-group contrast of session 2 versus session 1 revealed increased activation in several regions, including the left inferior/middle frontal gyrus, cingulate gyrus, and inferior parietal lobe during an untrained N-back working memory task. Increased activation in the left inferior/middle frontal gyrus was associated with improvements in attention and reasoning abilities, indicating some possible generalization of training effects.

Reality-monitoring

In a double-blind randomized controlled trial, our group investigated the behavioral and neural effects of intensive computerized cognitive training in schizophrenia on an untrained meta-cognitive reality monitoring task (Subramaniam et al., 2012). Reality-monitoring–the ability to distinguish self-generated information from externally-presented information–is impaired in patients with schizophrenia. Unlike healthy subjects, patients with schizophrenia do not show activation of the medial prefrontal cortex when performing the task, a region important for successful reality-monitoring decisions (Subramaniam et al., 2012; Vinogradov et al., 2008). Thirty-one patients with schizophrenia were randomized to 80 hours of either cognitive training (50 hours of the BFP plus 30 hours of visual processing training combined with social cognition training) or a computer games control condition. Before the intervention, patients showed no significant recruitment of the medial prefrontal cortex during the reality monitoring task (Figure 16.1A). By contrast, the 15 healthy comparison subjects showed activation of the medial prefrontal cortex that was significantly associated with accurate reality monitoring performance (Figure 16.1B). After the intervention, patients

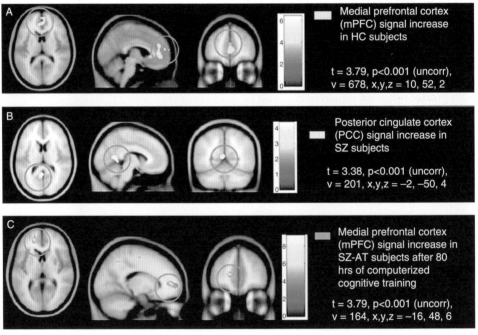

Figure 16.1. Whole brain fMRI analysis of reality-monitoring activity reveals signal increase within A: the medial prefrontal cortex (mPFC) in 15 healthy comparison subjects (HC); B: the posterior cingulate cortex, rather than the mPFC, in patients with schizophrenia (SZ) prior to computerized cognitive training; C: the mPFC in only the group of schizophrenia patients who completed 80 hours of active computerized cognitive training (SZ-AT), similar to the neural activation patterns observed in the HC sample. (Reproduced with permission from Subramaniam et al., 2012.) (See color plate section for colored image.)

in the cognitive training group showed improved reality monitoring that was associated with increased task-related activation of the medial prefrontal cortex, similar to the brain–behavior associations observed at baseline in the healthy subjects (Figure 16.1C).

These behavioral and neural improvements were not observed in control patients who completed 80 hours of computer games. Remarkably, patients who showed larger training-induced increases in medial prefrontal cortex activation during the reality monitoring task also revealed better real-world social functioning six months later. Results of this study indicate that intensive cognitive training of fairly basic cognitive processes can normalize brain–behavior associations during a non-trained higher-order reality monitoring task, so that they resemble more closely what is observed in healthy subjects.

Taken together, the fMRI data suggest that the higher-order behavioral and neural impairments in schizophrenia are not fixed and that, even during complex operations such as verbal working memory and reality-monitoring, they may be ameliorated by well-designed cognitive training interventions that target restoration of neural system functioning.

Voxel-based morphometry: improvements in neural structure

Voxel-based morphometry (VBM) allows investigation of volumetric changes in brain anatomy. In a recent study, Eack et al. (2010) showed that CET, which combines 60 hours of CogRehab integrated with approximately 70 hours of social-cognitive group sessions and individual coaching provided over a two-year period, was protective against gray matter loss in 30 outpatients with recent-onset schizophrenia. Patients who received CET showed preservation of gray matter volume over the two years of the study within the left hippocampus, parahippocampal gyrus, fusiform gyrus, and amygdala compared to the 23 outpatients who received enriched supportive individual therapy for the same period. Within the CET group, less gray matter decline in the left parahippocampal gyrus and fusiform gyrus and greater gray matter increases in the left amygdala were all associated with greater two-year improvement in social cognition/social behavior. Additionally, in the CET group, less loss of left parahippocampal gyrus and fusiform gyrus volumes were correlated with improvements in neurocognitive function. However, it is not clear whether these effects were mediated by the computerized cognitive training per se, or by the rich social skills training and enhanced therapeutic contacts of the psychosocial components of CET, as might be suggested by the gray matter preservation in neural structures critically important for social-emotional functions.

Neurobiological effects of computerized social cognition training in schizophrenia

In this section, we review prior research, which suggests that the neural impairments in schizophrenia are amenable to computerized social cognition training. For example, in 2010, Habel et al. used fMRI to examine the neural mechanisms of how computerized TAR could improve identification of the emotional aspects of facial expressions. Ten patients who completed nine hours of TAR exercises consisting of training recognition of six basic emotions showed increased activation in several regions – including the left middle and superior occipital lobe, the right inferior and superior parietal cortex, and bilateral inferior frontal cortices – as compared to 10 patients who did not receive TAR. Furthermore, these activation changes in patients who completed TAR exercises correlated with their behavioral improvement in emotion identification. Ten healthy control subjects activated the same occipital, parietal, and frontal regions, which also revealed increased activation in the TAR patients after nine hours of training. Taken together, the results suggest that the training induced better emotion recognition and more efficient neural activation of the systems underlying visual, attentional, and emotional evaluation functions in the patients who completed TAR.

More recently, in a double-blind randomized controlled trial, our group also investigated the behavioral and neural effects of intensive computerized cognitive and social cognitive training in schizophrenia on a facial emotion recognition task (Hooker et al., unpublished). Twenty-two schizophrenia participants were randomly assigned to either 50 hours of auditory-based cognitive training plus social cognition training (SCT), which consisted of exercises from the METT and SETT) (Eckman, 2003) and mind-reading (Baron-Cohen et al., 2003) programs, or to 50 hours of a placebo computer games condition (CG). We found a group by session interaction that was driven by the SCT subjects, who showed greater neural increases in two emotion-processing regions – including the superior temporal cortex and somatosensory-related cortex – as compared to the CG subjects. Furthermore, neural increases in these regions were correlated with behavioral improvement on emotion perception, as measured by the MSCEIT:perceiving emotions scores. Together, these findings suggest that combined cognitive and social cognitive training increased neural activation of the systems that supported better emotion recognition. Because facial emotion recognition has been shown to predict functional outcome even after accounting for the contribution of general cognition (Hooker and Park, 2002; Poole et al., 2000), these findings suggest that computerized cognition and social training interventions have the potential to improve quality of life for people with schizophrenia.

Psychophysical findings

What aspects of cognitive training are fundamental for optimal treatment response? Thus far, treatment duration, type of training, and participant characteristics have not shown a significant moderating effect on cognitive outcomes (Grynszpan et al., 2011; McGurk et al., 2007a; Wykes et al., 2011). Similarly, in our clinical trial of the BFP auditory training, we have not found a relationship between treatment duration or participant characteristics and change in cognition (unpublished data). However, we have found a significant association between psychophysical gains on an auditory discrimination training exercise and gains in verbal working memory and global cognition, but not visual cognition (Fisher et al., 2009).

In a more recent study, fourteen participants with schizophrenia completed separate BFP computerized training modules in auditory, visual, and cognitive control processes. Importantly, the progress in visual training as measured by improvement in basic visual processing strongly predicted improvement in visual memory but not in auditory or verbal measures (Surti et al., 2011). In contrast, the amount of time in visual training was not associated with improvements in visual memory.

These early results indicate that the ability to make progress in basic psychophysical components of training is more robustly associated with cognitive improvement than is the amount of time spent doing exercises. The results also suggest that progress in this form of training is domain-specific. It is likely that there is individual variation in psychophysical components of learning potential and/or cortical plasticity responses and that this will be a fruitful avenue for further investigation.

Serum biomarker and genetic findings

Serum compounds can serve as peripheral biomarkers of training-induced physiological changes and have the potential to predict response to cognitive training as well as to increase our understanding of biochemical processes that are recruited by different types of training. In our clinical trial of the BFP auditory training, we measured two compounds in the serum of participants before and after 50 hours of training: brain-derived neurotrophic factor (BDNF) (Vinogradov et al., 2009a) and D-serine (Panizzutti et al., personal communication). The BDNF is a neurotrophin that critically contributes to neuroplasticity, neurodevelopment, and neuronal function, and schizophrenia may be related in part to decreases in normal BDNF functioning (Buckley et al., 2007) – serum BDNF levels in adult schizophrenia patients are generally reduced compared with healthy controls (Buckley et al., 2007; Grillo et al., 2007; Pirildar et al., 2004; Rizos et al., 2008; Tan et al., 2005; Toyooka et al., 2002). Consistent with prior reports, we found significantly lower baseline serum BDNF levels in patients with schizophrenia relative to healthy control subjects (Vinogradov et al., 2009a). Subjects who received the BFP showed a significant increase in serum BDNF compared with subjects who were in the computer games control group, and after training, achieved mean serum BDNF comparable to healthy subjects.

Dysfunction of glutamatergic neurotransmission mediated by the N-methyl-D-aspartate (NMDA) receptors and D-serine (an endogenous receptor agonist), may also be involved in the pathophysiology of schizophrenia (reviewed in Labrie et al., 2012). Because animal studies indicate that learning and memory can affect the levels of D-serine (Vargas-Lopes et al., 2011), we asked whether training-induced cognitive gains would be associated with changes in serum D-serine levels. At baseline, we found reduced serum D-serine in schizophrenia subjects compared to healthy control subjects, consistent with previous findings in both serum and cerebrospinal fluid (Bendikov et al., 2007; Hashimoto et al., 2003; Panizzutti et al., personal communication). We also found a significant positive correlation between cognitive improvement and increases in serum D-serine in subjects who underwent 50 hours of the BFP exercises, but not in subjects who were in the computer games control condition (Panizzutti et al., personal communication). These results raise the possibility that D-serine is involved in the neurophysiological changes induced by BFP cognitive training in schizophrenia.

During this trial we also studied a serum correlate of cholinergic system functioning, another neuromodulatory system known to be critically involved in cognition and neuroplasticity. Schizophrenia is commonly treated with medications that have anticholinergic effects, and the anticholinergic activity of medications (as measured in the serum by means of radioimmunoassay, for example) is negatively associated with learning and memory in the elderly and in patients with schizophrenia (Minzenberg et al., 2004; Mulsant et al., 2003; Perlick et al., 1986; Tune et al., 1982). We measured serum anticholinergic activity in schizophrenia subjects and found that gains in global cognition after training were negatively correlated with their anticholinergic burden (Figure 16.2) (Vinogradov et al., 2009b).

Serum anticholinergic activity accounted for 20% of the variance in the change in global cognition independent of the effects of IQ, age, or symptom severity. These findings underscore the cognitive cost of medications that carry a high anticholinergic burden, and have implications for the design and evaluation of cognitive treatments for schizophrenia.

Finally, it is possible that common variants in genes known to influence cognition affect an individual's level of improvement from cognitive training. One small study investigated

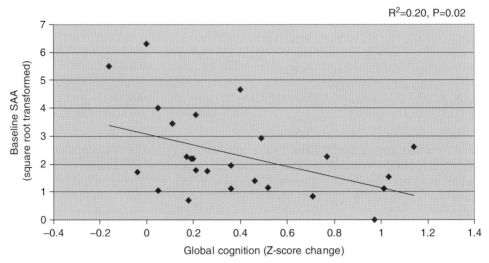

Figure 16.2. Serum anticholinergic activity is *negatively* correlated with cognitive improvement in schizophrenia and uniquely accounted for 20% of the variance in change in global cognition, independent of the effects of IQ, age, and symptom severity. (Reproduced with permission from Vinogradov et al., 2009b.)

the association between the COMT Val[158]Met polymorphism and neuropsychological improvement after 36 hours of Cogpack cognitive training in 27 patients with schizophrenia (Bosia et al., 2007). Patients with the COMT-Met allele made greater gains in cognitive flexibility than patients without the Met allele. In contrast, another study failed to observe a significant association between the COMT Val[158]Met polymorphism and cognitive improvement following therapist-led cognitive remediation therapy (Greenwood et al., 2011). In a recent pilot study, we genotyped 48 schizophrenia outpatients who had participated in our cognitive training studies using the BFP. We analyzed the association between the training-induced improvement in global cognition, and DNA variants in three genes known to show a relationship with cognitive performance: DISC1, COMT, and BDNF. Changes in global cognition after training were nominally associated with single nucleotide polymorphisms in the COMT and DISC1 genes. The strongest association was with COMT rs165599, a SNP previously associated with neurocognition in healthy subjects (Panizzutti et al., personal communication). It is probable that a wide number of gene variants that affect aspects of cognition or learning potential will play a significant role in determining the magnitude of patients' responses to cognitive training interventions.

What are important future directions for the field?

The behavioral and neurobiological evidence clearly indicates that individuals with schizophrenia benefit from computerized cognitive training. However, our ability to understand the meaning and implication of these findings is still in its infancy. Until we can systematically examine the effects of an intervention under carefully controlled and double-blind conditions, using well-defined cognitive, neurological, and functional outcome measures, and until we make a concerted effort to investigate the durability or sustainability of both behavioral and neurological effects, it will continue to be difficult to assess and compare the various cognitive training methods available to us.

As detailed by Vinogradov et al. (2012), there are several remaining questions for our field. First, how do we move our knowledge beyond nonspecific general behavioral improvements to specific and targeted gains in neural system functioning and behavior? Second, what elements of training are necessary and sufficient to generate robust and enduring neurobehavioral improvements? Third, what individual characteristics – inherent plasticity responses, mastery of a training task, or learning potential – determine the response to the treatment? Fourth, what limits response to treatment (e.g., medications, genotype) and how can we develop new approaches for these individuals? Fifth, what biological changes are driven by training and what are the implications for more sophisticated treatment approaches? Finally, future research of individuals at high-risk for psychosis is crucial to determine if cognitive training aids in preventing conversion to psychosis and/or mitigates further cognitive decline, resulting in significantly better clinical and functional outcomes for these young individuals.

Reference list

Adcock, R. A., Dale, C., Fisher, M., et al. (2009). When top-down meets bottom-up: auditory training enhances verbal memory in schizophrenia. *Schizophrenia Bulletin*, **35**, 1132–1141.

Baron-Cohen, S., Hill, J., & Wheelwright, S. (2003). *Mind Reading: The Interactive Guide to Emotions*. London: Kingsley Publishers.

Bell, M., Bryson, G., Greig, T., et al. (2001). Neurocognitive enhancement therapy with work therapy: effects on neuropsychological test performance. *Archives of General Psychiatry*, **58**, 763–768.

Bell, M., Bryson, G., & Wexler, B. E. (2003). Cognitive remediation of working memory deficits: durability of training effects in severely impaired and less severely impaired schizophrenia. *Acta Psychiatrica Scandinavica*, **108**, 101–109.

Bell, M., Fiszdon, J., Greig, T., et al. (2007). Neurocognitive enhancement therapy with work therapy in schizophrenia: 6-month follow-up of neuropsychological performance. *Journal of Rehabilitation Research and Development*, **44**, 761–770.

Bell, M. D., Zito, W., Greig, T., et al. (2008). Neurocognitive enhancement therapy with vocational services: work outcomes at two-year follow-up. *Schizophrenia Research*, **105**, 18–29.

Bendikov, I., Nadri, C., Amar, S., et al. (2007). A CSF and postmortem brain study of d-serine metabolic parameters in schizophrenia. *Schizophrenia Research*, **90**, 41–51.

Benedict, R. H., Harris, A. E., Markow, T., et al. (1994). Effects of attention training on information processing in schizophrenia. *Schizophrenia Bulletin*, **20**, 537–546.

Ben-Yishay, Y., Piasetsky, E., & Rattok, J. (1987). A systematic method for ameliorating disorders in basic attention. In M. J. Meier, A. L. Benton, & L. Diller (eds.), *Neuropsychological Rehabilitation*. New York, NY: Guilford Press, pp.165–181.

Bor, J., Brunelin, J., d' Amato, T., et al. (2011). How can cognitive remediation therapy modulate brain activations in schizophrenia? An fMRI study. *Psychiatry Research*, **192**, 160–166.

Bosia, M., Bechi, M., Marino, E., et al. (2007). Influence of catechol-O-methyltransferase Val[158]Met polymorphism on neuropsychological and functional outcomes of classical rehabilitation and cognitive remediation in schizophrenia. *Neuroscience Letters*, **417**, 271–274.

Bracy, O. (1995). *CogRehab Software*. Indianapolis, IN: Psychological Software Services.

Buckley, P. F., Mahadik, S., Pillai, A., et al. (2007). Neurotrophins and schizophrenia. *Schizophrenia Research*, **94**, 1–11.

Cavallaro, R., Anselmetti, S., Poletti, S., et al. (2009). Computer-aided neurocognitive remediation as an enhancing strategy for schizophrenia rehabilitation. *Psychiatry Research*, **169**, 191–196.

Chen, S. H., Thomas, J. D., Glueckauf, R. L., et al. (1997). The effectiveness of computer-assisted cognitive rehabilitation for persons with traumatic brain injury. *Brain Injury*, **11**, 197–209.

Combs, D. R., Adams, S. D., Penn, D. L., et al. (2007). Social Cognition and Interaction Training (SCIT) for inpatients with schizophrenia spectrum disorders: preliminary findings. *Schizophrenia Research*, **91**, 112–116.

Eack, S. M., Greenwald, D. P., Hogarty, S. S., et al. (2009). Cognitive enhancement therapy for early-course schizophrenia: effects of a two-year randomized controlled trial. *Psychiatric Services*, **60**, 1468–1476.

Eack, S. M., Greenwald, D. P., Hogarty, S. S., et al. (2010). One-year durability of the effects of cognitive enhancement therapy on functional outcome in early schizophrenia. *Schizophrenia Research*, **120**, 210–216.

Eckman, P. (2003). *Micro Expressions Training Tool and the Subtle Expressions Training Tool (METT AND SETT)*. Venice, CA: MOZGO Media.

Fisher, M., Holland, C., Merzenich, M. M., et al. (2009). Using neuroplasticity-based auditory training to improve verbal memory in schizophrenia. *American Journal of Psychiatry*, **166**, 805–811.

Fisher, M., Holland, C., Subramaniam, K., et al. (2010). Neuroplasticity-based cognitive training in schizophrenia: an interim report on the effects 6 months later. *Schizophrenia Bulletin*, **36**, 869.

Fiszdon, J. M., Bryson, G. J., Wexler, B. E., et al. (2004). Durability of cognitive remediation training in schizophrenia: performance on two memory tasks at 6-month and 12-month follow-up. *Psychiatry Research*, **125**, 1–7.

Foucher, J. R., Vidailhet, P., Chanraud, S., et al. (2005). Functional integration in schizophrenia: too little or too much? Preliminary results on fMRI data. *NeuroImage*, **26**, 374–388.

Friston, K. J. & Frith, C. D. (1995). Schizophrenia: a disconnection syndrome? *Clinical Neuroscience*, **3**, 89–97.

Frommann, N., Streit, M., & Wölwer, W. (2003). Remediation of facial affect recognition impairments in patients with schizophrenia:

a new training program. *Psychiatry Research*, **117**, 281–284.

Green, M. F., Penn, D. L., Bentall, R., et al. (2008). Social cognition in schizophrenia: an NIMH workshop on definitions, assessment, and research opportunities. *Schizophrenia Bulletin*, **34**, 1211–1220.

Greenwood, K., Hung, C.-F., Tropeano, M., et al. (2011). No association between the catechol-o-methyltransferase (COMT) val158met polymorphism and cognitive improvement following cognitive remediation therapy (CRT) in schizophrenia. *Neuroscience Letters*, **496**, 65–69.

Greig, T. C., Zito, W., Wexler, B. E., et al. (2007). Improved cognitive function in schizophrenia after one year of cognitive training and vocational services. *Schizophrenia Research*, **96**, 156–161.

Grillo, R. W., Ottoni, G. L., Leke, R., et al. (2007). Reduced serum BDNF levels in schizophrenic patients on clozapine or typical antipsychotics. *Journal of Psychiatric Research*, **41**, 31–35.

Grynszpan, O., Perbal, S., Pelissolo, A., et al. (2011). Efficacy and specificity of computer-assisted cognitive remediation in schizophrenia: a meta-analytical study. *Psychological Medicine*, **41**, 163–173.

Habel, U., Koch, K., Kellermann, T., et al. (2010). Training of affect recognition in schizophrenia: Neurobiological correlates. *Social Neuroscience*, **5**, 92–104.

Hashimoto, K., Fukushima, T., Shimizu, E., et al. (2003). Decreased serum levels of D-serine in patients with schizophrenia: evidence in support of the N-methyl-D-aspartate receptor hypofunction hypothesis of schizophrenia. *Archives of General Psychiatry*, **60**, 572–576.

Haut, K. M., Lim, K. O., & MacDonald, A. (2010). Prefrontal cortical changes following cognitive training in patients with chronic schizophrenia: effects of practice, generalization, and specificity. *Neuropsychopharmacology*, **35**, 1850–1859.

Hodge, M. A. R., Siciliano, D., Withey, P., et al. (2010). A randomized controlled trial of cognitive remediation in schizophrenia. *Schizophrenia Bulletin*, **36**, 419–427.

Hogarty, G. E. & Flesher, S. (1999). Developmental theory for a cognitive enhancement therapy of schizophrenia. *Schizophrenia Bulletin*, 25, 677–692.

Hogarty, G. E., Flesher, S., Ulrich, R., et al. (2004). Cognitive enhancement therapy for schizophrenia: effects of a 2-year randomized trial on cognition and behavior. *Archives of General Psychiatry*, 61, 866–876.

Hogarty, G. E., Greenwald, D. P., & Eack, S. M. (2006). Durability and mechanism of effects of cognitive enhancement therapy. *Psychiatric Services*, 57, 1751–1757.

Hooker, C. & Park, S. (2002). Emotion processing and its relationship to social functioning in schizophrenia patients. *Psychiatry Research*, 112, 41–50.

Horan, W. P., Kern, R. S., Shokat-Fadai, K., et al. (2009). Social cognitive skills training in schizophrenia: an initial efficacy study of stabilized outpatients. *Schizophrenia Research*, 107, 47–54.

Javitt, D. C., Shelley, A., & Ritter, W. (2000). Associated deficits in mismatch negativity generation and tone matching in schizophrenia. *Clinical Neurophysiology*, 111, 1733–1737.

Kasai, K., Nakagome, K., Itoh, K., et al. (2002). Impaired cortical network for preattentive detection of change in speech sounds in schizophrenia: a high-resolution event-related potential study. *American Journal of Psychiatry*, 159, 546–553.

Kawakubo, Y., Kasai, K., Kudo, N., et al. (2006). Phonetic mismatch negativity predicts verbal memory deficits in schizophrenia. *Neuroreport*, 17, 1043–1046.

Keefe, R., Vinogradov, S., Medalia, A., et al. (2012). Feasibility and pilot efficacy results from the multisite cognitive remediation in the Schizophrenia Trials Network (CRSTN) Study: a randomized controlled trial. *Journal of Clinical Psychiatry*. [Epub ahead of print].

Kurtz, M. M., Seltzer, J. C., Shagan, D. S., et al. (2007). Computer-assisted cognitive remediation in schizophrenia: what is the active ingredient? *Schizophrenia Research*, 89, 251–260.

Labrie, V., Wong, A. H. C., & Roder, J. C. (2012). Contributions of the D-serine pathway to schizophrenia. *Neuropharmacology*, 62, 1484–1503.

Light, G. A. & Braff, D. L. (2005). Mismatch negativity deficits are associated with poor functioning in schizophrenia patients. *Archives of General Psychiatry*, 62, 127–136.

Lindenmayer, J. P., McGurk, S. R., Mueser, K. T., et al. (2008). A randomized controlled trial of cognitive remediation among inpatients with persistent mental illness. *Psychiatric Services*, 59, 241–247.

Loong, J. (1988). *Progressive Attention Training*. San Luis Obisbo, CA: Wang Neuropsychological Laboratory.

Marker, K. R. (1987–2007). *COGPACK. The Cognitive Training Package Manual. Marker Software*. Heidelberg & Ladenburg. Retrieved from www.markersoftware.com

McGurk, S. R., Mueser, K. T., DeRosa, T. J., et al. (2009). Work, recovery, and comorbidity in schizophrenia: a randomized controlled trial of cognitive remediation. *Schizophrenia Bulletin*, 35, 319–335.

McGurk, S. R., Mueser, K. T., Feldman, K., et al. (2007b). Cognitive training for supported employment: 2–3 year outcomes of a randomized controlled trial. *American Journal of Psychiatry*, 164, 437–441.

McGurk, S. R., Mueser, K. T., & Pascaris, A. (2005). Cognitive training and supported employment for persons with severe mental illness: one-year results from a randomized controlled trial. *Schizophrenia Bulletin*, 31, 898–909.

McGurk, S. R., Twamley, E. W., Sitzer, D. I., et al. (2007a). A meta-analysis of cognitive remediation in schizophrenia. *American Journal of Psychiatry*, 164, 1791–1802.

Medalia, A., Dorn, H., & Watras-Gans, S. (2000). Treating problem-solving deficits on an acute care psychiatric inpatient unit. *Psychiatry Research*, 97, 79–88.

Medalia, A., Revheim, N., & Casey, M. (2001). The remediation of problem-solving skills in schizophrenia. *Schizophrenia Bulletin*, 27, 259–267.

Medalia, A., Revheim, N., & Casey, M. (2002). Remediation of problem-solving skills in schizophrenia: evidence of a persistent effect. *Schizophrenia Research*, 57, 165–171.

Minzenberg, M. J., Poole, J. H., Benton, C., et al. (2004). Association of anticholinergic load with impairment of complex attention and memory in schizophrenia. *American Journal of Psychiatry*, 161, 116–124.

Mulsant, B. H., Pollock, B. G., Kirshner, M., et al. (2003). Serum anticholinergic activity in a community-based sample of older adults: relationship with cognitive performance. *Archives of General Psychiatry*, 60, 198–203.

Nuechterlein, K. H., Barch, D. M., Gold, J. M., et al. (2004). Identification of separable cognitive factors in schizophrenia. *Schizophrenia Research*, 72, 29–39.

Panizzutti, R., Hamilton, S., & Vinogradov, S. (2012). Genetic correlates of cognitive training response in schizophrenia. *Neuropharmacology* [Epub ahead of print]

Penn, D., Roberts, D. L., Munt, E. D., et al. (2005). A pilot study of social cognition and interaction training (SCIT) for schizophrenia. *Schizophrenia Research*, 80, 357–359.

Penn, D. L., Sanna, L. J., & Roberts, D. L. (2008). Social cognition in schizophrenia: an overview. *Schizophrenia Bulletin*, 34, 408–411.

Perlick, D., Stastny, P., Katz, I., et al. (1986). Memory deficits and anticholinergic levels in chronic schizophrenia. *American Journal of Psychiatry*, 143, 230–232.

Pirildar, S., Gönül, A. S., Taneli, F., et al. (2004). Low serum levels of brain-derived neurotrophic factor in patients with schizophrenia do not elevate after antipsychotic treatment. *Progress in Neuro-Psychopharmacology and Biological Psychiatry*, 28, 709–713.

Poletti, S., Anselmetti, S., Bechi, M., et al. (2010). Computer-aided neurocognitive remediation in schizophrenia: durability of rehabilitation outcomes in a follow-up study. *Neuropsychological Rehabilitation*, 20, 659–674.

Poole, J. H., Corwin, F., & Vinogradov, S. (2000). The functional relevance of affect recognition errors in schizophrenia. *Journal of the International Neuropsychological Society*, 6, 649–658.

Popov, T., Jordanov, T., Rockstroh, B., et al. (2011). Specific cognitive training normalizes auditory sensory gating in schizophrenia: a randomized trial. *Biological Psychiatry*, 69, 465–471.

Ragland, J. D., Gur, R. C., Valdez, J., et al. (2004). Event-related fMRI of frontotemporal activity during word encoding and recognition in schizophrenia. *American Journal of Psychiatry*, 161, 1004–1015.

Ragland, J. D., Yoon, J., Minzenberg, M. J., et al. (2007). Neuroimaging of cognitive disability in schizophrenia: search for a pathophysiological mechanism. *International Review of Psychiatry*, 19, 417–427.

Rizos, E. N., Rontos, I., Laskos, E., et al. (2008). Investigation of serum BDNF levels in drug-naive patients with schizophrenia. *Progress in Neuro-Psychopharmacology and Biological Psychiatry*, 32, 1308–1311.

Roberts, D. L. & Penn, D. L. (2009). Social cognition and interaction training (SCIT) for outpatients with schizophrenia: a preliminary study. *Psychiatry Research*, 166, 141–147.

Russell, T. A., Chu, E., & Phillips, M. L. (2006). A pilot study to investigate the effectiveness of emotion recognition remediation in schizophrenia using the micro-expression training tool. *British Journal of Clinical Psychology/the British Psychological Society*, 45, 579–583.

Russell, T. A., Green, M. J., Simpson, I., et al. (2008). Remediation of facial emotion perception in schizophrenia: concomitant changes in visual attention. *Schizophrenia Research*, 103, 248–256.

Sacks, S., Fisher, M., Garrett, C., et al. (2012). Combining computerized social cognitive training with neuroplasticity-based auditory training in schizophrenia. *Clinical Schizophrenia and Related Psychoses*. [In press].

Sartory, G., Zorn, C., Groetzinger, G., et al. (2005). Computerized cognitive remediation improves verbal learning and processing speed in schizophrenia. *Schizophrenia Research*, **75**, 219–223.

Silver, H., Goodman, C., Knoll, G., et al. (2004). Brief emotion training improves recognition of facial emotions in chronic schizophrenia. A pilot study. *Psychiatry Research*, **128**, 147–154.

Subramaniam, K., Luks, T. L., Fisher, M., et al. (2012). Computerized cognitive training restores neural activity within the reality monitoring network in schizophrenia. *Neuron*, **73**, 842–853.

Surti, T. S., Corbera, S., Bell, M. D., et al. (2011). Successful computer-based visual training specifically predicts visual memory enhancement over verbal memory improvement in schizophrenia. *Schizophrenia Research*, **132**, 131–134.

Tan, Y. L., Zhou, D. F., Cao, L. Y., et al. (2005). Decreased BDNF in serum of patients with chronic schizophrenia on long-term treatment with antipsychotics. *Neuroscience Letters*, **382**, 27–32.

Toyooka, K., Asama, K., Watanabe, Y., et al. (2002). Decreased levels of brain-derived neurotrophic factor in serum of chronic schizophrenic patients. *Psychiatry Research*, **110**, 249–257.

Tune, L. E., Strauss, M. E., Lew, M. F., et al. (1982). Serum levels of anticholinergic drugs and impaired recent memory in chronic schizophrenic patients. *American Journal of Psychiatry*, **139**, 1460–1462.

Vargas-Lopes, C., Madeira, C., Kahn, S. A., et al. (2011). Protein kinase C activity regulates D-serine availability in the brain. *Journal of Neurochemistry*, **116**, 281–290.

Vinogradov, S., Fisher, M., & de Villers-Sidani, E. (2012). Cognitive training for impaired neural systems in neuropsychiatric illness. *Neuropsychopharmacology*, **37**, 43–76.

Vinogradov, S., Fisher, M., Holland, C., et al. (2009a). Is serum brain-derived neurotrophic factor a biomarker for cognitive enhancement in schizophrenia? *Biological Psychiatry*, **66**, 549–553.

Vinogradov, S., Fisher, M., Warm, H., et al. (2009b). The cognitive cost of anticholinergic burden: decreased response to cognitive training in schizophrenia. *American Journal of Psychiatry*, **166**, 1055–1062.

Vinogradov, S., Luks, T. L., Schulman, B. J., et al. (2008). Deficit in a neural correlate of reality monitoring in schizophrenia patients. *Cerebral Cortex*, **18**, 2532–2539.

Weiss, S. A., Bassett, D. S., Rubinstein, D., et al. (2011). Functional brain network characterization and adaptivity during task practice in healthy volunteers and people with schizophrenia. *Frontiers in Human Neuroscience*, **5**, 81.

Wexler, B. E., Anderson, M., Fulbright, R. K., et al. (2000). Preliminary evidence of improved verbal working memory performance and normalization of task-related frontal lobe activation in schizophrenia following cognitive exercises. *American Journal of Psychiatry*, **157**, 1694–1697.

Wexler, B. E. & Bell, M. D. (2005). Cognitive remediation and vocational rehabilitation for schizophrenia. *Schizophrenia Bulletin*, **31**, 931–941.

Wible, C. G., Kubicki, M., Yoo, S. S., et al. (2001). A functional magnetic resonance imaging study of auditory mismatch in schizophrenia. *American Journal of Psychiatry*, **158**, 938–943.

Wölwer, W. & Frommann, N. (2011). Social-cognitive remediation in schizophrenia: generalization of effects of the Training of Affect Recognition (TAR). *Schizophrenia Bulletin*, **37**, S63–70.

Wölwer, W., Frommann, N., Halfmann, S., et al. (2005). Remediation of impairments in facial affect recognition in schizophrenia: efficacy and specificity of a new training program. *Schizophrenia Research*, **80**, 295–303.

Wykes, T., Huddy, V., Cellard, C., et al. (2011). A meta-analysis of cognitive remediation for schizophrenia: methodology and effect sizes. *American Journal of Psychiatry*, **168**, 472–485.

Index